Change Leadership in Nursing

How Change Occurs in a Complex Hospital System

Mairead Hickey, PhD, RN, FAHA, is a nationally known nurse leader in academia and service. At the time this book was written, she was the chief nurse and senior vice president of Patient Care Services at Brigham and Women's Hospital in Boston, Massachusetts. She now holds the position of chief operating officer and executive vice president at Brigham and Women's/Faulkner Hospitals. Before returning to Brigham and Women's Hospital, Dr. Hickey was a clinical nurse specialist, associate professor, and chair of the graduate program for clinical nurse specialists at Yale University School of Nursing. Dr. Hickey has served nationally in a variety of nursing leadership positions, including as a director of the American Association of Critical Care Nurses, as a member of the Cardiovascular Nursing Council of the American Heart Association, and as a director of the Institute for Nursing Healthcare Leadership in Boston. She has participated on several national task forces to advance public policy and nursing practice and education. She has published widely in peer-reviewed journals, has an extensive record of national presentations, and has served on several editorial or review boards, including *Journal of Cardiovascular Nursing, American Journal of Critical Care, Nursing Clinics of North America, Nursing Research,* and others. She earned her bachelor's degree in nursing from Boston College, her MSN from Boston University, and her PhD from the University of Connecticut. She is a fellow in the American Heart Association.

Phyllis Beck Kritek, RN, PhD, FAAN, is a nationally known nurse-scholar and author, and is sought as a speaker, consultant, coach, and facilitator on conflict engagement; organizational/leadership development; gender, generational, and multicultural communications; and globalization. Dr. Kritek has published extensively in peer-reviewed journals and books and has produced two books: *Negotiating at an Uneven Table: Developing Moral Courage in Resolving Our Conflicts* (Jossey-Bass, 1994; 2001), and *Reflections on Healing: A Central Nursing Construct* (NLN Press, 1996). Dr. Kritek has served on the editorial board of several nursing journals and was the editor of *Nursing Forum* from 1989 to 1992. She has held a variety of academic leadership roles, including dean of nursing at Marquette University; founding doctoral program director and director of the Center for Nursing Research at the University of Wisconsin, Milwaukee; and Florence Thelma Hall Distinguished Professor in Nursing and founding doctoral program director of the University of Texas School of Nursing at Galveston. She earned her MSN and PhD degrees at the University of Illinois College of Nursing, and was awarded their Distinguished Nurse Alumna Award in 2000. Dr. Kritek is a Fellow of the American Academy of Nursing, and has served in a variety of professional organization leadership roles with the Community Health Accreditation Program (CHAP), NLN, NANDA, the Commission on Graduates of Foreign Nursing Schools (CGFNS), and the Society of Professionals in Dispute Resolution (SPIDR). She is a past recipient of a Kellogg National Leadership Fellowship, where she initiated her involvement in conflict engagement. Her international work has been as a consultant, educator, and group facilitator to health care communities in Canada, Mexico, Venezuela, Brazil, the Netherlands, the United Kingdom, Australia, China, India, and Iraq. In 2003, she resigned her academic position to create her sole proprietorship, "courage," to dedicate herself full time to providing conflict engagement services to health care professionals.

Change Leadership in Nursing

How Change Occurs in a Complex Hospital System

Brigham and Women's Hospital Nurses Tell Their Story

Editors

Mairead Hickey, PhD, RN, FAHA

Phyllis Beck Kritek, RN, PhD, FAAN

SPRINGER PUBLISHING COMPANY

NEW YORK

Springer Publishing Company, LLC
11 West 42nd Street
New York, NY 10036
www.springerpub.com

Acquisitions Editor: Allan Graubard
Composition: S4Carlisle Publishing Services

ISBN: 978-0-8261-0837-1
E-book ISBN: 978-0-8261-0838-8

12 13 14/ 5 4 3

The author and the publisher of this Work have made every effort to use sources believed to be reliable to provide information that is accurate and compatible with the standards generally accepted at the time of publication. Because medical science is continually advancing, our knowledge base continues to expand. Therefore, as new information becomes available, changes in procedures become necessary. We recommend that the reader always consult current research and specific institutional policies before performing any clinical procedure. The author and publisher shall not be liable for any special, consequential, or exemplary damages resulting, in whole or in part, from the readers' use of, or reliance on, the information contained in this book. The publisher has no responsibility for the persistence or accuracy of URLs for external or third-party Internet Web sites referred to in this publication and does not guarantee that any content on such Web sites is, or will remain, accurate or appropriate.

Library of Congress Cataloging-in-Publication Data
Change leadership in nursing : how change occurs in a complex hospital system / editors, Mairead Hickey, Phyllis Beck Kritek.
   p.; cm.
   Includes bibliographical references.
   ISBN 978-0-8261-0837-1 — ISBN 978-0-8261-0838-8 (e-book)
   1. Nursing services—Administration. 2. Leadership. 3. Organizational change. I. Hickey, Mairead. II. Kritek, Phyllis Beck, 1943–
   [DNLM: 1. Nursing Service, Hospital—organization & administration. 2. Leadership. 3. Nurse Administrators. 4. Nursing Care—organization & administration. 5. Organizational Innovation. WY 105]
   RT89 .C43
   362.17'3068—dc23

                                                                                    2011020935

Printed in the United States of America by Bang Printing

This book is dedicated to the nurses of the
Brigham and Women's Hospital:

those of the past on whose shoulders we stand,
those of the present who have made real
a vision toward excellence,
and those of the future
who will carry the vision forward.

Contents

PART IV: SUMMARY AND CONCLUSIONS: THE JOURNEY CONTINUES

Tables

Figures

Boxes

Contributors

Mary Absi, RN, BSN   Staff Nurse, Brigham and Women's Hospital, Boston, MA

Cheryl Avitabile, RN, MSN   Program Director, Central Education Programs, Center for Nursing Excellence, Brigham and Women's Hospital, Boston, MA

Phyllis G. Bailey, RN   Staff Nurse, Operating Room, Cardiac Surgery, Brigham and Women's Hospital, Boston, MA

Anne Bane, RN, MSN   Director, Clinical Systems Innovations, Center for Nursing Excellence, Brigham and Women's Hospital, Boston, MA

Barbara A. Bauman, RN, MS, MPA   Executive Director of Nursing, Surgical Services, Brigham and Women's Hospital, Boston, MA

Ellie Bergeron, RN, MSN   Program Director, Center for Nursing Excellence, Brigham and Women's Hospital, Boston, MA

Dorothy Bradley, RN, MSN   Program Director, Center for Nursing Excellence, Brigham and Women's Hospital, Boston, MA

Teresa Moore Buchanan, MBA, RN   Project Manager, ICU/Special Projects, Brigham and Women's Hospital, Boston, MA

Leo F. Buckley Jr., MBA   Executive Director of Business Services, Patient Care Services and Department of Nursing, Brigham and Women's Hospital, Boston, MA

Laurie Cairns, BS   Administrative Assistant, Center for Nursing Excellence, Brigham and Women's Hospital, Boston, MA

Diane Campbell, RN, BSN, ALM   Nurse Educator, Center for Nursing Excellence, Brigham and Women's Hospital, Boston, MA

Diane L. Carroll, PhD, RN, FAAN   Yvonne L. Munn Nurse Researcher, Institute for Patient Care, Massachusetts General Hospital, Boston, MA

Eloise Balasco Cathcart, MSN, RN, FAAN   Clinical Associate Professor and Coordinator, Graduate Program in Nursing Administration, New York University, College of Nursing, New York, NY; Consultant, Nurse Manager Role Development Program, Brigham and Women's Hospital, Boston, MA

Margaret Costello, PhD, RN   Nurse In-Charge, Brigham and Women's Hospital, Boston, MA

Pearl Cunningham, RN, BSN, MBA, CNOR   Nursing Director, Operating Room, Brigham and Women's Hospital, Boston, MA

Karyl Davenport, MSN, RN   Nursing Director, Burn/Trauma and Surgical ICU, Brigham and Women's Hospital, Boston, MA

Leslie A. DeLisle, MS, PMHCNS-BC   Program Manager, Psychiatric Nursing Resource Center, Brigham and Women's Hospital, Boston, MA

Patricia C. Dykes, RN, DNSc, FAAN   Senior Nurse Scientist, Center for Nursing Excellence, Brigham and Women's Hospital, Boston, MA; Instructor in Medicine, Harvard Medical School, Cambridge, MA

Elizabeth Eagan-Bengston, RN, MS   Assistant Nurse Director, Medical Cardiology, Brigham and Women's Hospital, Boston, MA

Mary Lou Etheredge, MS, PMHCNS-BC   Executive Director, Nursing Practice Development, Brigham and Women's Hospital, Boston, MA

Linda Evans, RN, MSN, CNOR   Research and Quality Specialist, Trauma and Burn Program, Brigham and Women's Hospital, Boston, MA

Katie Fillipon, RN, MS, OCN, FNP-BC   Nursing Director, Oncology and Clinical Services, Brigham and Women's Hospital, Boston, MA

Anne Furey, RN, MBA   Patient Education Program Director, Center for Nursing Excellence, Brigham and Women's Hospital, Boston, MA

M. Patricia Gibbons, RN, DNSc   Associate Chief Nurse, Department of Nursing, Brigham and Women's Hospital, Boston, MA

Shaun W. Golden, MSN, RN   Nursing Director, Neuroscience ICU, Brigham and Women's Hospital, Boston, MA

Denise Goldsmith, RN, MS, MPH   Executive Director, Informatics for Nursing and Patient Care Services, Center for Nursing Excellence, Brigham and Women's Hospital, Boston, MA

Hallie Greenberg, RN, MS-PREP, BC   Nurse Educator, Center for Nursing Excellence, Brigham and Women's Hospital, Boston, MA

Miriam Greenspan, RN, MS   Program Coordinator, Center for Nursing Excellence, Brigham and Women's Hospital, Boston, MA

Katherine Gregory, RN, PhD   Assistant Professor, Boston College, Haley Nurse Scientist, Center for Nursing Excellence, Brigham and Women's Hospital, Boston, MA

Yolanda B. Harmuth, RN, BSN   Nurse Educator, Center for Nursing Excellence, Brigham and Women's Hospital, Boston, MA

Carolyn M. Hayes, PhD, RN, NEA-BC   Executive Director, Oncology Nursing & Clinical Services, Brigham and Women's Hospital, Boston, MA; Senior Director, Patient and Family Programs, Dana-Farber Cancer Institute, Boston, MA

Nancy Hickey, RN, MS   Executive Director of Nursing, Emergency and Medical Services, Brigham and Women's Hospital, Boston, MA

Margaret Higgins, MSN, RN   Clinical Nurse Educator, Brigham and Women's Hospital, Boston, MA

Heather Hogan, RN, BSN   Staff Nurse, Brigham and Women's Hospital, Boston, MA

Ann C. Hurley, RN, DNSc, FAAN   Senior Nurse Scientist – Emerita, Brigham and Women's Hospital, Center for Nursing Excellence; Senior Investigator, Brigham and Women's Hospital, Department of General Medicine, Boston, MA

Ileana Jimenez-Garcia, MBA   Administrative Director of the Office for Multicultural Faculty Careers, Brigham and Women's Hospital, Boston, MA

Cynthia M. Jodoin, RN, BSN, MHA, OCN   Nursing Director, Hematology-Oncology-BMT, Brigham and Women's Hospital, Boston, MA

Martha K. Jurchak, RN, PhD   Executive Director, Clinical Ethics Service, Brigham and Women's Hospital, Boston, MA

Amy Kenefick, PhD, CNM, FNP-BC, APRN   Associate Professor, University of Connecticut, School of Nursing; Associate Professor, University of Connecticut, School of Medicine, Storrs, CT

Michael G. Kyller, RN, BSN, CCRN   Clinical Educator, Center for Diagnostic and Interventional Cardiology, Brigham and Women's Hospital, Boston, MA

Barbara E. Lakatos, DNP, PMHCNS-BC   Program Director, Psychiatric Nursing Resource Service, Brigham and Women's Hospital, Boston, MA

Diane R. Lancaster, PhD, RN   Former Executive Director, Quality Measurement & Improvement, Brigham and Women's Hospital, Boston, MA; Associate Chief Nurse, Evidence Based Practice Improvement, Cambridge Health Alliance, Somerville, MA

Kathleen Leone, BSN, MBA, RN   Nursing Director, Medical Intensive Care, Brigham and Women's Hospital, Boston, MA

Janice M. Little, MBA   Business Manager, Brigham and Women's Hospital, Boston, MA

Ellen Liston, RN, MSN   Program Manager, Nursing Practice Development, Brigham and Women's Hospital, Boston, MA

Cynthia F. Loring, RNC, MS   Clinical Nurse Educator, Brigham and Women's Hospital, Boston, MA

Carol Luppi, RN, BSN, ALM   Nurse Educator for Technology, Brigham and Women's Hospital, Boston, MA

De'Ann McNamara, RN, MS, CRN, ACNP   Clinical Educator, Interventional Radiology, Brigham and Women's Hospital, Boston, MA

Marsha J. Milone, RN, MSN/Ed   Nursing Director, Oncology and Clinical Services, Brigham and Women's Hospital, Boston, MA

Monique T. Mitchell, MS, PMHCNS-BC   Program Director, Psychiatric Nursing Resource Service, Brigham and Women's Hospital, Boston, MA

Eileen Molina, RN, MS   Nurse Director, Oncology Nursing/Pain and Palliative Care, Brigham and Women's Hospital, Boston, MA

Mary Lou Moore, MSN, RN   Executive Director, Cardiovascular Nursing, Brigham and Women's Hospital, Boston, MA

Laura Mylott, RN, PhD   Executive Director, Center for Nursing Excellence, Brigham and Women's Hospital, Boston, MA

Julie Nee, AS   Operations Project Coordinator, Brigham and Women's Hospital, Boston, MA

Patrice K. Nicholas, RN, MS, MPH, ANP, DNSc, DHL (Hon.), FAAN   Director, Global Health and Academic Partnerships, Center for Nursing Excellence, Brigham and Women's Hospital, Boston, MA

Patricia A. Normandin, DNP, RN, CEN, CPN, CPEN   Northeastern University and Simmons College Medical-Surgical, Obstetrics, Pediatric Nursing Instructor, Brigham and Women's Hospital, Boston, MA

Alice A. O'Brien, RN, MS   Nurse Director, Shapiro 8 and Cardiovascular Center, Brigham and Women's Hospital, Boston, MA

Eileen M. O'Connell, RN, MS   Nurse Administrator, Brigham and Women's Hospital, Boston, MA

Catherine Paccioretti, MS, RN   Nursing Director, Intermediate and ICU Float Pools, Brigham and Women's Hospital, Boston, MA

Maria Teresa Panizales, RN, MSN   Quality Program Manager, Center for Surgery and Public Health, Department of Surgery, Brigham and Women's Hospital, Boston, MA

Mary Pennington, RN, MSN   Nursing Program Director, Center for Nursing Excellence, Brigham and Women's Hospital, Boston, MA

Judith Perron, MSN, RN   Off Shift Nursing Administrator, Brigham and Women's Hospital, Boston, MA

Angellen Peters-Lewis, PhD, RN   Executive Director, Center for Women and Newborn's Nursing and Clinical Services, Brigham and Women's Hospital, Boston, MA

Patricia C. Powers, RN   Staff Nurse, Orthopedic Trauma, Operating Room, Brigham and Women's Hospital, Boston, MA

Matthew Quin, MSN, RN   Nursing Director, Cardiac Surgery, Brigham and Women's Hospital, Boston, MA

Patricia Reid Ponte, RN, DNSc, FAAN, NEA-BC   Senior Vice President, Patient Care Services and Chief Nursing Officer, Dana-Farber Cancer Institute, Boston, MA; Executive Director, Oncology Nursing & Clinical Services, Brigham and Women's Hospital, Boston, MA

Karen Reilly, MBA, RN   Nursing Director, CCU/Medical Cardiology, Brigham and Women's Hospital, Boston, MA

Patricia M. Reilly, RN, MSN Program Director, Integrative Care, Brigham and Women's Hospital, Boston, MA

Elvi Rigby, MSN, RN Off Shift Nursing Administrator, Brigham and Women's Hospital, Boston, MA

James Roche, RN, BSN, MEd Cardiovascular Nurse Educator, Brigham and Women's Hospital, Boston, MA

Elizabeth A. Samson, RN Staff Nurse, Brigham and Women's Hospital, Boston, MA

Catherine Saniuk, MSN, RN Clinical Educator, Cardiac Surgery, Ventricular Assist Device, Brigham and Women's Hospital, Boston, MA

Suzanne M. Silvernail, MSN, RN Nurse Director, Brigham and Women's Hospital, Boston, MA

Christine M. Smith, RN, MSN, PCCN Nurse Educator, Medical Nursing, Brigham and Women's Hospital, Boston, MA

Jacqueline Somerville, PhD, RN Senior Vice President of Patient Care Services and Chief Nursing Officer, Brigham and Women's Hospital, Boston, MA

Kristin Alt Styer, MSN, RN Quality Program Director, Perioperative Nursing, Brigham and Women's Hospital, Boston, MA

Sharon Swan, RN, BSN, MSN Clinical Nurse, Surgical Intensive Care Unit, Brigham and Women's Hospital, Boston, MA

Kim Ternavan, RN, MS/MBA Director of Critical Care Nursing, USC University Hospital, Los Angeles, CA

Neha A. Thakkar, MSN, FNP, RN Off Shift Nursing Administrator, Brigham and Women's Hospital, Boston, MA

Joyce Thomas-Browning, MS, RN Nursing Director, Thoracic Surgery ICU/Thoracic Intermediate Care, Brigham and Women's Hospital, Boston, MA

Sarah Thompson, MSN, RN Nurse Educator, Brigham and Women's Hospital, Boston, MA

Miriam Trainer, RNC, MS, IBCLC Nursing Director, CWN 9 and Lactation Support, Brigham and Women's Hospital, Boston, MA

Vincent M. Vacca, Jr., RN, MSN, CCRN Clinical Nurse Educator, Neuroscience Intensive Care Unit, Brigham and Women's Hospital, Boston, MA

Joan Vitello-Cicciu, PhD, RN, NEA-BC, FAHA, FAAN Executive Director, Perioperative Nursing and Clinical Services, Brigham and Women's Hospital, Boston, MA

Santina Wilson, RN, BSN Staff Nurse, Brigham and Women's Hospital, Boston, MA

Ronna Zaremski, RN, MSN, CCRN Clinical Nurse Educator, Brigham and Women's Hospital, Boston, MA

Foreword

*"Vision without action is merely a dream –
Action without vision just passes the time –
Vision with action can change the world."*

(Anonymous)

This extraordinary book by nurses at the Brigham and Women's Hospital (BWH) epitomizes this quotation. Led by Chief Nursing Officer Mairead Hickey, the Department of Nursing embarked upon a transformational journey that has re-shaped professional nursing practice and, in the process, has elevated patient care to a new level. Since its inception, BWH and its founding institutions, the Boston Lying In, Peter Bent Brigham, and Robert Bent Brigham Hospitals, have been known for their quality of care and spirit of innovation. BWH is consistently ranked among America's top hospitals. Yet as Dr. Hickey notes, the early 1990s was a diffi-cult time for nursing in the organization. The introduction of a service line approach separated nurses from each other. The administrative structure (with the chief nurse officer reporting to the chief operating officer) weakened nursing's voice. Role con-fusion among nursing leaders created uncertainty, and tensions existed around collective bargaining. During this period, I visited the organization and felt excep-tionally sad that things could not be different.

Enter Dr. Hickey, and the direction began to change. Starting with the nurses, she elicited their stories and launched a campaign that began with "finding and defining the good." She created new roles and an infrastructure and, more im-portantly, laid the foundation for a healthy work environment. Over the next 5 years, she worked with the nurses—staff nurses, directors, advanced practice nurses, community partners—to change almost every aspect of the Department of Nursing. Together, they created new partnerships and opportunities for the nurses. Collectively, they raised the voice of nursing at BWH. Reading now about the jour-ney of the past 5 years makes it seem so simple, yet the effort required for this trans-formation had to have been monumental.

As the coeditors note, this journey has relevance to clinicians, educators, admin-istrators, policy makers, and leaders of all levels. Its power lies in the vividness of the stories, the poignancy of the nurses' words themselves, and the recognition that nurses were fundamentally engaged in this transformation process. They had a leader with a vision, but as a proverb from the Iroquois Confederacy notes: "The leader is like a walking stick for the people to lean on, but it's the people who move the stick along."

The book's power also lies in two additional strengths. First, it is a wonderful resource book that outlines the steps a leader should take in transforming part, or all, of an organization. Separate chapters address specific issues that a nurse, or anyone else for that matter, can turn to for achieving a particular goal; taken together, they form a blueprint for action that guarantees success. Second, the book is an inspirational story that affirms, illuminates, and elevates nursing as the finest art. Reading the book, having been a nurse for more than 40 years, I was reminded again why I chose nursing and am so grateful for that choice. The nurses at BWH are to be profusely thanked for the gifts they have given us of their work and this book.

As a fitting endnote to this foreword, I had the opportunity of again visiting the hospital this past May—and the privilege of being the first Estrellita and Yousuf Karsh Visiting Professor in Nursing. The difference between my earlier visit and this one could not have been more profound. This time there was a vibrancy, an enthusiasm, and positive energy in the halls. I met with smiling and engaged nurses who were obviously busy but passionate about and proud of their work. Physicians and others talked eagerly about working with the nurses to improve patient care. Administrators spoke positively about the essential role of nursing within the organization. I felt exceptionally pleased that things were so different.

Joanne Disch, PhD, RN, FAAN
Clinical Professor and Director, Katharine J.
    Densford International Center for Nursing
    Leadership
Chair, Population Health & Systems
    Co-operative Unit
Katherine R. and C. Walton Lillehei Chair in
    Nursing Leadership
University of Minnesota, School of Nursing,
    Minneapolis, MN

Preface

*E*very preface orients. Ours is designed to answer the obvious questions: Why was this book written? Who wrote it? What is it about? How can it benefit a reader? Who will find it useful? Although there are many books, chapters in books, and journal articles that describe change leadership in nursing, we believe this book is unique. Eighty-eight people, nearly all nurses and nearly all colleagues in the same organization, tell their part of a larger story of a department of nursing's vision-driven change process. Each provides a unique perspective; all describe the same transformative process. Taken as a composite, the book documents the interrelatedness and synergistic impact of change leadership in nursing as reported by the nurses of Brigham and Women's Hospital. Viewed as a case study, it validates change leadership in nursing.

WHY THIS BOOK?

This is a book about nursing written by nurses for nurses, present and future. It's also for everyone they know who struggles to understand the work world of the practicing nurse, what we really do with our time, how we do it, and why. It provides a kaleidoscope of perspectives: Everyone tells a related story; everyone tells a unique story. If you're a nurse reading this book, you might want to buy a copy for that parent, partner, sibling, or great-aunt who simply never quite "gets" why you feel passionate about your job, why you want to improve your work world, and why you can't fully explain what you do for a living.

This is also a book about change: intentional, focused, persistent, practical change. It describes how a nurse leader, making common cause with a group of nurse leaders, attentive to the potential found in every nurse, can shift an organization's sense of itself and its culture. No single perspective prevails: they all count. No change stands alone: they are all part of the fabric of a larger commitment to a shared vision. The change assumes partnerships, synchronicities, and the opportunistic attention to possibility. Those who made it happen took the scholarship of change, leadership, and nursing practice and wove it into the fabric of a process. If you are interested in change, this book describes how all those theories play out in the real world. You might want to share it with others who seek constructive and affirmative change in their work worlds.

This book intends to inform. It suggests that there are gains to be had in breaking some old habits and patterns, that you can translate research into action. This change emerged not from attention to "what's wrong" but to a systematic invest-ment in "the good." The critical role of leadership is apparent throughout the book, and yet the change emerges from the expertise, dedication, and engagement of all participants in the process. Voice, visibility, vision, and values show up and make their statement. Experimentation with everything from engaging novice nurses to improving signage becomes an opportunity to create better nursing practice and a better practice world. Every author is clear: The primary beneficiaries of all this change are the patients and families who seek care at BWH. Metrics are resources to be mined and are balanced with an insistence on the qualitative forces that shape the caring, compassionate, deeply ethical soul of nursing.

WHAT IS THIS BOOK ABOUT?

The editors conceived the beginning and the end of this book. In Part I, Phyllis Kritek issues an invitation to you as the reader to share in our journey and Mairead Hickey tells the nuanced story of beginning the journey: its precursors, her vision and intent, the processes she set in motion, and the reasoning behind the actions she took. Part IV includes a summary of the book and an opening to the next stage of the journey, provided by the new BWH Chief Nursing Officer, Jacqueline Somerville.

Parts II and III are quite different. They were "designed" by the authors them-selves, from novice to expert, who stepped forward, willing to tell their part of the story. From staff nurse to executive director, these nurse authors describe their part in the journey of change, and do so in their own voice, from their individual perspective. Sometimes groups joined together to tell the story, sometimes a single person set out to reflectively provide a narrative. From this "volunteer" community of storytellers with stories to be told, we crafted the structure of Parts II and III, let-ting the stories themselves determine how we structured the book.

Part II is largely told from the perspective of those who had the greatest respon-sibility for creating the conditions for change: directors and executive directors who took responsibility for institution-wide initiatives that would make it possible for the Department of Nursing to pursue a transformative vision: *Excellent care to patients and families, with the best staff, in the safest environment.* Starting from the rigorous process designed to "find and define" the good, nurse leaders and consultants participated in a range of efforts to create a healthy work environment, develop nurse leaders, sup-port reflective practice, and create the structures necessary for all nurses to have voice. Emphasizing evidence-based practices, the Center for Nursing Excellence launched a myriad of changes and initiatives essential to the pursuit of excellence. The associate chief nurse, M. Patricia Gibbons (Trish), moved among the projects seamlessly, both catalyzing and supporting them. Evolving from traditional and fragmented nursing relationships to professional collaborative ones ensured attention to quality, and in-novative programs and practices shifted the quality enterprise to change at the point of care grounded in real-time data dissemination and usage.

Section A of Part III describes institution-wide changes, first in setting stan-dards and essential policies for excellent care. The use of narrative integrated throughout the change process gives voice to nurses and provides a path to reflec-tive practice. Advanced practice nurses (APNs) take on new roles that change both care and resource management, bolstered by evidence of impact. Consistent with nursing's leadership in the ethics of caring, attention to the moral challenges faced by nurses and patients are explored and addressed. The ubiquitous expansion of technology in health care is reframed, and the primacy of clinical practice drives these changes. A myriad of new partnerships and new partners emerge and become essential to the synergies that move the change process forward. Rigorous collaborative research and publication of seminal findings intensify the commitment to evidence-based professionalism. The humanizing impact of integrative practices gains visibility, acceptability, and effect.

In Section B of Part III, nurse authors describe service area and program changes. The intensive care unit directors combine forces to make changes that benefit all, staff and patients. A complex and challenging move is described, providing details about how the vision shaped both planning and execution. One unit's efforts to mirror the changes instituted by the Department of Nursing in their world is described, including the introduction of the patient and family voice in unit self-improvement. Finally, as the change processes moved forward throughout the hospital, nursing roles changed with them. The impact of a vision to ensure this change is documented.

Part III, Section C, provides a forum for reflective voices, describing change process from a personal, individual perspective, through narratives that tell the reader what it seemed like for these nurse authors as they experienced the change process. Leadership roles, nurse educator contributions, and the engagement of nurses in the expanding global initiatives of BWH provide focal points of reflection and sharing. The final voice in Part III is provided by Leo Buckley, an engaged participant and observer, who synthesizes much of what is implied throughout Part III: why nurses aspire to work at BWH. He is able to stand back, observe the whole, and share his sense of affirmation of the story. These final voices point to the end point of this story of change, the summary in Part IV, and the opening to the next journey unfolding as the book ends.

WHAT IS THIS BOOK GOOD FOR

Brigham and Women's Hospital is part of an intense hub of health care research, policy, power, and politics. There are several of these hubs in the United States, and what they do makes a difference. We believe this book can make a difference. We are not suggesting replication or imitation. Rather, we believe this book can catalyze others to create the change they desire. While others ponder the impact of the diverse shifts in health care in the United States, nurses will be busy making the changes happen that best serve patients, families, and communities. This book describes what that looks like, and provides templates that are at once pragmatic and transformative.

WHO WILL FIND THIS BOOK USEFUL?

When you write a book, it helps to picture your reader. Here are some of the readers we pictured:

- The persons wondering if nursing is for them, if they would like the work, what it's really like
- The beginning nursing student imagining the future, eager to hear from "real nurses" doing "real nursing" and how they go about making things better

- The nursing master's student envisioning a role as change agent, as someone who, with a new set of competencies and a new credential, wants to use these to make a difference to improve patient care
- The nursing DNP student edging toward the capstone project and looking for a menu of great ideas worth exploring
- The nursing PhD student curious about a program of research embedded in the intense immediacy of the delivery of nursing care
- The nurse educator, attentive to the needs of nursing students and their desire and need to study and envision their careers through the lens of clinical nurses doing real-world nursing
- The aspiring nurse leader looking for colleagues, for others who have imagined the path toward excellence and could provide some good, practical ideas for how to proceed
- The established nurse leader who knows there is always more to do and more that can be done, and welcomes the stimulus of another's story of leadership

We think there is no other book that tells nursing's story quite this way: one change process shared by many, variable and comprehensive in the number and nature of the stories told, rich in the array of storytellers. You'll find the pragmatism of quality control enlivened by creativity, the expansion of evidence-based practice to include descriptions of excellence in nursing practice, the sharp nexus when scholarship meets practice with openness, the power of measurement and the power of narrative. Nurses will recognize nursing in this book, not as we fantasize it, but as it is: extraordinary in its commitment and complexity and always challenged to get better.

This book is a snapshot of a moment in time when a community of nurses, sharing a journey of change, changed themselves and their work world. They are willing to tell their story, to give voice to nurses and nursing through that story. They are not going to promise right answers, or sell their version of reality—but we know you will learn from them.

Acknowledgments

Mairead Hickey would like to make the following acknowledgments:
This book reflects our journey as nurses at Brigham and Women's Hospital (BWH). Speaking for the entire Department of Nursing, I would like to acknowledge several individuals and groups who have been so important to making this book a reality:

Phyllis Kritek, who as our consultant, observer, colleague, and friend, provided validation of our work and inspiration to our department. This book was her initial idea, and as co-editor, teacher, and nursing leader, she generously offered many gifts to us throughout our journey.

Brigham and Women's Hospital, an institution where clinical and administrative leaders and employees create the environment in which patients and families receive the very best care. It was through the commitment to patient care of Dr. Gary Gottlieb, then president of BWH and now chief executive officer of Partners HealthCare; Dr. Betsy Nabel, president of BWH; Dr. Andy Whittemore, chief medical officer; and Kate Walsh, then chief operating officer; that BWH nurses make their unique contribution to patients and families.

The leaders of the BWH Department of Nursing, who are shaping a practice environment in which nurses reliably "know their patients and ensure patients feel known by their nurses." Within the leadership team, Dr. Trish Gibbons, associate chief nurse, was a fierce advocate for the work and position of nurses in patient care. Mary Lou Etheredge, RN, executive director of Nursing Practice, elegantly created the pathway for nursing practice to grow, and the Nursing Executive Board and nursing directors passionately ensured that the conditions of nursing practice were vibrant and sustainable. Julie White, as an administrative assistant, managed any logistical issue on any day, giving all authors the space to be creative.

Finally and most importantly, the community of nurses at BWH, who provide excellent care to patients and families each and every day and tirelessly advance the work of the discipline of nursing.

On a personal note, there are two people I would like to acknowledge. First, my mother, Louise Hickey, RN, who as a chief nurse modeled and taught me what it is to be an authentic leader. Second, my husband Bob, who fulfills my spirit with love, motivation, energy, and wise counsel.

Phyllis Kritek would like to make the following acknowledgments:

I would first like to acknowledge my co-editor, Mairead Hickey, whose vision, courage, commitment, and competence made the change described in this book a reality; those same qualities made the book a reality. Trish Gibbons provided grounding in realism and possibility and Julie White managed logistics and communication with grace and skill. My anchor at the Brigham, Mary Lou Etheredge, fulfilled her role with compassion, clarity, and wisdom and has my admiration and gratitude. Our authors, from novice to expert, were energetic, committed, often grateful, and forgiving.

At Springer Publishing, our editor, Allan Graubard, championed and understood this project and provided superb expertise. His guidance was inerrant, even when I wished otherwise, and was expressed with patience and persistence. Christina Ferraro managed the process efficiently, creating a path to completion. Rose Mary Piscitelli, our production manager, was superb: competent, responsive, and consistently helpful.

My friends are the wind beneath my wings. The "Women Who Go to the Water," as always, cheered me on: Eleanore Kirsch, Janet Krejci, Shelly Malin, and Sue Pinkerton. Phyllis Waters and Poldi Tschirch are my touchstone with what counts, and Sara Looney has been, as always, the wise woman. Barbara Nichols and Gloria Smith ensured that I view reality with a wide-angle lens. Deb Gerardi and John Godon were my local support, providing encouragement and a patient ear to my frequent ruminations.

My motivation to create a better world for the next generation is always crystallized by those I most cherish: my daughters, Patricia Kritek and Rebecca Kritek, aka Trish and Becky; my grandchildren, Alex, Grady, and Riley Mormon; and their father, Shannon Mormon. This inner circle of the future keeps me focused on what matters and why it should matter to me.

PART ONE

An Invitation to Our Readers

The Invitation

Phyllis Beck Kritek

---

*C*hange happens. It can be intentional, planned, and implemented with attentiveness and purpose. It can be shaped by a myriad of initiatives and supported both through resources and interpersonal care and affirmation. This book grew out of a series of conversations about change, about nurses making a difference, about the challenge of excellent patient care provided by nurses who were given vision, voice, autonomy, and engaged leadership. The conversations concluded with a commitment.

I was occasionally a participant, more often an observer, entering and exiting the arena of change, noticing, commenting. While present, I served as a consultant on creating professional work environments. The work itself provided a measure of the change process. It also afforded me the experiences that validated the change. Our conversations turned to sharing the lessons learned. We realized that we could provide other nurse leaders, aspiring nurse leaders, and nursing students with a window into health care today in one of its most challenging venues. Our story would be descriptive, not prescriptive.

We nurses are often reminded that we have failed to tell our story. We also tend to tell it in fragments, one or another manuscript in a journal describing one dimension of what is possible when good nurses do good work. Sometimes a great nurse leader shares his or her lessons learned, though those who shared in the process may have a limited opportunity to give perspectives that enrich the story. Often academic nurses tell the story of nursing. Less often do we hear the voice of nurses who do the work of nursing full time.

Our conversations became responsive to all these realizations: We could tell nursing's story in a unique way. We could tell it as a composite, bringing in a rich array of perspectives, many voices, and points of view from throughout the nursing department. We could tell the story as those who lead, design, organize, supervise, and give the care tell it. And in telling the story, we could unveil the subtle interactions among initiatives, how a change in one space interacts with other changes, and how the synergistic whole is quite different from the narrative about a single part. Diversity enriches, and our story would validate that truism.

Mairead Hickey, the co-editor of this book, initiated a change process as the new Chief Nursing Officer of Brigham and Women's Hospital in Boston,

Massachusetts. Hers is the first story in the book, and sets the stage for the unfolding of the varied narratives that tell a more complex, complete, and compelling story. Mairead used the metaphor of journey, integrating every change and development into this larger and more open-ended metaphor, making it possible for the Department of Nursing to adapt while staying focused, to respond to crises while sustaining forward progress, to stay on the journey.

One nurse leader can make a difference. A diverse group of nurses can make common cause with that leader and create the change they choose. We do not posit that we have the "right" or "best" stories to tell, only that nursing collectively benefits from shared templates of possibility. We do not posit the perfect, but rather tell the story of what is possible in a collective investment in the perfectible. Health care environments are complex adaptive systems: If you pursue adaptation with intent, you become the change you wish to see. Change is a given: It's what you do with it that counts.

I will be guiding you through the book, weaving the voices of nurses into a single story. I will point out signposts along the journey, indicate linkages among the diverse voices, offer reflections that emerged for me as I observed a complex, challenging, high-profile hospital's nurses make good on their commitment to the vision they shared.

1

Beginning the Journey

Mairead Hickey

In 2005, I had the great good fortune of being appointed chief nursing officer (CNO) of Brigham and Women's Hospital (BWH), a 763-bed tertiary and quaternary academic medical center, affiliated with Harvard Medical School, in Boston, Massachusetts, that is dedicated to patient care, teaching, research, and community health. Like every new CNO, I was proud of my appointment and excited by the opportunities it offered. After the first blush of excitement, however, I began to reflect more soberly on my dual responsibilities as a senior executive of the organization and chief of the discipline of nursing (Cathcart, 2008; Clifford, 1998). I recognized my accountability for integrating the goals of nursing and the institution and for creating a culture and environment that ensured patients and families of excellent nursing care and nurses of opportunities to practice in a meaningful and accountable way.

Fortunately, there is a rich and growing body of literature that CNOs can turn to that describes what nurses require to provide excellent care and achieve positive patient outcomes. I found myself referring to that literature frequently in my first weeks and months. It provided guidance as I met with BWH clinical nurses to learn about the joys and challenges of their practice, and with both nurse and non-nurse leaders to learn about the institution's support and expectations for the Department of Nursing (DON). What I learned through these conversations not only gave new meaning to the literature, but also shaped our work, as we developed a vision and goals for the DON, and mapped out a plan for creating a healthy environment for nurses, patients, and families at BWH. In this book, I am joined by nurses throughout BWH in describing our journey toward achieving our department vision: *Excellent care to patients and families, with the best staff, in the safest environment.*

I begin our story in this chapter by discussing what we have learned from the research on healthy work environments for nurses and describing the nursing practice environment at BWH when I became CNO. I also describe the process we used to lay the foundation for an environment in which our vision could come alive. Central to this process was the active participation of nurses from every role and setting. Through focus groups, staff meetings, community forums, committees, and one-on-one discussions, nurses throughout the organization participated in defining a vision and goals for the DON, establishing priorities for change, and evaluating our progress toward developing an optimal environment for nurses, patients, and families.

Engaging so many nurses in this work meant we received a constant stream of feedback, new ideas, and suggestions about new directions to explore. The result was a dynamic process, one that was marked by occasional backtracking and frequent course corrections as we defined what the department's vision looked like in operational terms. Although at times complex and often challenging, I believe our participative approach accounts for our success in developing an infrastructure that allows us to support and advance nurses and nursing practice, and ensure excellent outcomes for patients and families today and in the future. It was this participative approach that made writing our story possible, because it became not just my story but the story of every nurse in our department.

Although we have achieved a great deal, our journey is not over, because the DON at BWH, like departments of nursing everywhere, will continue to change and evolve in synchrony with the broader organization and health care environment and the needs of our patients and families. Nevertheless, we believe the values and infrastructure we have established position us to meet future challenges. Though every department of nursing is unique, nurse leaders in today's health care organizations face many of the same issues and can learn a great deal by studying one another's stories and experiences. It is for that reason we have written this book. It is my hope that our story of what we have done at BWH, and what we have learned and accomplished to date, will be helpful to nurse leaders, aspiring nurse leaders, and student nurses who share our commitment to creating the very best environments for nurses to practice and for patients to receive care.

SUPPORTING THE ESSENTIAL WORK OF NURSES

As nurses, we are all members of a professional community united by a tradition of practice dedicated to the care of patients and families. Since Florence Nightingale, nurses have been joined by a shared understanding of caring and what it means to be a nurse. As stated so elegantly by Virginia Henderson and Gladys Nite in their landmark book, *The Principles and Practice of Nursing*, as nurses we have the unique privilege of entering the lives of individuals when they are most vulnerable and "assisting individuals (sick or well) with those activities contributing to health, or its recovery (or to a peaceful death) that they perform unaided when they have the necessary strength, will, or knowledge" (1998, p. 14). With this privilege, however, comes the responsibility of ensuring that the nursing care we provide is appropriate to each patient's needs and wishes and is grounded in the best available knowledge. Since Nightingale's time, the practice of nursing has evolved and matured, and today is based on a rich body of scientific information, experiential knowledge, and a code of ethics (American Nurses Association, 2001) that requires us to respect the dignity and worth of every individual.

Even as nursing practice continues to evolve, the focus on patients and families remains central, grounding the way nursing care is delivered in many settings. The nurse-patient relationship is at the core of professional nursing practice and serves as the basis of relationship-based nursing models that have set the standard for the delivery of nursing care for years (Clifford, 1980; Manthey, 1973, 2006). These models emphasize nurses' professional accountability for patient care and assign nurses responsibility for developing, implementing, and overseeing plans of care for their patients and advocating for patient and family needs. For the models to be successful, practices and systems supporting professional judgment and decision making by nurses, protecting the nurse-patient relationship, and ensuring nurses' ongoing professional development must be in place. Developing these systems and creating an environment that supports the work of nurses and that facilitates caring practices are fundamental responsibilities of nursing departments and nursing leadership (Benner, 2001; Cathcart, 2008). These responsibilities shaped my study of the nursing literature and guided my leadership decisions.

I learned that nurse leaders seeking to create optimal work environments for nurses can learn much by examining our growing body of nursing research. It has now been more than 25 years since the American Academy of Nursing's original Magnet hospital study (McClure, Poulin, Sovie, & Wandelt, 1983) examined characteristics of hospitals that excel at attracting and retaining nurses. Through the study, the authors identified key characteristics of work environments that promote nurses and nursing practice, and that support nurses' efforts to influence patient care and achieve optimal patient outcomes. These characteristics include a patient-centered focus and philosophy of caring; leaders who are visible and accessible; opportunities for direct-care staff to participate in planning and decision making; support for nursing autonomy and ongoing professional development; and strong, quality programs focused on addressing and correcting problems in the practice setting (Coile, 2001; McClure et al., 1983).

The original Magnet hospital study set the stage for research and dialogue about healthy work environments for nurses and patients that continues today. Over the past decade, for example, Aiken and colleagues have conducted numerous studies examining the relationship between the work environment of nurses and nurse and patient outcomes. They have demonstrated that appropriate staffing and organizational and managerial support for nursing are associated with higher levels of patient and nurse satisfaction, lower rates of nurse burnout, better nurse ratings of quality of care, and lower rates of patient mortality and failure to rescue (Aiken, Clarke, & Sloane, 2002; Aiken, Clarke, Sloane, Sochalski, & Silber, 2002; Vahey, Aiken, Sloane, Clarke, & Vargas, 2004). The quality of the nurse practice environment is especially important, with better patient and nurse outcomes found in environments characterized by strong nursing leadership and support, collegial relationships among nurses and physicians, and ongoing staff development and quality management efforts (Aiken, Clarke, Sloane, Lake, & Cheney, 2008). The education level of nurses also makes a difference, as demonstrated by studies in surgical settings where higher proportions of baccalaureate nurses were associated with lower rates of patient mortality and failure to rescue (Aiken, Clarke, Cheung, Sloane, & Silber, 2003).

The work environment of nurses is also a primary focus of the Institute of Medicine (IOM). In its 2003 report, *Keeping Patients Safe: Transforming the Work Environment of Nurses* (IOM, 2003), the IOM highlighted the relationship between the quality of nurses' work environments and patient safety. The report placed particular emphasis on the role of nurse leaders, calling on nurse leaders to adopt a transformational style of leadership: engaging with staff in pursuing jointly held goals, while also ensuring appropriate staffing and supporting nurses in acquiring knowledge and skills needed to practice safely and to communicate and collaborate with members of the health care team.

A number of nursing organizations have built on this evolving body of work to create guidelines for developing healthy work environments for nurses. The American Nurses Credentialing Center (ANCC), for example, provides a framework through its Magnet Recognition Program® for developing work environments that promote nursing excellence (ANCC, 2008). Similarly, the American Association of Critical Care Nurses (AACN) has defined *Standards for Establishing and Sustaining Healthy Work Environments* (AACN, 2005). These standards highlight the importance of skilled communication, true collaboration, effective decision making, appropriate staffing, meaningful recognition, and authentic leadership.

Each of these sources was helpful in conceptualizing the journey I was beginning.

THE ROLE OF THE CNO

As CNOs, we are challenged to create a culture and environment that support nurses and nursing practice and ensures excellent nursing care for patients and families. We can best achieve that goal by building on the evidence presented in the literature, the standards recommended by professional organizations, and our own insights and experiences. Another critical responsibility involves interpreting nursing practice to the organization through our comportment, the language we use to describe the work of the clinical nurse, and the strategies we develop to promote and support nursing within the institution (Cathcart, 2008). Through our words and actions, we can help the organization better appreciate how expert nursing practice makes a qualitative as well as quantitative difference in the care experience and the outcomes of care for patients and families.

In operational terms, I believe the role of the CNO and the department of nursing encompasses three overlapping realms or areas of responsibility:

- *Organizational operations*   This includes ensuring appropriate staffing and the availability of appropriate resources to meet patient and family needs 24/7. It also requires jointly leading and participating in organizational planning and quality and safety efforts.
- *Nursing practice*   This includes engaging nurses in shaping the practice environment, giving nurses the support they need to develop in their own practice so that they can provide evidence-based, patient- and family-centered care. It also requires ensuring that nurses never feel "alone" in their practice, or unsupported while caring for patients and families.
- *Professional practice environment*   This includes creating and maintaining a culture and programs and resources that support nurses' ongoing learning and professional development, while promoting nursing scholarship, reflective practice, collaboration, and authentic leadership.

I found that this conceptualization of the role of the CNO and DON provided me with a useful framework for developing an infrastructure to meet organizational demands and advance and support nurses and the professional discipline of nursing.

In the next section, I describe our first steps toward developing this infrastructure. These steps began in my first month as CNO, and involved a discovery process through which I assessed each of the three realms I described above and gained an understanding of the culture, structure, and operations of BWH and the DON. Although my description presents a methodical and fairly linear story, it is perhaps important to note that we engaged in this shared discovery process while contending with the demands and crises that shape the complex and challenging health care systems nurses work in today. We quickly learned that staying focused on our change goals was itself an essential skill in moving forward on our journey.

ASSESSING THE ENVIRONMENT

Based on my earlier experiences as a clinical nurse, nurse researcher, and administrator at BWH and elsewhere, I came into the CNO role with a vision of what I personally believed was necessary to achieve the very best patient outcomes through the work of nurses. I also realized that a healthy work environment for nurses had to be built on a foundation that is strong enough to sustain the cycles of change in health care delivery, and that represents a fit—and hopefully a synergy—between what nurse leaders and clinical nurses value and want to accomplish and what the institution will accommodate and support over time. Before charting a course for the DON at BWH, I knew I first had to learn more about the institution from my new perspective as CNO, particularly about its expectations regarding patient care, the care environment, and the role, position, and authority of nurse leaders and the clinical discipline of nursing. I also had to learn about the DON, including how it was structured and positioned within the organization, the quality of nursing care, and the vision, values, and expectations held by clinical nurses.

I realized the best way to acquire this understanding was by talking to the individuals who knew BWH best: the leaders who guided its operations and the clinical nurses who provided care day in and day out, 24/7. I thus embarked on a discovery process. Over the course of 3 months, I spoke with every nursing leader and many non-nursing leaders and met with clinical nurses throughout the institution. I also was able to begin crafting the relationships that were essential to our future efforts at change.

Institutional Assessment

As noted, BWH is a 763-bed tertiary and quaternary academic medical center, affiliated with Harvard Medical School, that is dedicated to patient care, teaching, research, and community health and service. BWH was created in 1980 when the Peter Bent Brigham Hospital, the Robert Breck Brigham Hospital, and the Boston Hospital for Women merged to become the Affiliated Hospital Center, later named Brigham and Women's Hospital, one of the largest hospitals in the New England region. Before the merger, each of the founding institutions enjoyed many years of local and national prominence. The roots of the Boston Hospital for Women, for example, stretch back to 1832 with the founding of the Boston Lying-In Hospital, one of the nation's first maternity hospitals; the Peter Bent Brigham and Robert Breck Brigham Hospitals were founded in 1911 and 1914, respectively. The three institutions were the site of many groundbreaking clinical advances, including the use of antiseptic techniques in childbirth; successful use of the "iron lung" in the treatment of polio; the development of methods to collect, store, and transfuse blood; and the first successful human organ transplant.

Today, BWH is recognized for its quality of care, an extensive research enterprise supported by more than $500 million in funding, highly competitive training programs, advancements in patient safety, and innovations in health care technology and informatics. The hospital is also a co-founder of Partners HealthCare System, the largest integrated health care delivery network in New England. With approximately 44,000 inpatient admissions and 950,000 ambulatory visits each year, BWH meets the needs of patients throughout Boston, Massachusetts, the New England region, and beyond. Key to our success is our 12,000 employees, 3,100 of whom are nurses.

In the 1990s, BWH, like hospitals throughout the United States, went through a period of deep cost-cutting and restructuring spurred in part by intense competition related to managed care and efforts to contain hospital expenditures. During this time, the hospital's leaders introduced a service line structure that gave administrative vice presidents of service lines broad authority for budgeting and managing costs, including some costs relating to nursing personnel. This had serious implications for the CNO and DON, who lost financial control over significant nursing resources yet remained accountable for nursing practice. As they worked to balance nursing and administrative needs, nurse leaders experienced role confusion, while programs to advance nursing practice suffered and clinical nurses grew increasingly aligned with their service lines rather than the DON.

In 2004, 1 year before I became CNO, the situation changed when the hospital's president restructured the executive reporting relationships. The CNO now reported directly to the president rather than the chief operating officer (COO). This put the CNO on an equal footing with the COO and chief medical officer (CMO). The CNO also regained a good deal of budgetary control. With these changes, the CNO and DON were in a position to reestablish and strengthen their relationship with clinical nurses and to develop a professional community and practice environment that transcended service line boundaries.

In my early discussions with the hospital's leaders, I focused on gaining a deeper understanding of the leaders' perspectives, expectations, and commitment to the chief nurse role and the DON. What I heard from the president and COO was reassuring. Both individuals had previously practiced in institutions with strong nursing departments and understood the essential role nurses play in patient care and on the care team. They viewed the DON as central to the organization's mission-critical work—providing excellent patient care—and expected the CNO to partner with them and the CMO, as appropriate, on administrative and clinical initiatives. They also voiced their commitment to having all nurses positioned in the DON and responsible to the CNO for nursing practice, countering prior decisions that had nurses in selected service lines reporting to non-nurse service line administrators. At the same time, they expected leaders in the DON to ensure that nurses were wholly committed to patient care, the care team, and the quality of care in the institution.

While talking to other senior leaders, however, I found that though the majority appreciated the contributions of individual nurses and nurse leaders, their understanding of nursing as a professional discipline, and of how the DON helped the organization achieve its mission and strategic goals, was more limited. In part, this was because of their infrequent interactions with nurses, since clinical nurses rarely participated on organizational committees and few nurse leaders served as committee chairs. Unless they worked with nurses on the clinical units, leaders and staff in non-nursing departments had few opportunities to witness the wisdom and expertise nurses have to offer.

Departmental Assessment

From my earlier experiences in the DON, I knew that patient care and clinical practice are central to the department's identity. So, too, is a commitment to nursing education. Until 1985, BWH was home to the Peter Bent Brigham School of Nursing, and many of the school's graduates still practiced on the units. Since then, BWH has become the hospital of choice for many schools of nursing in the region, with over 1,000 graduate and undergraduate nursing students completing clinical rotations in the hospital each year. Collective bargaining has also played a role in shaping nursing's identity, as BWH nurses have been represented by a collective bargaining unit for more than 40 years.

As already noted, in the 15 years before I was appointed CNO, the BWH DON had weathered significant challenges stemming from organizational restructuring. Throughout this time, however, nurse leaders and staff had demonstrated creativity and leadership in supporting the hospital's continued growth, even though programs to advance nursing practice and the professional discipline of nursing received only limited organizational support.

One primary goal during my discovery phase was to meet with as many nurses as possible and learn about nursing practice and patient care through their stories. Here, I was guided by the principles of appreciative inquiry, a philosophy and strategy for change that emphasizes identifying the good in an organization, and building on it to envision and then achieve an ideal or "what might be" (Watkins & Cooperrider, 2000). These two merged approaches—reaching out and finding the good—became the bedrock of the change process described in this book.

Discovering the good in BWH nursing required being present with nurses and meeting them in their own settings on the inpatient units and ambulatory areas where they provided care. It also required that I remain open to hearing what nurses had to say while clarifying, for myself, who they were, what made them proud, what they wanted their practice to look like, and what their concerns were. Ultimately, I met with hundreds of nurses on the patient care units, in focus groups, and through meetings with groups and individuals; nurses, in fact, from every level and in every role, including clinical nurses, nurse educators, nurses-in-charge, nurse managers, and nurse directors. These meetings provided me with a data-rich assessment, and established a pattern of sharing information based on mutual trust and respect.

Through my observations and conversations I witnessed examples of amazing teamwork and interdisciplinary collaboration, met nurses who were engaged in innovative nursing research, and heard of many instances of exquisite patient- and family-centered care. I also learned of the tremendous pride BWH nurses took in their work and the care they provided to patients and families. This was a universal theme voiced by nurses in every role and setting. I realized that this strength would serve us all well in our shared journey.

As nurses shared their thoughts about their practice, the DON, and the institution, other themes also began to emerge. These were focused on what nurses wanted as nursing professionals at BWH, including:

- To "be heard" and involved in decisions that affected their practice and the care of patients and families
- To be actively involved in shaping the clinical practice environment (e.g., systems, technology, supplies, and other resources)
- To be supported by the presence of their managers
- To have opportunities to develop professionally and engage in scholarship
- To actively engage in interdisciplinary communication about patients and families
- To continue to have conversations with the chief nurse

In addition to identifying these themes, I also learned that while examples of nursing excellence could be found throughout the institution, they tended to occur in isolation and were usually unknown to nurses in other areas, as nurses had few opportunities to discuss nursing practice and share experiences across unit boundaries. Additionally, the systems, practices, and processes that were in place to support nursing practice varied markedly depending upon a range of variables, including the time of day, the day of the week, the unit, and the manager. Many nurses also seemed unfamiliar with the concept of nursing as a professional discipline with a social contract and responsibilities, and with being part of a broader nursing community that extended beyond the boundaries of their unit. They were similarly unclear about what they could expect of the CNO and the role and purpose of the DON, and noted that meeting with me represented their first experience speaking with the chief nurse.

While I realized there was much work to be done, I was motivated by the energy and pride I had witnessed in my discussions with nurses. I also believed I had acquired a sound understanding of nursing's position within the organization and had begun to formulate priorities at the institutional level. One priority was to focus on ensuring that leaders of non-nursing departments developed a deeper understanding of the discipline of nursing and of the critical role nurses and the DON play in ensuring safe, effective, patient-centered care, and 24/7 operations. To that end, I consistently shared with my BWH leader colleagues our progress toward the changes we set out to achieve. I also wanted to facilitate broader nurse participation in organizational decision-making groups and to promote the development of nurse-physician leadership partnerships to oversee clinical areas, where appropriate. I believed that such partnerships, already in place in several areas of the institution, promote the interdisciplinary collaboration that is essential for patient safety and care improvement (Ponte, 2004). I expected, however, that these and other changes would evolve naturally as a more pressing and important priority was addressed: developing a professional practice environment where the discipline and practice of nursing could thrive and continually grow and develop to meet patient and family needs. Addressing this priority required engaging nurse leaders and clinical nurses, and having them work with me to examine where we were as a department and to define a vision for the future.

DEVELOPING A VISION FOR THE DEPARTMENT OF NURSING

Throughout my initial discovery period, I had been meeting with the Department of Nursing's Nurse Executive Board (NEB), made up of the nursing executive directors, that is, nurses providing leadership in specific clinical areas or with department-wide responsibilities. I turned to members of this group to help me evaluate what I heard in my conversations with nurses, and to use this information and the literature regarding nursing practice development and professional practice environments to identify changes we needed to make and begin sketching out near- and long-term plans.

As noted earlier, I knew that examples of nursing excellence were present throughout the organization; however, because excellence occurred in pockets, the possibility that a patient and family would receive excellent nursing care varied depending on the nurse, the unit, unit leadership, and other factors. The executive directors and I agreed that our most critical challenge (Figure 1.1) was to move from this current state of *high variability* to a state of sustained *high reliability*, where every BWH patient and family was assured of receiving excellent nursing care throughout their care experience, and every nurse consistently demonstrated excellent practice. This required strengthening aspects of the work environment and developing a professional practice environment. More specifically, we wanted to create an environment distinguished by a culture of openness, transparency, and collaboration; authentic nursing leadership; nurse participation in decision making; and systems to support nurses in their practice and to nurture continued learning, advancement, and scholarship.

FIGURE 1.1 *BWH Department of Nursing Model of Change Process*

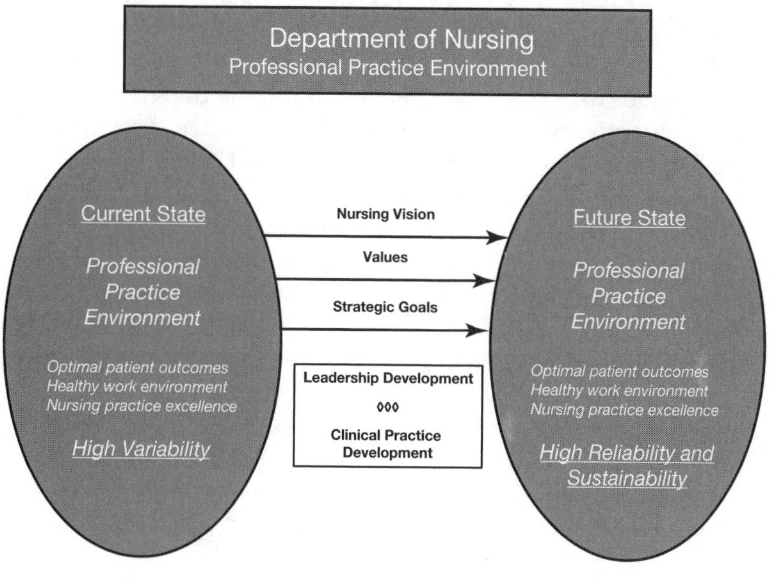

A critical first step, we agreed, was to develop a department vision to unify nurses across the organization and guide change. As a start, a group of us worked to review what nurses had said during my meetings with them and identify essential themes. Once again, nurses' pride in the care they provided patients and families was apparent, as was their desire for a work environment that promoted their professional development and supported them in delivering safe and excellent care. Building on nurses' words and statements, we drafted this vision statement for the DON: *to provide excellent care to patients and families, with the very best staff, in the safest environment.* We also identified the values that supported this vision and drafted the following statements to describe them:

- Respectful partnerships among patients, families, and caregivers are the foundation of care.
- Individual and collective accountability are essential to achieve our mission.
- All who seek, provide, or support delivery of care in our diverse community deserve our sensitivity, compassion, and respect.
- Excellent practice is evidence based and is characterized by creation, application, and evaluation of knowledge.
- Consistency, fairness, and integrity are essential in developing and mentoring staff.
- Interdisciplinary teamwork is essential to excellent care.

The first group to review the vision and values statements was the full membership of the NEB, which also reviewed the underlying qualitative data and the themes from which the vision and values were derived. In addition to validating the vision and values, NEB members helped organize the themes into department goals. The goals identify guiding principles for the professional practice environment we wanted to create in terms meaningful to practicing nurses. They include the centrality of the nurse-patient relationship; nurse participation in shaping the environment; inter- and intraprofessional collaboration; and support for nursing practice, professional development, and scholarship.

With the NEB, I recognized that the true test of the vision, values, and goals was how they were received by nurses in the organization: whether nurses agreed that these statements reflected their beliefs and role in patient care, and whether they motivated nurses to become partners in taking the department to a new level. Three months after the start of my initial discovery phase, I again began meeting with nurse leaders and clinical nurses in meetings and open forums and on patient care units to discuss the vision, values, and goals and whether they resonated with nurses' experiences and beliefs. I also presented them in what was to become an annual "State of the Nursing Department" address, which was open to all nurses in the organization and gave us an opportunity to reflect together on where we were as a department and what we wanted to become. Establishing this feedback loop became an essential practice in sustaining relationships of trust, collaboration, and change.

Feedback from nurse leaders and staff obtained through these forums was consistently positive, with many nurses stating that they felt well represented by the vision, values, and goals. We also received the endorsement of the hospital president and the COO, who reaffirmed their belief in the importance of a strong DON. Their support was critical to all of our work, including the next phase, which involved strengthening elements of the department's core infrastructure and positioning the department to turn its vision into a reality.

PREPARING THE ENVIRONMENT FOR CHANGE

With the department vision, values, and goals established, we then faced the challenge of sorting out our next steps. The vision itself helped us stay on track. In dialogues with nurses throughout the organization, we continually posed two questions: *What does the vision look like in operational terms? How will we know when we've achieved it?* Feedback from nurses on the meaning of excellent care and what was needed to ensure the best nurses and safest environment was critical in prioritizing the next steps. We also found it helpful to recall the DON's three main realms or areas of responsibility: day-to-day operations, nursing practice, and the professional practice environment. The vision clarified what we were striving for, while the departmental realms provided a framework for evaluating our core infrastructure and identifying elements that needed strengthening and development. As we dealt with the day-to-day challenges of our responsibilities, we were able to concurrently frame the decisions we made through our vision and values and thus further our goals.

In early 2007, having completed the first steps in our shared journey, I worked with members of the NEB to map out an initial strategic plan for the DON. Our intent was to ensure that we had the expertise, structures, and systems required to meet our immediate obligations in each realm and also begin work on achieving our longer-term goals. The plan identified foundational systems that needed strengthening, such as those required for financial management, nurse recruitment and retention, and quality and safety monitoring and management. It also identified other priorities. These included strengthening the department's leadership structure and leadership development capabilities; creating mechanisms for engaging clinical nurses in shaping the practice environment; and developing structures and processes to support learning and promote innovation, scholarship, and inter- and intraprofessional collaboration. Some of the early initiatives launched to address these priorities are described in the following sections.

Strengthening Leadership Structure and Development

A strong leadership team is critical for ensuring effective day-to-day operations and an environment that supports healthy nursing practice. My goal was to have an executive team that would partner with me to achieve the department's goals. Concurrently we would model authentic leadership behaviors by remaining open to new ideas, welcoming opportunities for collaboration, and fostering leadership among nurses in all roles. As a precursor to emphasizing this focus in our department goals, I had already broadened the executive leadership team as the change process evolved. I created several new roles:

■ Associate Chief Nurse, to provide leadership in overseeing aspects of clinical operations, nursing practice, and patient care, and to help strengthen the department infrastructure

- Executive Director, Quality Measurement and Reporting, to provide leadership on clinical quality processes and patient outcomes
- Executive Director, Nursing Practice, to lead efforts aimed at understanding the characteristics of excellent nursing practice and conditions required to support it
- Executive Director, Nursing Professional Development, to advise us on the most effective and appropriate methods for supporting ongoing learning in contemporary nursing practice
- Executive Director, Nursing Academic Partnerships and Global Health, to facilitate partnering with university-based schools of nursing and global communities and to create innovative clinical education programs and experiences

The creation of these roles expanded our leadership capacity to meet our goals. With this expanded leadership team in place, we were then able to create initiatives within the strategic plan that furthered our commitment to leadership development and clarity. We identified a subgroup tasked with reviewing and clarifying role descriptions for other key leadership positions, including the nurse manager and clinical director roles. We reaffirmed the importance of NEB in facilitating dialogue, planning, and oversight among executive nurse leaders and developed additional structures to ensure effective communication among the broader nursing leadership team. We launched initiatives to promote ongoing leadership development and help nurse leaders acquire skills needed to create a healthy practice environment for clinical staff. We took steps to expand the involvement of nurse leaders on organizational committees and other interprofessional structures that influence clinical operations and decision making in the organization. As a result of this work, the titles "Nurse Director" and "Nurse Manager" were changed to "Executive Director, Nursing" and "Director, Nursing," respectively, to be congruent with leadership titles of interprofessional colleagues within the institution.

Engaging Clinical Nurses

Underlying our department vision, values, and goals was our commitment to ensuring that the voice and perspective of clinical nurses guided our efforts to reshape the practice environment. Involving clinical nurses in decision making, and partnering with them to define care standards, policies, and practices, promote a sense of community and shared accountability and help nurses appreciate their role as "member-participants in nursing's tradition of practice" (Benner, 2001, p. vi). Nursing committees are an especially effective way to ensure nurse involvement. In 2007, the NEB chartered five nursing committees: Standards, Policies, and Procedures; Patient and Family Education; Safety, Quality, and Care Improvement; Informatics and Clinical Innovations; and Practice. The leadership team and I agreed that 50% of each committee's members would be clinical nurses.

To ensure that the voices of other nurses would also be heard, I worked with nurse leaders to formalize plans for continuing my weekly meetings with nurses on patient care units and in focus groups. These forums had proved critical to helping me establish relationships with clinical nurses and to gaining insight into what nurses need to develop professionally and to deliver excellent care. To support nurses in attending these sessions, we agreed to schedule dates ahead of time so that nurses could factor the meetings into their work flow. This public investment in structured opportunities to give voice to nurses was a central factor in moving forward on our goals and ensuring widespread nursing commitment to those goals.

Supporting Learning and Promoting Innovation, Collaboration, and Scholarship

The DON had in place a number of programs designed to meet nurses' learning and professional development needs. Of these, some were recognized for innovative techniques, whereas others relied on longstanding practices that had not been critically examined for years. A key element of our strategic plan involved bringing these programs together under a single umbrella by launching the Center for Nursing Excellence (CNE). From the start, the CNE was envisioned as an engine of innovation and a hub that would integrate nursing education, research, professional development, and innovation in support of clinical practice. In addition to being a resource for clinical nurses, the CNE would serve as a home for nursing scholars, researchers, and clinical staff.

IMPLEMENTING CHANGE

The structures, programs, and practices I have described here are just a sampling of the changes we introduced and continue through the present. They also tell the story from my perspective. In the next sections of this book, nurse leaders and clinical nurses describe these and other changes in more detail and discuss what it was like to be part of the change process. Although I have described beginning the journey and our intent as we set out, theirs is the story of making it happen, of implementing change.

By the end of 2007, we had reached a milestone. Change had been set in motion. We knew where we were going and why—and we were progressing steadily. Although we were still a good way from achieving the department vision, nurses throughout the organization had begun to view themselves as members of a professional community, and an ever-widening circle of nurses was committed to, and directly involved in, our effort to build a strong, healthy practice environment—to ensure *excellent care to patients and families, the very best nurses, and the safest environment.*

REFERENCES

Aiken, L. H., Clarke, S. P., Cheung, R., Sloane, D., & Silber, J. (2003). Educational levels of hospital nurses and surgical patient mortality. *Journal of the American Medical Association, 290,* 1617–1623. doi:10.1001/jama.290.12.1617

Aiken, L. H., Clarke, S. P., & Sloane, D. M. (2002). Hospital staffing, organization, and quality of care: Cross-national findings. *Nursing Outlook, 50*(5), 187–194.

Aiken, L. H., Clarke, S. P., Sloane, D. M., Lake, E. T., & Cheney, T. (2008). Effects of hospital care environment on patient mortality and nurse outcomes. *Journal of Nursing Administration, 38*(5), 223–229. doi:10.1097/01.NNA.0000312773.42352.d7

Aiken, L. H., Clarke, S. P., Sloane, D. M., Sochalski, J., & Silber, J. H. (2002). Hospital nurse staffing and patient mortality, nurse burnout, and job dissatisfaction. *Journal of the American Medical Association, 288,* 1987–1993. doi:10.1001/jama.288.16.1987

American Association of Critical Care Nurses. (2005). AACN standards for establishing and sustaining healthy work environments: A journey to excellence. *American Journal of Critical Care, 14,* 187–197.

American Nurses Association. (2001). *Code of ethics for nurses with interpretive statements.* Silver Spring, MD: Author.

American Nurses Credentialing Center. (2008). *Application manual: Magnet Recognition Program.* Silver Spring, MD: Author.

Benner, P. (2001, Commemorative ed.). *From novice to expert.* Upper Saddle River, NJ: Prentice-Hall.

Cathcart, E. B. (2008). The role of the chief nursing officer in leading the practice: Lessons from the Benner tradition. *Nursing Administration Quarterly, 32*(2), 87–91. doi:10.1097/01. NAQ.0000314536.91122.8b

Clifford, J. C. (1980). Primary nursing: A contemporary model for delivery of care. *American Journal of Hospital Pharmacy, 37,* 1089–1091.

Clifford, J. C. (1998). *Restructuring: The impact of hospital organization on nursing leadership.* Chicago, IL: American Hospital Publishing.

Coile, R. C. (2001, July 1). Magnet hospitals use culture, not wages, to solve nursing shortage. *Journal of Healthcare Management.* Retrieved from http://www.allbusiness.com/management/3604699-1.html

Henderson, V., & Nite, G. (1978). *The principles and practice of nursing* (6th ed.). New York, NY: Macmillan.

Institute of Medicine. (2003). *Keeping patients safe: Transforming the work environment of nurses.* Washington, DC: National Academies Press.

Manthey, M. (1973). Primary nursing is alive and well in the hospital. *American Journal of Nursing, 73*(1), 83–87.

Manthey, M. (2006). Leadership for relationship-based care. *Creative Nursing, 12*(1), 10–11.

McClure, M. L., Poulin, M. A., Sovie, M. D., & Wandelt, M. A. (1983). *Magnet hospitals: Attraction and retention of professional nurses.* Kansas City, MO: American Nurses Association.

Ponte, P. R. (2004). Nurse-physician co-leadership: A model of interdisciplinary practice governance. *Journal of Nursing Administration, 34,* 481–484.

Vahey, D. C., Aiken, L. H., Sloane, D. M., Clarke, S. P., & Vargas, D. (2004). Nurse burnout and patient satisfaction. *Medical Care, 42*(2 Suppl.), 1157–1166.

Watkins, J. M., & Cooperrider, D. L. (2000). Appreciative inquiry: A transformative paradigm. *Journal of Organizational Development Network, 32,* 6–12.

PART TWO

Creating the Conditions for Change

2

Finding and Defining the Good

Mary Lou Etheredge and M. Patricia Gibbons

The vision for the Department of Nursing (DON)—*to provide excellent nursing care to patients and families with the very best staff in the safest environment*—was developed after months of conversations between the chief nursing officer (CNO), Mairead Hickey, and the clinical nursing staff at Brigham and Women's Hospital (BWH). The vision resonated with nurses in all roles and throughout the organization because it reflected nurses' hopes, values, and beliefs. Among nurse leaders, it sparked a dialogue about beginning the process of creating an environment in which the vision could be achieved. In the spring of 2006, the CNO challenged nurse leaders to focus specifically on two questions: *What does excellent nursing care at Brigham and Women's Hospital look like?* and *How do we ensure excellent care for every patient?*

As nurse leaders on the Nurse Executive Board (NEB), we knew these were critical questions, because their answers would provide a roadmap for the work on which we were to embark. By defining what excellent nursing care at BWH looked like, the DON would be positioned to build on the pockets of excellence that we believed were already present in the organization and create an environment in which every patient and family received excellent care. Our intention was to support all nurses in developing their practice to provide that care.

On the surface, the question of what excellent nursing care looked like at BWH appeared easy to answer. All of the nursing directors (formerly called nurse managers) and executive directors could point to examples of excellent practice in the organization and to excellent nurses. After considering the questions more deeply, however, we realized that our understanding of excellent nursing care at BWH was limited, as it was based largely on anecdotes and on assumptions we had developed from observing various individuals and groups of nurses in the institution. We realized that to truly understand what excellent nursing care looked like, we had to go to the source: to the nurses in every part of the organization who consistently provide excellent care and are identified as role models by their peers.

We decided to launch the "Finding and Defining the Good" initiative, with the goal of describing what excellent nursing care looks like at BWH as articulated by nurses known for giving excellent care. The CNO appointed me (MLE), as the executive director of nursing practice development, to lead the initiative. A team of nurse leaders, including the associate chief nurse (MPG) and the director of perioperative nursing, joined me in planning and implementation. The CNO remained engaged in the work and supported our progress, underscoring the importance of this work and ensuring widespread support among the nursing leadership team.

DEVELOPING A PLAN FOR FINDING AND DEFINING THE GOOD

To develop a plan for finding and defining the good, the work team employed the principles of appreciative inquiry. As noted in Chapter 1, *appreciative inquiry* is a philosophy and change strategy that involves identifying the best of "what is" within an organization, and using that to envision and achieve an ideal, or "what might be." Appreciative inquiry methods were first modeled at BWH by the CNO as she met with nurses throughout the hospital and incorporated their input into the department's vision. Appreciative inquiry methodology differed from former change methods in that it demanded the active engagement of staff at every level and shifted the focus from identifying what is wrong to embracing and building on what is right and what might be.

To fully understand what excellent care looked like at BWH, we needed to hear from nurses throughout the organization. Additionally, involving many clinical nurses in the *discovery* phase of the appreciative inquiry process laid a foundation for widespread participation in subsequent phases: *dreaming,* or envisioning what is possible; *designing,* or co-constructing the ideal environment; and achieving *destiny,* in this case, a healthy environment for patients and families that could be sustained reliably into the future. The discovery phase of appreciative inquiry also relies on storytelling and on individuals sharing facts and feelings about what is working best in the organization. This type of approach explores the facets and dimensions of an organization or construct and facilitates the identification of key themes. With more than 3,000 nurses in multiple clinical areas, finding a way to capture and analyze stories and descriptions of excellent care and practice from nurses throughout the institution was a daunting challenge. We met this challenge through the following multistep process:

Step 1: *Unit-based focus groups*   The nurse directors conducted focus groups in their units/areas. The focus groups consisted of nurses recognized by peers, colleagues, and supervisors as providing excellent care to patients and families.

Step 2: *Analysis*   Comments obtained from the focus groups were analyzed to extract themes. The themes, we found, mirrored those in the literature (notably Benner's work).

Step 3: *Review and validation by clinical nurses*   Clinical nurses reviewed the themes and responded to the question, "Did we get it right?"

Step 4: *Clarification and refinement*   Though not originally planned, a fourth step was ultimately added, and involved small-group discussions with recipients and honorees of the Essence of Nursing Award. (This award, given annually to a clinical nurse or nurse-in-charge [NIC], recognizes nurses who represent the ideals of the nursing profession and the best of BWH nursing. See Chapter 7.) The purpose of these discussions was to uncover, through the nurses' narratives, how they made a difference to patients and families, eliciting greater detail about the characteristics of excellent nursing practice that may typically escape notice and remain invisible.

Unit-Based Focus Groups

Asking the nursing directors to conduct the focus groups on their units offered key advantages. First, unit-based focus groups enabled meetings to be held at a time convenient for clinical nurses, making it easier for more nurses to participate. Engaging staff from one unit or area meant the groups could focus on aspects of practice and conditions that uniquely contributed to excellent care from their specific perspective. Finally, focus groups led by nurse directors gave clinical nurses and directors an invaluable opportunity to talk about unit-specific practice and patient and family care. The conversation between nurse directors and staff shifted from operations and "what is not working" to patients, families, and care. For BWH nursing, this was a significant cultural shift.

At the same time, conducting unit-based focus groups raised a number of logistical challenges. These involved ensuring consistency in the focus group questions and format, preparing and supporting the nurse directors as focus group leaders, and helping them select appropriate staff members for participation. In collaboration with nurse directors, we developed and implemented a plan to address each of these challenges.

To ensure a consistent approach, we developed the following four questions the directors posed to their groups:

1. What does good care look like on this unit?
2. What contributes to your ability to provide good care?
3. What does good care look like from the patient's perspective?
4. How frequently are you able to provide good care?

We developed a focus group toolkit for the nurse directors/focus group leaders that included flip charts, markers, sticky notes, and the focus group questions. Additionally, we met with the nurse directors in small groups to discuss tips and techniques for conducting the focus group sessions, answer the leaders' questions, and provide guidance on selecting clinical nurses for participation. When needed, we held focus group simulations, using role-playing to better prepare the leaders for conducting a session.

When offering guidance about selecting nurses for participation, we asked the nurse directors to choose nurses who were recognized by their colleagues for giving excellent care; who demonstrated a high level of knowledge, skill, and comportment; and whom the nurse directors would want to provide care for themselves or their own families. In addition to relying on their own assessments, the directors were encouraged to obtain recommendations from unit educators and other nurses on staff. They were asked to include at least three or more nurses in each session and to involve at least 10% of their staff in the focus group process. Nurse directors conducted more than one focus group if they wished. When directors completed their focus groups, we reconvened to debrief. All commented on how positive it was to talk about patients and practice with their nurses and how pleased they were to have conversations with clinical nurses about patient care and focus on "the good." The debriefings and enthusiasm of the nurse directors invigorated all of us.

The unit-based focus groups were conducted over a period of 3 months. In the end, all but three (out of more than 30) clinical areas held at least one group, and more than 300 clinical nurses (more than 10% of all BWH clinical nurses) participated. The process yielded a tremendous quantity of data: Approximately 1,000 recorded comments were delivered to us for analysis.

Analyzing the Focus Group Data and Reviewing and Validating the Findings

After the last focus group was conducted, we reviewed and analyzed the data. In the process, we consulted intermittently with a qualitative researcher, as well as a nurse known for her knowledge of nursing practice, the work of Patricia Benner, and how excellent care is demonstrated in clinical settings.

We analyzed the data in two ways. Each individual reviewer first reviewed each data point multiple times. The reviewers as a group then convened to examine the data. Through this process, common themes began to emerge. Ultimately, the following four themes were identified, each describing a different dimension of excellent nursing care at BWH:

- Relationship with patients and families
- Relationship with the team
- Communication
- Environment

We then turned to the nursing literature, and to Benner's work in particular (Benner, 2001; Benner, Kyriakidis, & Stannard, 2000; Benner & Wrubel, 1989), to develop operational definitions and descriptors for each theme, using the individual comments obtained through the focus groups as points of comparison (Table 2.1). For example, for the theme "Relationship with patients and families," the following definition was developed: *Being in partnership with patients and families provides the framework for the caring relationship, and through caring practices the central work of nursing occurs.* The descriptors identified for this theme—involvement, healing relationship, maximizing the patient's participation and control in his or her own recovery, and teaching-coaching—further clarified the scope of the theme and how it is manifested in the practice of excellent BWH nurses.

The four themes, with their definitions and descriptors, were presented to three groups consisting of nurses who had participated in one of the original unit-based focus groups. All three groups confirmed that the themes, definitions, and descriptors were accurate in their representation of what had been said, proposing only minor wording changes.

Taken as a composite, the definitions and descriptors describe how excellent nurses at BWH approach patient care and interact with their environment. Excellent nurses at BWH view the patient and family as central, which is the basis of all their care decisions. They are present for the patient and see the patient as a real person with a life, culture, and relationships that precede and extend beyond an episode of care. Acting as a guide, excellent nurses purposefully use clinical knowledge, forethought, and skilled know-how to respond to and manage the changing clinical needs of their patients. These BWH nurses bring this fundamental understanding of the patient to the care team and work collaboratively to ensure an integrated approach to care.

TABLE 2.1 *Focus Group Themes*

Theme	Descriptors	Representative Comments
Relationship With Patients and Families:		
Operational Definition: Being in partnership with patients and families provides the framework for the caring relationship, and through caring practices the central work of nursing occurs.	Involvement: Interpersonal engagement or relational connection between the nurse and patient/or family (Benner). Healing relationship: Creating a climate for and establishing a commitment to healing. Mobilizing hope for the nurse as well as for the patient. Finding an acceptable interpretation or understanding of the illness, pain, fear, anxiety, or other stressful emotion. Assisting the patient to use social, emotional, or spiritual support (Benner). Maximizing the patient's participation and control in his or her own recovery. There are two components: (1) sensing a patient's strength, drive, desire, and ability to improve and (2) mobilizing these forces in the relationship between the nurse and the patient. In some cases it may also entail serving as a patient advocate (e.g., arguing against a potentially harmful technological intervention in favor of the patient's ability to control and improve his or her condition without the intervention). In situations like these, nurses used their relationship with the patient to elicit the patient's own involvement and control. There is a determined effort to maximize the patient's control over his or her life (Benner). Teaching coaching: Nurses provide benchmarks and timetables to the (hospitalized) patient who does not know what to expect during the course of an illness. So nurses, when possible, forewarn patients what to expect, correct misinterpretations, and offer explanations for the bodily changes. Thus, nurses become experts in coaching a patient through an illness (Benner).	"Here for patient" "Bonds with patient and family" "Presence of the nurse to be sure someone is always looking out" "RN is interested in the patient not as a diagnosis but as a person" "Knowing I made a difference" "Active listening" "Listen, clarify" "I know the patient better than anyone in the room"

(continued)

TABLE 2.1 *Focus Group Themes (continued)*

Theme	Descriptors	Representative Comments
Relationship With Team: *Operational Definition*: Expert nurses at BWH position themselves as partners with all members of the team in order to orchestrate the patient/family care and treatment. They are aware of strengths/weaknesses of team/environment and stay engaged and involved to get the patient what is needed.	Team building: Developing a community of attentiveness, skill, and collaboration. In order to develop sufficient practical knowledge, know-how, and common understanding about practice and roles, common expectations must be built (Benner). Agency: Ability to act upon or influence a situation (Benner). The skilled know-how of clinical leadership and the coaching and mentoring of others: Facilitating the clinical development of others; coaching others in interpreting, forecasting, and responding to patients transitions; bridging the gaps in patient care; building and preserving collaborative relationships; transforming care delivery systems (Benner).	"Cohesive" "Sets the tone for the rest of the nurses" "Teamwork, jump in when someone needs help" "Courage" "Being proactive to prevent escalation of problems" "Shares knowledge" "Teach by example"
Communication: *Operational Definition*: Based on their knowledge of the patient, their clinical grasp and understanding of the clinical situation and desired outcomes of care, BWH expert nurses stay in partnership with patients and families and engage with team members in a dialogue best characterized as open, honest, and collaborative. Knowing that patients need team-based care for the best outcomes, the expert nurse works to understand the specific contributions of each discipline and engages in behavior that promotes and preserves the functioning of the	Team building and community development inherent in caring work require attentiveness and work: Work that is so essential it is the very fabric that holds together the possibility for acting in a social world. The fabric of feeling, culture, and convention that sustains trust and communication is always fragile and vulnerable. It not only has to be preserved from damage and destruction, but must be shielded from mere indifference or neglect. Comportment: Refers to style and manner of acting and interacting, which includes gestures, posture, and stance (Benner).	"Open, easy communication with team" "Strong communication across services" "Quick communication" "Communication with families and each other on care team" "Calm"

team. Through consistent insight into their own and others' behaviors, these nurses communicate and build relationships by offering, and being open to, constructive feedback and advice.

Environment:

Operational Definition: At BWH, the expert nurses demonstrate commitment to a practice environment that is mutually respectful and supportive. They value visible and knowledgeable leadership that facilitates their ability to provide care. These nurses foster clinical inquiry, function autonomously, and assume responsibility for their own professional development. Though expert nurses recognize and acknowledge the importance of having systems and processes in place, they don't allow the absence of such systems/processes to act as barriers to providing care.

Designing nurses' work so that that they have the continuity and context for developing trusting relationships and astute clinical judgments based on knowing their patients provides the safest care (Benner).

"Assignment—Keeping same assignments, continuity of care and assignment, know the patients"

"Inspiring leaders"

"Positive unit energy"

Clarification and Refinement

The themes, definitions, and descriptors provided an essential window into what excellent nursing care looks like at BWH, and into the conditions required for nurses to provide excellent care. However, we believed that the dialogue was just beginning. In particular, we wanted to further hone in on the specifics of how these nurses' excellent practice developed and how they make a difference for patients and families. To gain insight into these areas, we invited nurses who in the past 3 years had been honorees or recipients of the BWH Essence of Nursing Award to assist us.

The Essence of Nursing Award is the DON's highest honor. It recognizes clinical nurses who represent the ideals of the nursing profession and the best of BWH nursing. Peers, colleagues, managers, patients, and families submit nominations for the award. Eleven of the 15 "Essence Nurses," representing a cross-section of clinical areas and specialties, participated in this process. We consulted with Patricia Hooper Kyriakidis, co-author with Patricia Benner and Daphne Stannard, of *Clinical Wisdom and Interventions in Acute and Critical Care: A Thinking-in-Action Approach* (2000), who helped ensure that we captured accurately and comprehensively what the Essence Nurses were telling us.

In small groups, the Essence Nurses were asked to talk about memorable situations from everyday practice when they made a difference for a patient or family. As these nurses described how they came to know the patient, we asked them to include details about the care they provided, the concerns they had, and how the situation unfolded. We coached them to offer as much detail and specificity as possible. The stories they shared illustrated the powerful bond that excellent nurses develop with their patients and the blend of knowledge, compassion, and skill that are the hallmarks of their practice.

Each group session was audiotaped and then transcribed verbatim for in-depth analysis by an interpretative team composed of clinical, content, and methodological experts who helped ensure that we captured, accurately and comprehensively, what the Essence Nurses had discussed. Guided by Patricia Hooper Kyriakidis, and using an interpretive phenomenological methodology (Benner, 1996), the interpretive team reviewed and interpreted each story in detail for themes and aspects of excellent practice (Packer & Addison, 1989). Our goal was to uncover all of the pervasive principles and characteristics of excellent nursing practice at BWH. The interpretation process involved thematically coding and describing the common, everyday habits and practices demonstrated by these Essence Nurses. Through this process, 49 themes were identified as common and pervasive across the nurses' practice. An additional 25 themes emerged that were more specific and enabled clearer articulation of the pervasive themes.

As noted by Benner, this type of interpretive approach yields a "manageable yet rich description of actual nursing practice" (Benner, 2001, p. 39). Individual nursing responses can have different meanings depending upon their context. Involving interpretive team members in the unpacking process, who have a clinical understanding and experiential knowledge like that of the storytellers, better ensures that the storyteller's concerns and intentions are more fully understood and best interpreted. Benner notes, "Usually one or two best interpretations emerge because the meaning of the situation is maintained rather than stripped away to objectified, context-free traits or behaviors" (Benner, 2001, p. 40). In contrast to a checklist approach, the description of nursing practice that emerges is vivid, holistic, and more complete.

The interpretive team then clustered the 49 themes that shared commonalities. Each cluster enabled us to define five characteristics of excellent nursing practice at BWH:

- Knowing the patient and family and having them feel known and cared for
- Making clinical judgments based on specific patient needs, resolving patient concerns, and anticipating likely probabilities
- Working with and leading others to act responsibly and courageously in a timely manner on the patient's/family's behalf
- Caring practices, including interactions and interventions, that are guided by strong notions of good care, moral responsibility, and respect for person/family/loved ones
- Staying attentive, in tune, and responding to the specific patient's clinical and teaching needs when things are and are not going well

We then presented these five characteristics to a small group of the Essence Nurses, all of whom had participated in the narrative groups, asking them to review the characteristics and respond to the question: "Did we accurately interpret what you told us about your practice?" The nurses affirmed that the five characteristics reflected what they had told us. We were pleased to see that the original four themes emerged as part of the characteristics.

Later, in November 2008, we further validated the characteristics when we introduced them to the newly formed Practice Committee. Members of the Practice Committee included nurses in all roles (clinical nurses, educators, directors) representing each area of the hospital (35 members) who were selected by their directors for giving excellent care to patients and their families. This committee also affirmed that the five characteristics accurately reflected excellent nursing practice at BWH. We gained additional confidence when we noted that the characteristics of excellent practice uncovered in BWH nurses' narratives embodied all of the essential aspects of nursing practice described by Benner, Tanner, and Chesla (1996) and Benner et al. (2000), aspects now validated with more than 35 years of research influenced by Benner's work. With this validation, the DON formally adopted the four themes and five characteristics.

KEY LESSONS AND NEXT STEPS

In combination, the initial four themes of excellent nursing care and the five characteristics of excellent nursing practice identified by the nurse focus groups and the narrative groups provide a clear and compelling picture of what excellent nursing care is at BWH. For nurse leaders and staff alike, the findings were especially compelling because they were founded on the actual practices of BWH clinical nurses—insights that were ultimately validated by the nursing literature.

The results of the Finding and Defining the Good initiative gave our vision meaning in a more concrete way and became the foundation for the department's efforts to create a professional practice environment for patients, families, and nurses. In particular, the results directly informed the work of the Practice Committee, which was charged with developing strategies for "preserving and extending the good" that we had found and for supporting nurses in acquiring skills and the integrated clinical knowledge needed to provide excellent care. Leadership development also became a priority to support nurses in providing excellent care. Initiatives were launched to clarify leadership roles and to support nurse leaders at all levels in acquiring skills needed to function as strong leaders of the clinical discipline of nursing at the local and departmental level. Other initiatives were launched to help nurse leaders and staff continue their examination of practice and the nurse-patient/family relationship. Appreciative inquiry, the focus group process, and the narrative groups had given nurses a newfound appreciation for what they could learn by examining their experiences and sharing insights with one another. As a result, they were eager for additional opportunities for dialogue and reflection.

A variety of factors contributed to the success of the Finding and Defining the Good initiative. Among the most important was the ongoing engagement and support of the CNO. From the start, the initiative remained a top priority for her. This in turn kept it a top priority for every member of the NEB. Appointing the director of nursing practice to lead the initiative was another key to its success. In addition to ensuring that the initiative remained on the front burner, the DON imbued it with a deep respect for the clinical work of nurses, a respect that was mirrored by every person who became involved in the initiative.

We also believe that the design of the initiative was important. By validating the results of focus groups and narrative sessions with the staff nurses and with findings from the literature, the process took on a rigorousness that we believe is not often found in service settings. Involving nurses and directors from nearly every unit was also key. Not only did they contribute to the validity of the findings, but it also helped nurses throughout the organization develop enthusiasm for finding approaches to our emergent challenge to "preserve and extend the good" in ways that would benefit patients and families as well as staff.

The authors acknowledge the following persons who made substantive contributions to the work and outcomes described in this chapter: Peggy Doyle, MS, RN; Karen Dick, PhD, RN; and Mary Ellin Smith, MSN, RN.

REFERENCES

Benner, P. (Ed.). (1996*). Interpretive phenomenology: Embodiment, caring and ethics.* Thousand Oaks, CA: Sage.

Benner, P. (2001). *From novice to expert: Excellence and power in clinical nursing practice* (2nd ed.). Menlo Park, CA: Addison Wesley.

Benner, P., Kyriakidis, P., & Stannard, D. (2000). *Clinical wisdom and interventions in acute and critical care: A thinking-in-action approach.* Philadelphia, PA: W.B. Saunders.

Benner, P., Tanner, C., & Chesla, C. (1996). *Expertise in nursing practice: Caring, clinical judgment, and ethics* (1st ed.). New York, NY: Springer Publishing.

Benner, P., & Wrubel, J. (1989). *The primacy of caring.* Menlo Park, CA: Addison-Wesley.

Packer, M.J., & Addison, R.B. (1989). *Entering the circle: Hermeneutic investigation in psychology.* Albany, NY: SUNY Press.

3

Creating a Healthy Work Environment

Angelleen Peters-Lewis, Mary Lou Etheredge, Joan M. Vitello-Cicciu, Mary Lou Moore, and Nancy Hickey

Our systematic efforts at "finding and defining the good" did more than provide us with an understanding of excellent nursing practice at Brigham and Women's Hospital (BWH) (Chapter 2); it also drew our attention to the environment of care. The Department of Nursing (DON) executive leadership team members recognized that this area required our concurrent attention. A healthy work environment that is supportive and respectful is a necessary prerequisite of a professional practice environment and of nursing excellence. Without such an environment, nurses' ongoing professional development and their ability to provide excellent care and achieve optimal patient outcomes can be seriously constrained. In January 2008, the Nurse Executive Board (NEB) committed to developing a healthy work environment as a foundational step in creating a professional practice environment, and embarked on a multifaceted process to define and implement a plan of action.

The concept of our DON working together as a unified collective to advance patient care and practice development was relatively new for us. Prior to Mairead Hickey's appointment as our chief nursing officer (CNO), some nurses and nurse leaders reported to administrative vice presidents in service lines and were thus outside the purview of the DON. This resulted in fragmentation that inhibited the development of our discipline and our identity as a professional community. However, we decided that our history would not inhibit our plan to build a professional practice environment. In this chapter, we describe our work to identify key elements of a healthy work environment at BWH, to examine these elements within the context of our ongoing work, and to establish priority areas and a comprehensive action plan.

UNDERSTANDING HEALTHY WORK ENVIRONMENTS

As nurse executives in a busy academic medical center, we acknowledged that activities related to patient care operations took up significant amounts of our time and attention. We realized we would need to structure for and commit to a deliberate exploration of healthy work environments. To meet our commitment, we designated our monthly Advancing Nursing Practice (ANP) meetings as the optimal arena to begin exploring principles and elements of healthy work environments. ANP meetings bring us together as a nurse executive team for the express purpose of engaging in discussions about nursing practice, practice development, and strategies to advance the discipline of nursing. As a first step, we examined how healthy work environments are described in the literature, and found compelling evidence that validated our commitment and offered helpful guidance. We discovered mounting evidence that a healthy work environment is linked to safe patient care, patient satisfaction, and nurse satisfaction and retention (American Hospital Association, 2002; Aiken, Clarke, Cheung, Sloane, & Silber, 2003; Aiken, Clarke, Sloane, Lake, & Cheney, 2008; Kramer & Schmalenburg, 2008).

Of particular interest to us was the work of the American Association of Critical Care Nurses (AACN). This organization has played a lead role in advocating for work environments that support and foster excellence in patient care and that are safe, healing, humane, and respectful of the responsibilities, needs, contributions, and rights of all individuals, including patients, their loved ones, and nursing staff (AACN, 2005). The AACN identified six essential *standards* for establishing and sustaining a healthy work environment: skilled communication, true collaboration, effective decision making, appropriate staffing, meaningful recognition, and authentic leadership. For each standard, AACN also identified *critical elements*, consisting of structures, processes, programs, and behaviors, required for the standard to be achieved. These elements had particular appeal and resonance for us and began to shape our planning.

ESTABLISHING PRIORITIES FOR ACTION

Through our literature review, we gained a clearer understanding of the elements of a healthy work environment. Our next step involved reviewing the elements and establishing priority areas where we would focus our attention. Through an iterative process involving vigorous debate and dialogue, we reached consensus on the following areas: *skilled communication, collaboration, authentic leadership, meaningful recognition, appropriate staffing,* and *educational preparation of nurses in all roles*—priority areas that to a high degree reflected the AACN list of essential elements. We also agreed to stay focused on practice excellence as a core emphasis.

We realized that our priorities were part of a larger process of transformative change and that some of our priorities were already the focus of other substantive initiatives. The Center for Nursing Excellence (CNE) was redesigning our DON practices around nursing education (Chapter 6). Nursing literature supports the relationship between an educated nursing workforce, patient outcomes, and a healthy work environment (Aiken, Clarke, & Sloane, 2002; Aiken et al., 2003; AACN, 2005). As a leadership group, we took pride in the fact that the number of BSN-prepared nurses within BWH continued to increase. This progress led the NEB, within the last 2 years, to create a position statement establishing the BSN as a requirement for entry into nursing practice for newly licensed nurses. The document we developed explaining our requirement of a BSN for our newly licensed nurses communicates our values about formal education to our BWH clinical nurses and the larger community. As a DON, we also take pride in the longevity and experiential knowledge of nurses, including those who may not have advanced degrees but demonstrate a deep commitment to lifelong learning. Thus, we were also dedicated to creating a description of an educated workforce that honored a senior staff who demonstrated this commitment. An engaged learner in an environment that supports curiosity and continuous education characterizes lifelong learning. This principle was integrated into the DON definition of educational preparation for nurses, demonstrating our deep commitment to lifelong learning and our investment in creating opportunities for this learning.

We also realized that the CNE was catalyzing initiatives on meaningful recognition for our nurses, integrating this into their goals that were focused on education, research, scholarship, and global health care (Chapter 7). Practice excellence had been explored and articulated through our process of "finding and defining the good" (Chapter 2). Therefore, we focused on the remaining priority areas: collaboration, skilled communication, authentic leadership, and appropriate staffing.

Our plan was to share our recommendations for priority areas with nursing leadership (nurse directors and program managers) and obtain their feedback, consensus, and support in developing and implementing an action plan. Before engaging with the larger nursing leadership team, however, we agreed that it was important to first develop an operational definition, an explanation of what we meant by each concept. We wanted to respect the integrity of the AACN's seminal work while making the concepts applicable to the BWH culture. We believed that adapting the definitions and embedding them within the context of BWH would help this work resonate and be more easily embraced by members of the nursing community. We developed the following definitions for this purpose:

- *Collaboration*   The ability to form partnerships for the greater good that are based on mutual goals, honor the philosophy of patient- and family-centered care, and perhaps most importantly, are guided by discipline-specific knowledge.
- *Skilled communication*   Is contextual and must be guided by a commitment to be respectful, engage in ongoing dialogue, demonstrate civility, and embrace openness to varying points of view. It is imperative that the mode of communication be appropriate for the situation.
- *Authentic leadership*   For this priority area, we identified the following descriptors: congruence among expressed values, integrity, courage, and the ability to communicate value for nursing knowledge. These descriptors only begin to reflect the rich discussion that surrounded this area, or our appreciation for the importance of authentic leadership in establishing and advancing a healthy work environment (see Chapter 20.1).
- *Appropriate staffing*   A dynamic, complex phenomenon that reflects both quantitative and qualitative factors. For us, appropriate staffing is not based solely on a predetermined ratio. Rather, nurse leaders determine appropriate staffing based on census, acuity (including psychosocial variables), clinical judgment, and the experience of the clinical nurse.

After developing these definitions, we celebrated briefly and reflected on our accomplishment of identifying priority areas before deciding on next steps. We realized that in order to achieve a meaningful level of advancement, our areas of focus had to be clear, realistic, and achievable. Developing an action plan aimed at fully advancing all the priority areas seemed unrealistic, so we decided to further refine the list. To guide our decisions, we assessed our strengths as a department of nursing and our accomplishments to date, and identified the areas that would really propel us forward on the journey toward co-creating, with clinical nurses, a professional practice environment. We were comfortable with our judgment that appropriate staffing was already being addressed. We had a robust staffing program, embraced by nursing leadership, that included a consistent and unified message regarding staffing to clinical staff.

We agreed that skilled communication and true collaboration are interdependent. Listening, being open to the ideas and suggestions of others, and communicating clearly are fundamental to the collaborative process. For this reason, in April 2008 we began our intentional journey as a leadership community to refine our communication skills. To help guide us on this journey, we invited Phyllis Beck Kritek to BWH. She has offered us guidance, observations, and ongoing learning about healthy work environments, conflict engagement, and leadership development. Her ongoing engagement and coaching have made an invaluable contribution to the successes we have achieved. While focusing on communication skills, we continued to narrow our list of priority areas, now three: *collaboration*, *authentic leadership*, and our continued attention to *practice excellence*. In the fall of 2009, we were ready to move on to our next step: igniting a passion for acting on these priority areas among the nurse director group.

ENGAGING NURSE DIRECTORS IN DEVELOPING AN ACTION PLAN

As we made plans to reach out to the nurse directors, we also realized that continued leadership at the executive level was essential for ensuring transformation and progress within each service and program area in the DON. Each nurse executive was therefore assigned to one of the three priority areas and charged with developing a more comprehensive and detailed definition that further framed the area within a BWH context. Our plan was to share these definitions with nurse directors at our next monthly Leadership Seminar. We agreed that we had already developed a comprehensive definition for *practice excellence* through our "finding and defining the good" initiative. Once more working toward greater clarity, we generated more refined definitions of the two focal priorities that would shape our work with the directors:

Authentic leadership: Authentic leadership is the ability to embody and demonstrate professional values and beliefs, make decisions guided by values, exhibit courage, and motivate and inspire others to engage in advancing the work of the discipline in creating a professional practice environment. Authentic leaders are reflective practitioners who engage in ongoing self-assessment aimed at understanding their ability to influence individuals and groups and how others experience them. Authentic leaders serve as role models and achieve their work through skilled communication, team building, strategic thinking, creativity, leading change, serving others, and building professional partnerships.

True collaboration: True collaboration is the concerted effort of individuals and groups to attain a shared goal. Collaboration exists in outcomes exceeding that which any one person could achieve individually. Collaboration involves engaging in open dialogue to confront issues, exploring underlying concerns, and combining insights to shape a richer understanding and/or approach. This "collective wisdom" acknowledges, embraces, and facilitates interdependence. It is built on intradisciplinary and interdisciplinary partnerships based on mutual respect, trust, shared vision and decision making, and common goals.

We were now ready to present our work and the operational definitions to nurse directors at the Leadership Seminar, which we viewed as the optimal venue for our plan. The Leadership Seminar is an important monthly forum that brings together the chief and associate chiefs of nursing, nurse executive directors, nurse directors, and program directors. As the DON leadership community, we engage in collective learning, work toward gaining consensus, and validate and further refine the DON's current and future work. Through the Leadership Seminar, nurse leaders have worked together to articulate the work of leadership, develop a common language, promote consistency in leadership practice, develop and refine leadership skills, build trust, and solve common problems. Mairead Hickey has used the seminars to challenge us as a leadership community to move from a state of high variability to one of high reliability, and to apply what we are learning in the practice environment. We have invited nationally recognized nurse leaders, in addition to Phyllis Beck Kritek, to the seminars to advance our collective learning. Kathleen McCauley, former AACN president, BWH Visiting Scholar, and Professor and Associate Dean at the University of Pennsylvania, shared her insights during nurse recognition week. Patricia Hooper Kyriakidis, noted scholar and researcher on practice development and how expert practice is demonstrated in clinical settings, has been an ongoing guide of the Practice Committee and of our work to "preserve and extend the good." Our purpose in bringing the priority areas for a healthy work environment to the Leadership Seminar was to engage the nursing leadership team in dialogue, and obtain their validation and help in developing actionable goals.

The Leadership Seminar group embraced the concept of a healthy work environment and the selection and definitions of the three priority areas. The discussion was lively and generated much excitement within the group. Mairead Hickey noted that the next step for advancing the three areas was developing actionable goals. She invited the members of the Leadership Seminar to form work teams focused on authentic leadership, true collaboration, and practice excellence, and to collaborate on defining goals that would guide the work as we moved forward.

Over the next several months, the work teams, in combination with the larger seminar group, focused on identifying skills and education required to help all members of nursing leadership fully integrate each area into their leadership practice. The outcomes of our work are displayed in Box 3.1. The work teams also developed statements that made our commitment to authentic leadership, true collaboration, and practice excellence among clinical nurses explicit, and identified criteria or evidence for assessing our success in incorporating each priority area into leadership practice.

BOX 3.1 *Priority Areas for a Healthy Work Environment: Commitment Statements, Evidence of Progress, and Required Skills*

Authentic Leadership

Commitment Statement

I believe that authentic leadership is essential for excellence in patient care. The nursing leadership at BWH and I are committed to developing all leadership practices to ensure we are able to continuously inspire others; support growth, learning, and scholarship; be powerful advocates for patients and families and mentors to staff; and champions for change with courage, transparency, integrity, and self reflection.

Evidence

- Trusting relationships
- Safe environment to engage in open dialogue about practice and patients. How could I have handled this situation differently?

Skills

- Staying in dialogue
- Building relationships
- Self-reflection
- Courage
- Engagement

True Collaboration

Commitment Statement

We commit to providing excellent patient- and family-centered care through true collaboration that is intentional, respectful, reflective, and accepting of diversity of thought.

Evidence

- Proper e-mail etiquette (25% decrease in volume, increased employee satisfaction with IT communication)
- Conflict resolution through verbal collaboration (use more effective words, explore "trigger" words, conduct at least one appreciative inquiry workshop on use of affirmative words/language)
- Mentoring and coaching in conflict resolution
- Explore and define huddle and staff meeting components
- Service-/unit-/department-specific huddles
- Form leadership book club with membership

Skills

- Use of silence/reflection
- How to stay in conversation when conflict/divergence emerges

Practice Excellence

Commitment Statement

Our commitment is to preserve and promote the nurse-patient/family relationship.

Evidence
- Assignments that are guided by continuity to preserve the nurse-patient/family relationship
- Nurse director presence for "intentional" surveillance (engagement and involvement to know your staff, patients, and climate on the unit)
- Creation of shared vision (leading and managing change)

Skills
- How to develop staff for practice development
- Stages of practice development

NEXT STEPS

The work of ANP and the Leadership Seminar was foundational and continues to guide our efforts to create and sustain a respectful, supportive, and healthy environment for nurses at BWH. We were collectively shifting our nursing culture, creating a professional practice environment that integrated the best practices of our discipline with the unique character and characteristics of BWH. We had transcended the fragmentation that characterized our previous structure and practice and realized that we were developing our unique identity as a BWH professional nursing community. Nurse leaders engaged in intensive learning to ensure that the skills defined for each priority are embedded in our leadership practice. We have also developed and introduced a Nurse Director Development Program. This program will be used to guide nurse directors in examining their own leadership style and abilities and help them acquire new leadership skills. It is our intent to continue to use these and other initiatives to empower nurse leaders to create and sustain a work environment that benefits patients, families, and nurses and helps us achieve the DON vision: *Excellent care to patients and families, with the best staff, in the safest environment.*

REFERENCES

Aiken, L. H., Clarke, S. P., Cheung, R., Sloane, D., & Silber, J. (2003). Educational levels of hospital nurses and surgical patient mortality. *Journal of the American Medical Association, 290,* 1617–1623.

Aiken, L. H., Clarke, S. P., & Sloane, D. M. (2002). Hospital staffing, organization, and quality of care: Cross-national findings. *Nursing Outlook, 50*(5), 187–194.

Aiken, L. H., Clarke, S. P., Sloane, D. M., Lake, E. T., & Cheney, T. (2008). Effects of hospital care environments on patient mortality and nurse outcomes. *Journal of Nursing Administration, 38*(5), 223–229.

American Association of Critical Care Nurses. (2005). AACN Standards for establishing and sustaining healthy work environments. *American Journal of Critical Care, 14*(3), 187–197.

American Hospital Association [AHA], Commission on Workforce for Hospitals and Health Systems. (2002). *In our hands: How hospital leaders can build a thriving workforce.* Chicago, IL: American Hospital Association.

Institute of Medicine, Board on Health Care Services, Committee on the Work Environment for Nurses and Patient Safety. (2004). *Keeping patients safe: Transforming the work environment of nurses* (A. Page, Ed.). Washington, DC: National Academies Press.

Kramer, M., & Schmalenberg, C. (2008). Confirmation of a healthy work environment. *Critical Care Nurse, 28*(2), 56–63.

4

Strengthening the Practice of Nursing

Eloise Balasco Cathcart and Katie Gallagher Fillipon

The BWH Department of Nursing's (DON) vision of providing "excellent care to patients and families, with the best staff, in the safest environment" comes alive within the relationship between the patient and the clinical nurse. Practice is the core of the nursing profession's work; the roles of administration and education are important in that they support this central endeavor. Patient care is also the mission-critical work of the organization, so assuring that the clinical nurse is supported to practice well and that the environment is fit for the practice are essential account-abilities of the Chief Nursing Officer (CNO) and the nursing leadership team.

THE PRACTICE OF NURSING

Thus, early on in the process of implementing the vision, we began to speak about the work of the clinical nurse engaged in the direct care of patients and families as a *practice*. At every opportunity, we recognized nursing as one of the central practices required to ensure quality and safety in the care of patients hospitalized at BWH. Refining our collective understanding of nursing as a practice became a central focus of our process of change.

A *practice* is an integrated web of knowledge, skill, and ethical comportment; all must be simultaneously present and continuously strengthened in particular situations over time for the practice to grow and flourish. Having a practice is more complex than mastering tasks and techniques or applying theory to a particular situation (Benner, Tanner, & Chesla, 2009).

We believed that the clinical nurses who would be leaders in making this vision a reality would be expert practitioners, able to see in a particular situation *what* is needed to be done for the patient and family, and knowing *how* to do it in ways that were respectful of the patient's and family's concerns. These nurses would always work toward achieving what was both right and good for the patient, and could be depended upon to build trust with the patient and family. They would also be instrumental in creating excellent practice communities on the units where they worked, where knowledge and values that the group deemed important would shape the culture, style, and habits of practicing nurses and hold out a vision of practice for new nurses.

A practice has a particular kind of knowledge, "skilled know-how," embedded within it which practitioners of nursing acquire through experiential learning and knowing the patient. For experiential learning to occur, the nurse must be attuned to the patient and be able to read what is going on in the particular situation, be open to having his or her predetermined understanding of the situation turned around, and be able to reflect on what has happened and what has been learned (Benner, Sutphen, Leonard, & Day 2010). For this reason, the practice itself is a continuous source of clinical knowledge development and skill acquisition for the nurse.

It follows, then, that the patient care setting is a place where learning is inextricably linked to the delivery of patient care, a fact that has profound implications for nurse administrators and unit educators. Learning the skilled knowledge of the practice requires tolerance for error; thus a healthy work environment characterized by respect and civility that is supportive of young practitioners is a prerequisite for learning how to be an excellent nurse (Shirey, 2006). The challenge for nurse managers is how to connect nurses and patients in relationships that ensure the best care for patients and maximum experiential learning for the nurse while protecting the safety of both (Cathcart, 2008). Our understanding of these imperatives shaped our initiatives that were focused on strengthening nursing practice.

Patricia Benner used the Dreyfus Model of Skill Acquisition to describe how nursing practice evolves from the detached, rule-driven, analytic thinking of a new nurse to the highly efficient and effective situation-driven practice of the expert nurse (Benner, 1984). As a nurse progresses to a new level of practice, the clinical world is seen with new eyes, and how the nurse understands his or her moral agency changes as well.

Advanced beginners focus on task completion within the time demands of clinical practice, and learn to use and adapt rules and theoretical knowledge in concrete situations. Their mode of thinking is primarily analytic; they tend to be preoccupied with solving tasks at hand and are most comfortable following prescribed procedures. Their performance is mostly normative and mostly safe; they understand moral agency as the responsibility to get the patient through the day and accomplish all the tasks and procedures that are required (Chan, Brykczynski, Malone, & Benner, 2010).

Expert practitioners, in contrast, make intuitive links between seeing the salient issues in the situation and responding to them in ways that are efficient and effective. The expert uses engaged practical reasoning and a sophisticated perceptual grasp to see what needs to be done for the patient, and can move in quickly to meet the patient's needs without going through a time-wasting process of considering alternative solutions (Benner et al., 2009). The expert nurse sees the ethical demand of practice as that of authentically engaging with the patient and family to walk with them through the experience of illness, with the intent of restoring health and preserving dignity in whatever way is meaningful for the particular patient.

As a step in the development from advanced beginner to expert, the nurse becomes a competent practitioner. This developmental phase is critically important, because the nurse begins to see the inherent possibilities within the practice while at the same time coming face-to-face with the suffering, vulnerability, courage, and resilience that are all part of the human condition (Benner et al., 2009). These issues were hidden from the advanced beginner, who was primarily concerned with getting the patient safely through the day. At the competent stage, the nurse realizes the limitations of theory and rules in prescribing the correct intervention for a given situation, and sees that his or her judgment is critical to assuring a good outcome for the patient. This can be a time of great awakening for the nurse as well as a time of great anxiety, and safe passage into this important "competent" phase of practice development still depends on learning acquired from working alongside more experienced nurses. The competent nurse's inability to see or interpret a salient clinical sign or symptom is corrected by others' experiential wisdom and skill of seeing (Benner et al. 2010).

Through the creative use of clinical narrative, we were able to initiate supportive learning experiences for nurses designed to assist them through this progression toward increased competence. As written by Katie Gallagher Fillipon, this clinical narrative illuminates how clinical knowledge and moral agency developed in a young nurse who had approximately 2 years of clinical experience and whose practice was progressing to the competent phase:

> The day that she came was a busy day, I remember that. Her husband came up before her with a ton of belongings and I was trying to help him wipe down movies and clothes and load them into a room. He looked just like a kid; his eyes were wide and scared. All the bone marrow transplant (BMT) family members look like that the first day, like they have just stepped onto a foreign planet where you can only interact through masks and gloves and clothes delivered in zip-lock bags.
>
> When she wheeled onto the floor after having her Hickman catheter placed, the first thing she wanted to do was eat. I tried to start teaching her about what to expect, but quickly came to realize that she apparently knew even more than I did. She was the polar opposite of many of our patients— she was talking about chromosome structure and protein derivatives and I was trying to tell her about dietary restrictions.
>
> She was 28 and I was 24. In her, I could see myself so clearly, which was scary. She could have been me and just as easily I could have been her.
>
> At 18, she was diagnosed with aplastic anemia. Ten years later she had converted to myelodisplastic syndrome. She had searched for a transplant match for almost a year when the option of a double cord transplant became available to her. Her disease had been a battle she fought silently and alone. She lost her mother at a young age and her father is in his 70s. Soon after diagnosis, she became pregnant with a son. Everyone advised her to abort the baby, that it was too dangerous, but she resisted and her son is now 10.
>
> Her husband and her son are her whole world. She never cried. She never showed weakness. She was a model of strength and willpower. For the first month she was with us, she sailed through. We got to know her family and they knew us. We decorated her room for her son's 10th birthday—we helped arrange a special Thanksgiving dinner for her—we crossed off the days on her calendar and waited for her counts to return. In the back room, we would worry for her—she was never sick enough. In my gut, I knew something wasn't right, and then the day after Thanksgiving, I left her with a fever

of 105 rigoring off the bed. She was scared, her husband was scared and we knew something was wrong.

Less than a week later we found out that she had rejected both cords, which had never happened on this protocol at the Brigham. She was profoundly neutropenic and in danger of developing a major infection, but what was worse was the devastation: the prospect of another 30 days in the hospital, isolated, apart from her family.

We did our best to keep her motivated, assured her that they would find two more cords, that they would come up with a new treatment plan, that it would work, even though we didn't know if it would. We encouraged her to walk, to eat, and to believe that it had all happened for a reason.

As Christmas approached, we decided to decorate the unit. Above each door, we hung the words *love* and *faith*, and above her door we hung the word *HOPE*. As we decorated the pod, we thought of making things a little brighter for her.

They did find new cords and they came three days before Christmas. They were like an early present for all of us. Her counts did come back about 30 days later, and the day she left, we cried for her and with her. She told us she couldn't have done it without us, but I will never forget the lessons she taught me.

When she arrived, she knew everything there was to know about transplant and I had wondered what I would have to offer her. But what she helped me to remember was the reason I became a nurse. It's about more than rattling off facts and changing central line dressings. It's about sitting with someone for 10 extra minutes, hanging Happy Birthday signs for a 10-year-old, and helping people find hope when they have lost it.

This narrative set the stage for a conversation between the nurse and an expert interviewer who guided the nurse toward articulating the increased skill and knowledge embedded in her practice and recognizing the value and worth of her work with this patient and her family. As such, it creates the conditions for strengthening the practice of nursing. The exchange that follows provides a template for this process. Our conversation reflects our respective roles, Eloise Cathcart as interviewer and Katie Fillipon as the reflective nurse chronicling her expanding competence.

Interviewer: What did you learn from the experience of caring for this patient?

Nurse: When I met this patient, I really saw myself for the first time in another patient. I had treated many older patients, but this was the first time I think I was really faced with my own mortality and I think also the first time I may have been able to see that patients are really no different than we are. I think I was changing in the way that I practiced and was reaching a point where I could walk into a room and no longer saw the equipment but saw the person and it was allowing me to really become a "nurse" in a very meaningful way.

By recognizing aspects of herself in this young patient, the nurse gets in touch with her common humanity and is able to see her young patient as a real person, with a real life shaped by hopes, joys, fears, and concerns. The nurse's understanding of what this patient's life has been like and what this particular illness and hospitalization mean for her help the nurse to imagine how she might make a difference in a way that is more significant than solely managing the technical aspects of the patient's care. She is beginning to see that being a nurse is more profound than mastering tasks and getting through the day; that the practice offers the opportunity to make a real difference in the life of another human being. The nurse's sense of moral agency—her understanding of why she is there—is changing and she is able to see the possibility of venturing into a place of authentic engagement with this patient in her unique experience of illness. The nurse is beginning to acquire the skill of involvement, without which one cannot achieve expertise in the practice (Benner et al., 2009).

Interviewer: What was hard for you in taking care of this patient?

Nurse: When I knew in the morning that her cords had not engrafted, this was one of the most difficult days for me. We were waiting all day for the Attending to come over and talk to her about the news, they were trying to put a plan together so they would have something hopeful to share. This was only the second time we did a double cord transplant on the unit, but my fear was almost more for her spirit because I knew her and what was important to her and it was her family and it felt like she was being robbed of time with them. I felt like we were taking the wind out of her sails and I was really scared it was going to break her.

Knowing this patient and what is important to her sets up what matters to the nurse. Despite the clinicians' lack of experience with this cutting-edge medical procedure, the nurse's fear is that the patient's world will collapse under the burden of continued separation from her family. She knows that the patient's "husband and her son are her whole world." The nurse's concern becomes preserving the patient's ability to be a wife and mother, which constitutes her personhood and gives meaning to her life. By protecting the dignity and personhood of this patient, the nurse is living out one of the focal caring practices of nursing and strengthening her own understanding of what it means to be a nurse (Benner et al., 2010).

Interviewer: What helped you to get through this time of caring for this patient?

Nurse: I think what was so important about this time was actually the concept of a team. To be a strong care provider, you have to work in a supportive environment, which I did. We had so many doubts about this patient but we all believed in her and when it was hard to walk in that room with a smile and talk her through her anxiety we could rely on one another to talk about our fears for her so she would never see or feel any of that. What was critical at this time was knowing this patient; she was strong-willed and stubborn and had a tough exterior, you had to chip through it to get to what was inside and that was critical because she needed to talk about how scary this was so that she could focus on getting better and not keep everything bottled up. Also, what got me through this time was the wisdom of nurse mentors who had been doing this work for years and years. These mentors always told me that when a patient gets chemotherapy and doesn't get sick, you should know it is a bad sign. This came from years of experience and from knowing their patients.

The nurse tells us how the support of colleagues helped bolster her courage and ability to tolerate and bear witness to the unfair losses and tragedies that this patient experienced (Charon, 2001). The staff's shared understanding of good practice and of what was important in the care of patients on this unit shaped the ways in which they worked together to offer each other guidance and respite from the demanding work of caregiving with critically ill, bone marrow transplant patients. The practice community served as a place of renewal for the nurse, so that she in turn was able to support the patient in maintaining hope and excavating her fears. It also served as a repository of the clinical wisdom of more experienced nurses who had cared for many patients in similar situations, and this experientially gained clinical knowledge sensitized the nurse to the fact that something was wrong with the patient—not unlike an early warning sign of impending disaster.

Interviewer: What did writing this narrative and reflecting on this experience mean to you?

Nurse: When I wrote this narrative, I had no idea that it meant anything. When I shared it with my peers, they told me I had done a good job with this patient, and I began to believe that maybe I could make a difference. Looking back, this was the first time I remember leaving everyday and knowing why I was doing what I was doing. I could see that by forming relationships with patients, I could be a nurse in a completely different way.

The validation that comes from peers helps this young nurse to recognize the value and worth of her work and reinforces her sense of competence and mastery. The nurse's understanding of good practice is not a matter of individual preference, but "is socially constituted and embedded within the discipline as well as within the norms and mores of the particular unit on which the nurse practices" (Benner et al., 2009, p. 215). Narrative gives voice to this nurse's experience, tells what it was like for her to care for this patient, and describes the ways in which her practice grew from this experience. Narrative helps to preserve and extend the caring practices that are foundational to nursing practice and that may be at risk in cultures focused on efficiency, effectiveness, and productivity (Cathcart, 2008).

Living out a vision that encompasses excellent care requires nurses to authentically engage with patients and families to achieve healing, restore dignity, and make complex medical treatments safe and effective (Cathcart, 2008). Such exquisite work is more complex than simply performing tasks and treatments; it depends upon the presence of highly skilled caring practices reliably lived out by nurses who understand the power inherent in the practice and are committed to achieving expertise. The realization of this vision is ultimately dependent upon strong nursing leaders who respect the work of clinical nurses as critical to the DON's mission, understand and support the ways in which clinical knowledge develops, and hold open organizational space for these caring practices to be articulated and flourish. It was this commitment and support that moved the BWH DON to strengthen practice through a focused and fostered process of change.

REFERENCES

Benner, P. (1984). *From novice to expert: Excellence and power in clinical nursing practice.* Menlo Park, CA: Addison-Wesley.

Benner, P., Sutphen, M., Leonard, V., & Day, L. (2010). *Educating nurses: A call for radical transformation.* San Francisco, CA: Jossey-Bass.

Benner, P., Tanner, C., & Chesla, C. (2009). *Expertise in nursing practice* (2nd ed.). New York, NY: Springer.

Cathcart, E. (2008). The role of the chief nursing officer in leading the practice: Lessons from the Benner tradition. *Nursing Administration Quarterly, 32*(2), 87–91.

Chan, G., Brykczynski, K., Malone, R., & Benner, P. (2010). *Interpretive phenomenology in health care research.* Indianapolis, IN. Sigma Theta Tau.

Charon, R. (2001). Narrative medicine: A model for empathy, reflection, profession and trust. *Journal of the American Medical Association, 286*(15), 1897–1902.

Shirey, M. (2006). Authentic leaders creating healthy work environments for nursing practice. *American Journal of Critical Care, 15*(3), 256–267.

5

Ensuring the Voice of the Nurse: Designing, Developing, and Implementing a Committee Structure

Barbara Bauman, Ellen Liston, Anne Bane,
Denise Goldsmith, Ann Furey, and Diane R. Lancaster

*I*n the summer of 2006, members of the Brigham and Women's Hospital (BWH) Nurse Executive Board (NEB) embarked on an exploration of our existing and desired shared governance infrastructure. We wanted clinical nurses to be actively and deeply engaged in the actual work of the department, and sought to create an infrastructure that would ensure this. We had been charged by our Chief Nurse Officer (CNO) Mairead Hickey to develop the right structure for doing the work that we determined was essential to the Department of Nursing (DON). Included in this charge was the expectation that we would create a reporting-out process to the nursing community.

Before moving to developing the right structure, our first action was to consider our vision, our values, and our experiences to date with accomplishing essential work of the department. Upon reflection, we realized that many past successes within the DON had been realized through formal committees, task forces, and work groups. We were also committed to designing systems, structures, and processes to ensure that the collective voice of all nurses would be heard within an environment that fostered clinical inquiry, collaboration, and continuous learning. Therefore, we proposed a committee structure to respond to our CNO's charge.

We envisioned that the primary work of committees would be to provide forums in which the expertise of nurses influenced and shaped the nursing practice environment. Further, we determined that the primary work of nurses in leadership positions would be to establish and implement processes and systems that operationalized committee decisions.

Based on these two fundamental premises, we developed the following guiding principles for developing the committee structure:

1. Nurses from direct care, leadership, and executive roles are involved.
2. Membership will ensure appropriate expertise and clinical area representation.
3. Evaluation of goals is part of each committee's work.
4. Because safety and quality are components of good-quality care, patient safety and practice development are shared responsibilities of all roles.

5. Mentoring and coaching are core components of committee work.
6. Committees will be supported through leadership and other resources.
7. When appropriate, committees will be linked to the director of the relevant nursing departmental program.
8. Accountability for implementation is the work of leadership.

As discussion continued, the notion of "critical threads" emerged. *Critical threads* were essential themes, concepts, or considerations that we committed to weaving throughout all the work of all the committees. The critical threads we identified are:

1. Department vision and goals
2. Regulatory compliance
3. Evidence-based practice
4. Staff education plan
5. Operational feasibility and impact
6. Communication plan, including key stakeholders
7. Program evaluation

We recognized that not all work of the department would (nor should) be done through committees. There are programmatic initiatives within the department that have defined processes and goals, such as orientation and training/education for new technology implementation. We decided that this committee structure would be designed to accomplish work in five key strategic areas:

- Nursing Practice
- Quality, Safety, and Care Improvement
- Patient and Family Education
- Informatics and Clinical Innovations
- Standards, Policies, and Procedures

Each committee would be co-chaired by a clinical nurse and a nurse leader (either director or educator), and membership would be configured so that at least 50% of the members on each committee were clinical nurses. Membership was to be evenly distributed across clinical divisions and specialty areas. Each committee also would have one or two advisors, who were senior nursing leaders, either Program Directors or Executive Directors in the DON. The co-chairs and advisors would become our Nursing Coordinating Committee (NCC). They would meet monthly to review and coordinate the activities of all the committees. The NCC was co-chaired by the Associate Chief Nurse, the Executive Director for Practice Development, and a nursing director. All committees would report into the NCC, which reports to the NEB. The NEB would thus become the final approval body for committee recommendations.

   The systematic work of creating our desired infrastructure completed, we presented the guiding principles, structure, and initial committee charges to the NEB in fall of 2006. With their formal approval, we set ourselves to the next task: developing the proposed infrastructure that would activate the committees and their work. Advisors further refined committee charges, selected the first co-chairs, and determined the detailed membership of each committee. After consulting

FIGURE 5.1 *Nursing Committee Structure*

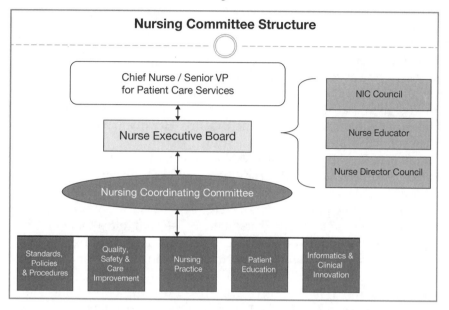

with nurse directors regarding what would work best with staff schedules, the meeting schedules were set, rooms booked, and administrative support and resources obtained. The advisors and NCC co-chairs developed a formal process for requesting and approving clinical nurses to be committee members. Co-chairs attended a formal educational session, conducted by the advisors, on how to set up and run effective meetings. The fall of 2007 marked the formal kickoff of the new committee structure. What follows are brief reflections on the work of the past 3 years, authored by the advisors with contributions from the co-chairs of each committee (Figure 5.1).

PRACTICE COMMITTEE

Advisor: Ellen Liston, RN, MSN

The Practice Committee, co-chaired by Mary Beth Mondello and Alice O'Brien, has 40 members; 65% are clinical nurses, and 35% are in nursing leadership roles. This committee was charged with providing input to nursing leadership about what needed to be in place so that each BWH nurse had the opportunity to achieve excellence and each patient would receive excellent care with high reliability rather than variability. We knew that excellent practice existed. Prior to the formation of the Practice Committee, excellent clinical nurses at BWH had been identified and, from their narratives, five characteristics of excellent practice had been uncovered in a process we called "Finding and Defining the Good" (Chapter 2). The Practice Committee's work would therefore focus on preserving and extending that excellence in practice.

Historically, when talking about excellence in nursing practice, the BWH culture had framed discussions around compliance, technology, and assessment/documentation of competency. Therefore, conversations about excellence in patient care with the focus on the nurse/patient/family relationships and practice development would be new. The committee needed to be prepared for this work. We sought the assistance of Patricia Hooper Kyriakidis, who brought to the committee her knowledge of the stages of practice and practice development, and her experience with the richness that narratives bring to understanding and affirming the complex and experiential nature of nursing practice. Her availability to the committee proved to be invaluable.

The first task of the committee was to confirm the characteristics of excellent practice that had been uncovered from the narratives of expert nurses at BWH. For the purpose of validation, the committee was asked, "Do the characteristics accurately reflect excellent nursing practice at the BWH?" The answer was yes, but recommendations for changes in the language were offered. The committee thought some of the wording was too academic to be accessible to the typical nurse caring for patients (e.g., clinical instead of critical thinking, comportment instead of behaviors). However, oversimplifying the wording diluted the breadth, depth, complexity, and meaning of the rich practices uncovered in the nurses' narratives. To move our nursing culture from a technical to a professional mindset, clear, accurate language was important. After lively dialogue about the meaning and significance of what had emerged in BWH nursing practices, we adopted the language of the characteristics to reflect and preserve the richness of the practice as well as the scholarly interpretive work employed to define them. We more fully appreciated the reason for the concern after we increased our understanding about the stages of clinical development, from beginner to expert. We gained a fuller knowledge of the foundational work that provided scientific support for the five BWH characteristics. This education was highly interactive, and situated in the context of specific patient situations so that the committee members heard the voice, intent, and concerns of the nurse through narratives. Through this process, members gained a deeper understanding of the origin of and complexity articulated in the characteristics and how they appear at the different stages of practice. They came to appreciate that excellence can be present at each stage of practice when there is constant learning. There was also a better understanding of expert practice.

Next, in order to grasp the extent of the need for clinical development, the committee was asked, "What percent of nurses on your unit would you choose to care for you or a family member?" The committee acknowledged that the majority of nurses would benefit from further clinical development to gain the experiential expertise defined in the five characteristics of excellent nurses (e.g., collaboration, clinical leadership). Patricia Hooper Kyriakidis explained that this was not a surprise, as little post-undergraduate clinical education focuses on developing key practical aspects identified in the characteristics, such as engagement, skillful interactions with patients and families, or moral agency, leaving nurses to depend on trial-and-error learning. Drawing on the same rich literature resources that guided the "Finding and Defining the Good" initiative described in Chapter 2, we were able to find support for our decisions that was evidence-based and tested.

We then used the appreciative inquiry process to elicit and describe the supports and/or conditions that needed to be in place to give every BWH nurse the opportunity to develop expertise and every patient the opportunity to receive expert nursing care. After careful consideration, the committee detailed the supports and conditions required for the advancement of practice. These were grouped into five themes:

- An effective nurse manager
- Supportive colleagues
- A culture of learning
- An assurance of adequate and equitable resources
- Conducive strategies and conditions

We reviewed available nursing literature, once more drawing heavily on the resources that shaped the "Finding and Defining the Good" initiative, and working to identify what constitutes a healthy work environment. The readings, made available to committee members, validated for us that our themes were consistent with current nursing research. However, the committee's voice was weighted as more meaningful and the need to act made it more urgent.

The Practice Committee takes great pride in its accomplishments: confirming the characteristics of excellent practice, becoming knowledgeable about the stages of practice, estimating the prevalence of the necessary clinical development, and identifying the supports and conditions necessary to support excellent practice. This committee's work has informed and shaped the ongoing development of several programs, including our Nurse Director Role Development project designed to further develop the nursing directors as clinical leaders of the discipline at the unit level; our nursing Leadership Seminars, which provide a forum for the collective learning of all nurses in leadership roles; and our Acute Care Documentation Project, a system-wide initiative to convert current paper documentation of patient care to an automated electronic format.

The committee has faced unfamiliar challenges that differ from those confronting most other committees. Unlike committees that are charged to produce something tangible, such as revised policies or new safety protocols, this committee's work has been less tangible and more qualitative in nature. Issues that result in variability in the quality of care are discussed; recommendations that may result in achieving high reliability in quality of care are offered. Communicating the content of these discussions has been ongoing with nursing leadership; however, conveying this to clinical staff has been a challenge. Committee members are surveyed regularly about the methods they have utilized to share this work with their colleagues. Some members, with mixed results, have utilized staff meetings and communication boards. Time at committee meetings is reserved for coaching members on engaging colleagues in conversations about practice development and hearing about their successes and failures. It is a continuous process for the committee, and it is teaching us how best to communicate and advance this qualitative work.

Another challenge for this committee is differentiating the work of the committee from the work of leadership. Adoption and implementation of this committee's recommendations are most often the work of leadership. Some experience delays and uncertainty as lack of progress. Committee members are reminded that changing a culture is slow and that specific outcomes will be hard to measure in the short term. We reinforce with committee members that they are indeed influencing the leadership and shaping the direction of the DON.

Their voice continues to guide the evolving excellence of nursing practice at BWH and the quality of care on which patients and their families can rely.

INFORMATICS AND CLINICAL INNOVATIONS COMMITTEE

Advisors: Anne Bane, RN, MSN and Denise Goldsmith, RN, MS, MPH

The Informatics and Clinical Innovations Committee was co-chaired by Heidi Doucette, RN, CNRN, and Carol Booth, RN, MSN. It has 36 members, of which 74% are clinical staff nurses and 26% are either nurse educators or have nursing leadership roles. The primary purpose of the Committee is to insure that nursing practice drives technology related decisions, thereby supporting and enhancing the clinical nurse's role in caring for patients while promoting patient and staff safety. To achieve this objective the committee agreed upon a set of primary functions. The committee will:

- Serve as a forum for review and approval of new information system technologies which impact the clinical nurse, including informing the design, configuration, implementation and ongoing support of new technologies and clinical information systems.
- Serve as a forum for feedback and continuous improvement for existing technologies in use at BWH.
- Identify criteria related to the selection of new technologies and clinical information systems with an emphasis on critical human factors and the workflow of the clinical nurse.
- Provide user-testing expertise for BWH clinical systems.
- Provide information and feedback to the Information Systems Steering Committee that makes decisions around project budgeting and funding.

Through structured focus groups, work flow analysis activities or listening to guest presentations followed by group discussions the committee has provided feedback and direction for many BWH initiatives, including:

- Acute Care Documentation (ACD) project
- Smart Pump Drug Library development and validation
- Laboratory Order Communication
- Patient Education TV
- Pharmacy/eMAR (electronic Medication Administration Record) downtime support

The establishment and communication of meeting etiquette ground rules was a crucial first step to our success. It helped to clarify the role of member, co-chair and advisor, and the responsibility of each within the context of the committee work. While the committee advisors were seasoned meeting facilitators, the co-chairs were not. Advisors coached the co-chairs on how to develop reasonable time frames for agenda topics. We also developed and implemented a structured template with clear timelines to help guide guest presentations. To help establish the positional authority of the co-chairs the advisors found it best to be seated towards the back of the room so that eye contact between member and co-chairs was encouraged.

We continue to struggle with two main issues; outspoken committee members and communication of the committee work. To address the former we have had to have side bar conversations with members taking more than their fair share of air time, and focus during the meeting on encouraging our less active members to participate. To address the latter we have instituted a "take away" set of information that members distribute to their units.

Prior to the establishment of this committee no forum existed for clinical nurse/end-user feed back on new technologies that were introduced into their workflow. This committee provides clinical nurses at the bedside access to BWH employees whose job it is to purchase and/or support new information technologies. This was a new phenomenon in our organization. While the cultural shift of seeking out end-user feedback was slow at first, we now find that the committee is highly sought after to provide feedback prior to, during and after new technology purchase and implementations. It is clear that providing a forum for end-user feedback on new clinical systems as well as current issues/problems leads to a more accurate and timely solution. Additionally nurses feel more valued and now view themselves as part of the solution.

Members report that sharing their work with each other "inspires others in the room" and that it is a "great motivator". A very important theme we found in the evaluation feedback was that there was "sharing of ideas in a non-judgmental setting", that "we are listened to and that our opinions matter". They believe that what they do "impacts the bedside nurse in a positive way" and they are "actually solving problems and improving care". One member summed up nicely her thoughts on the work; "Work we do will have far-reaching impact on BWH nursing in the future".

PATIENT AND FAMILY EDUCATION COMMITTEE

Advisor: Ann Furey, RN, MBA

The Patient and Family Education Committee was co-chaired by Deb Moody, RN, BSN, and Cindy Loring, RN, MSN. It is comprised 22 members; 51% are clinical nurses; the other 49% are nurse leaders and the director of the Patient and Family Library. Additionally, we include a provision for ad hoc committee members when the work of the committee requires expertise from other disciplines. The committee charges provide the foundation for our goals and objectives, and include:

- Providing feedback into the DON patient education policies, procedures, and standards based on best practices and Joint Commission standards
- Providing input into the goals of the Patient Education program
- Making recommendations for necessary educational resources
- Providing input and feedback on new technologies and media that can support the delivery of patient education
- Advising on the development needs of staff

The initial priority of the committee was to provide adequate patient education resources to staff nurses. Because we have all clinical areas represented on the committee, an initial brainstorming session about needed resources served as an organizational-wide needs assessment. Our purpose was to ensure that staff had the necessary patient education resources.

Orientation of the members was an important first step in our focus on patient education. The Joint Commission emphasizes the need to provide patients with written materials that are current, accurate, and have approximately a sixth-grade reading level. They advocate reinforcing print materials with verbal instruction to improve patient comprehension and compliance with the plan of care. Our committee member orientation included education on health literacy and appropriate education materials for patients, in part shaped by these guidelines. This orientation prepared us as a committee to begin pursuing our goals and meeting our charges.

The committee has engaged in a number of activities over the 3 years since its inception. Some that were highly significant include:

■ Identifying and evaluating electronic resources that currently exist on the hospital intranet and determining which would be useful for staff nurses and could be included on the Patient Education Website

■ Providing feedback on the new BWH interactive TV system as a patient education tool

■ Providing feedback on the purchase of a patient education database by evaluating content to determine that an adequate breadth of topics was available to meet the needs of multiple clinical areas and evaluating the content for accuracy and relevancy

■ Advising on the process of educating and documenting anticoagulation therapy and infection control

■ Advising on the best course of action to take when a change in insurance coverage altered the availability of diabetes glucometers and created a significant impact on a nurse's glucose monitoring teaching

The work of this committee has provided those of us involved with many valuable lessons. Some of the most important include our conviction that:

1. Broad representation of nurses from all clinical areas is essential to facilitate the work of the committee.
2. The percentage of staff nurses serving on the committee should always be greater than 51%, to ensure that their voice is present in the work.
3. Representation of several nursing roles is important. The attendance of nurse directors, nurse educators, and staff nurses allows all perspectives to inform the committee's work.

For others who hope to create a comparable initiative, we offer the following advice:

■ CNO support is essential. When nurses participate in committee work, it is at a cost to their unit budgets, and requires nursing director effort to ensure that nurses scheduled for meetings are adequately covered on the unit.

The BWH practice of ensuring staff nurses' participation in committee work away from patient care has been successful because it has strong executive support.

■ It is important to respond to nurses' requests and demonstrate how their feedback has shaped decisions. It is both empowering and satisfying to nurses to know that their voices have made an impact.

■ Patient education committees are often multidisciplinary. At BWH, our committee is a nursing committee. This has allowed us to focus on nursing practice as a means to provide quality patient education.

QUALITY, SAFETY, AND CARE IMPROVEMENT COMMITTEE

Advisor: Diane R. Lancaster, RN, PhD

The Quality, Safety, and Care Improvement (QSCI) Committee was co-chaired by Mary Antonelli, RN, MPH, and Stephanie Capello, RN, BSN. It has 19 members; 58% are clinical nurses and 42% are nurses in leadership roles. In designing this committee, we were challenged to create a balanced relationship between the governance role of the committee and the operational responsibilities of the quality department's program directors in our newly formed quality program.

Because the members of this committee are a group of exquisitely talented nurses whose usual method of operation is to jump right in with both feet to solve an issue, the group struggled at first to accept that this was not the expectation. It took about 18 months for the committee to become comfortable with the notion that the primary role of each member was to ensure that the voice of the nurse is heard and serves to inform the system and process improvement initiatives that were underway or in development; essentially, that their role and that of the committee was one of representational governance and not program administration. In addition, the committee co-chairs consistently reminded staff at each meeting that their voice is critical to identify and advise on safety or quality-of-care issues they experience during their everyday bedside practice before such issues become patterns or trends. Framing their role and contribution in this way was an intentional strategy used by the co-chairs to help staff develop a stronger value for prevention as a key intervention in a quaternary academic medical center.

Having the committee co-led by a staff nurse and one of the quality program directors during its first 3 years was an effective mechanism by which the staff co-chair had a role model and mentor to learn and grow from. By the end of her 3-year term, our staff nurse co-chair was able to assume the lead for running the meetings, developed superb skills in agenda management and item follow-up, and served as a role model for other committee members in the communication and application of project findings on her unit. In an effort to ensure that all committee members had opportunity to bring forth issues for discussion, she proposed and implemented the "open circle" concept. This is a standing agenda item that occurs either at the start or end of each meeting during which members are encouraged to share innovative work occurring on their units or to identify process or systems issues that affect patient safety and/or care.

The primary functions of the committee are to:

- Review data from related hospital committees to identify trends pertinent to nursing practice and patient outcomes
- Identify and recommend department systems and processes in need of improvement to advance patient outcomes and nursing practice
- Utilize reliable and valid data to support clinical decision making and development of clinical innovation
- Identify patient and staff education needs related to quality and safety initiatives
- Identify need for new or revised policies, procedures, and guidelines based on quality and safety project findings
- Provide staff with reliable and valid data to empower their clinical decision making and assist with development of clinical innovations
- Review departmental and unit-based performance on nurse-sensitive outcome measures and identify opportunities for improvement

To accomplish its work, the QSCI committee interfaces with a broad range of hospital functions and task forces. Some examples include:

- Ergonomics related to ceiling lift use, education, staff injury, patient satisfaction
- Biomedical Engineering Department, to revise repair tag policies and procedures to enhance staff use and provide a process for reliable identification of broken equipment
- Drug Safety Committee, to review medication-related issues trended out of the safety report system

In summary, the department owes much to the lessons it was taught by this inaugural group of committee members, and will continue to reap those benefits for many years to come.

STANDARDS, POLICIES, AND PROCEDURES STEERING COMMITTEE

Advisor: Barbara Bauman, RN, MS, MPA

The Standards, Policies, and Procedures Steering Committee is co-chaired by Cindy Jodoin, RN, MHA, and Sharon Swan, RN, BSN, MSN(c). It has 23 members, of which 61% are clinical nurses and 39% are nurses in leadership roles. A more in-depth description and discussion of this fifth committee is provided in Chapter 9. This detailed account of one committee's structure and work provides a closer look and better understanding of the actual "nuts and bolts" of starting up, growing, and sustaining a large committee in a complex acute care hospital environment. We believe our work provides a valuable exemplar of a change process guided by a vision.

6

The Center for Nursing Excellence: Setting the Table

Laura Mylott, Patrice K. Nicholas, and M. Patricia Gibbons

When our new Brigham and Women's Hospital (BWH) chief nurse, Mairead Hickey, articulated the departmental vision to "provide excellent care, with the best staff, in the safest environment," she also promised that as change occurred, no nurse would feel alone in his or her practice. Her intent was to open up possibilities to refine and extend excellent nursing practice; allow for innovative thinking; and create safety for patients, families, and nurses as new models of practice emerged and were tested. Early on she envisioned a Center for Nursing Excellence (CNE) as a core vehicle to bring about the necessary level of transformational change in the clinical area.

Merging two existing traditional programs—staff development and nursing research—the CNE was created in 2007. To signal the key role that the CNE would play in achieving the goals of the Department of Nursing (DON), the Associate Chief Nurse, Patricia Gibbons, assumed the position of Executive Director of the CNE and appointed two directors of nursing to newly established positions: one for innovation in clinical teaching and evidence-based practice (Laura Mylott), and one for global health and academic partnerships (Patrice Nicholas). Both directors brought scholarship to clinical nursing practice and led initiatives designed to foster engagement and partnership with clinical staff. We created the pioneering team that made the CNE a central resource in our process of change and transformation.

Our first task was to bring the new CNE staff together to explore how they would integrate education, research, professional development, and innovation to support clinical nursing practice. Our intent was to ensure stability in existing programs while opening up possibilities for new and creative ways of meeting the needs of clinical staff. It was precisely this focus on integration and advancement of nursing practice that began to signal the change to come. Eight goals were then developed to guide the CNE's work with clinical staff (Box 6.1).

We knew change was necessary both within the newly created center and in the center's relationship to clinical and leadership staff. An early internal assessment of the CNE revealed that although individual staff members and some programs were highly valued, the emergent "Center" was seen as distant and detached from the real world of clinical practice. In turn, center staff experienced a lack of

---

BOX 6.1 *Inaugural Goals of the Center for Nursing Excellence*

1. Support the successful transition of experienced clinicians and newly licensed nurses into nursing practice and as members of an interdisciplinary team at BWH.
2. Create orientation and development programs for unlicensed staff who provide care to patients and families, and support clinicians in their work.
3. Use evidence-based and innovative teaching strategies to guide teaching practices, assuring excellence in the teaching of both practicing nurses and nursing students.
4. Utilize innovations in technology to enhance patient safety, expedite the work of the clinical nurse, improve documentation processes, build simulated clinical environments for learning, and seamlessly integrate these innovations into practice.
5. Establish a center for evidence-based research so that nursing practice at BWH reflects the current best science, experiential learning, and clinical knowledge development.
6. Promote the integration of healing and integrative care therapies into the practice of nurses.
7. Partner with colleges of nursing to discover better ways to educate nursing students, seamlessly integrate students across their professional education, and identify the critical role of BWH's clinicians in that endeavor.
8. Develop a global health agenda based on a culturally competent approach that incorporates the roles of clinical nurses and educators to promote health, reduce disease disparities, and improve treatment outcomes.

---

connection to clinical managers, a connection which they needed to ensure that programs designed to support clinical nurses were relevant and grounded in the realities of clinical practice. Both groups functioned in parallel silos and missed the opportunity for dialogue and collaboration. As we looked to the future, we believed successful change would require new relationships, both within and outside the CNE, and the development of a strong sense of nursing community within the nursing department. We believed that the basis of these relationships should be a common vision clearly describing where we were going as a clinical department of nursing and how the CNE might help to get us there. Finally, we knew that doing this work would have the best possibility of success if it were framed as a strategic priority of the chief nurse. These insights shaped our early initiatives.

We were confident that staying engaged, as well as bringing the right people together who could stay in conversation and ask the right questions, would generate the creativity needed to imagine a new Center for Nursing Excellence (Cooperrider, Whitney, & Stavros, 2008). We realized that a call for change would be enhanced by early successes that could be celebrated to build credibility and momentum (Kouzes & Posner, 1995). We recognized that a large number of stakeholders who could create the desired future needed to be engaged in the process. For these reasons, we chose a Future Search planning process as our change strategy (Weisbord & Janoff, 2000). The chief nurse and associate chief nurse sent a personal letter inviting 60 individuals to participate. The invitation set the stage for this important work:

> This year's Department of Nursing Strategic Plan identified some work we need to accomplish over the coming years. The Center for Nursing Excellence is critical to our mission. The Center's goal is to merge education, research, professional development, and innovation to develop nursing practice, support

the care of patients and families and advance the discipline of nursing. It is now time for us to think about how the CNE of the future should look. To that end, we would like to invite you to join us with the Center staff in a strategic planning process to assure right programs, talent and ideas as we move forward for a successful future. (M. Hickey & M. P. GIbbons, personal communication, invitational letter to BWH staff, 2007)

LAUNCHING THE FUTURE SEARCH

In January 2008, we launched our Future Search conference, entitled "Tomorrow's Center for Nursing Excellence." More than 60 staff members, representing all roles and clinical areas within the DON, actively participated in the 4-day program. The Future Search conference itself was an intervention. Never before had a group like this come together to listen, learn, and create a vision for change. For the center staff, it took courage to hear and remain open to the ideas of a group representing the broad nursing community, and for the community it took faith that its voice would be heard and that its opinions mattered. The two objectives of the conference were to:

- Build partnerships that would inform programs of clinical knowledge development, skill acquisition, and scholarship
- Describe ways in which the CNE could become a core element in all DON efforts to advance nursing practice and improve patient and family care

Using this action-planning tool, we described historic and global trends, travelled to the present, and finally created an ideal future based on a shared vision. Through the guidance of an expert facilitator, all teams managed themselves; the energy in the room was powerful, creative, and deeply moving. Many staff reported that they had never participated in a process that was so energizing, nor had they ever been asked their opinions on matters of importance.

Out of this conference, a set of strategies was proposed that focused on building partnerships between the CNE staff and the nursing community. Our goal was

> to strengthen the quality of nursing practice, clinical innovation, scholarship, teaching and leadership to improve outcomes of care. The intent of these partnerships would be to assure that all programs designed to advance clinical knowledge development, skill acquisition and scholarship are clinically relevant, grounded in clinical and scientific knowledge and evidence-based best practices, conform to sound principles of program design and pedagogy and utilize state-of-the-art technology. (BWH Center for Nursing Excellence, 2008)

Together the nursing community identified five areas as priorities in shaping the future of nursing practice at BWH and created tasks for each. The areas were renewal, schools of nursing, nurse-designed technology, communication, and patient care assistant (PCA) role development. Each task force was given a charge and was co-led by a CNE staff member and a professional nurse from the nursing community, reinforcing the commitment to partnership. Members were selected based on interest identified at the conference; other members were added as appropriate.

Each of these groups achieved outcomes and reported out to the larger community. More than anything, the Future Search conference served as a catalyst for rapid change and set in motion a new way of forming relationships to move the DON's agenda forward. By sharing an experience that created the beginnings of a new center on behalf of the entire nursing community, we were well on our way to the next phase of our work.

DEVELOPING NEW PARTNERSHIPS AND STRATEGIES FOR LEARNING

Energized and informed by the new intradisciplinary dialogue that the Future Search conference inspired, the CNE staff partnered with clinical staff and leadership to begin a process of evaluating existing educational programs, acting upon the priorities identified in the Future Search, and responding to new challenges. Although we knew that clinical staff and nurse leaders valued individuals in the CNE for their knowledge, mentoring, and project management skills, we saw an opportunity to enhance the educational value of existing programs.

We identified several factors here. At that time, most planned educational programming taught by CNE staff supported orientation and Basic and Advanced Cardiac Life Support (ACLS/BLS). Traditional didactic teaching methods in the classroom emphasized "things to know" as opposed to "how to think" (Benner, Sutphen, Leonard, & Day, 2010). Opportunities for application of new knowledge and hands-on practice were limited. As class size was unpredictable, with participants from various clinical settings and roles, the lecture format was frequently used with across-the-board content—a "one size fits all" approach. Staff had limited opportunities to accommodate different learning types and generational differences.

Each RN orientation program provided a mentored clinical practicum that paired small groups of newly hired nurses with one CNE educator in a clinical unit (designated an *orientation pod*). Opportunities for contextually based, peer-supported learning, and acculturation (Benner et al., 2010) were supported in this model and valued by participants, CNE staff, clinicians, and leaders. While aspects of this program were highly successful, it simply could not meet the growing demand for new nurses based on increased patient volume. Consequently, hiring dates for new nurses were delayed, with nurse directors highly dissatisfied as a result. In addition, new nurses were anxious to get to their home units and expressed dissatisfaction at having to "start over again" and build new relationships with colleagues.

We all agreed that we wanted to maintain the strengths of evidence-based, experiential learning opportunities and to include these strategies in all our programs. We also wanted to be responsive to existing concerns and accommodate the volume of new hires to support hospital growth. We realized that experiential learning and team building occurred best when the new nurse was partnered with a knowledgeable clinical nurse mentor. We were committed to redesigning the program to meet organizational needs, by placing the preceptor-nurse dyad at the core, while preparing and surrounding our new nurses with the right supports to promote clinical knowledge development and transition into the BWH practice environment.

Our planning also was shaped by the exponential growth in the amount of clinical and informational technology used in the clinical care environment. In the recent past, CNE staff had successfully led and supported the design and translation of technology into clinical practice. We learned that true partnership with the end user (the clinical nurse or the PCA) in the design, teaching, implementation, and evaluation phases was essential for success. We recognized the opportunity to integrate this approach into all programs. We were invested in expanding the clinicians' involvement in all our programs and in learning how to effectively teach technology both in the classroom and in the clinical environment. We wanted this investment to support caring clinical practices, with the patient at the center of nursing practice. We wanted our patients to feel known by their nurses.

CONTEXT AND CATALYSTS FOR CHANGE

It is important to note that our change was occurring within the broader context of an array of DON changes. Our goal in the CNE was to lead and manage program redesign while maintaining the ability to innovate. As we prepared to convene task forces, we included representatives from all roles in nursing to study educational programs or develop new programs. The CNO's vision of engaging the voice of the clinical nurse in shaping the practice environment offered us different ways of thinking and talking about clinical practice and of conversing as a nursing community. CNE staff participated as both leaders and members in these DON initiatives, with the intended result of strengthening collegial relationships, enriching the work, and including diverse perspectives and expertise. These experiences fostered new learning and a new colleagueship that helped prepare the CNE staff and the clinical community to make evidence-based, culturally compatible changes. Both clinical staff and leadership shared not only how they learned, but also reframed what they needed to know.

Within the CNE, the new acquisition of high-fidelity simulation equipment provided an exciting opportunity to learn about innovative experiential teaching strategies. Simulation is participant-focused, and offers reflective learning opportunities, contextual relevance, and immediate feedback. It is also an excellent method for learning how to communicate more effectively, to work together in teams, and to practice using clinical and information technology in real time without putting patients at risk—all priority learning needs for clinicians and important for quality patient outcomes. As CNE staff learned these new ways of teaching in partnership with clinicians as content experts, it informed their practice and they began replacing lecture with "low-fidelity" teaching/learning strategies such as role playing, reflective discussion, and problem-based teaching methods. A shift from teaching facts to teaching how to reason, problem solve, prioritize, delegate, negotiate, resolve conflict, be culturally aware, and achieve consensus began to occur.

IMPACT OF PROGRAM REDESIGN AND NEW INFRASTRUCTURE

We were able to initiate the changes we had sought. Over a period of 3 years, we redesigned the fundamental educational programs that support transition (orientation), as well as preceptor and charge-nurse role development. We initiated a new simulation program. Through this redesign process, both CNE staff and the clinical community began to realize that while traditional educational programs have value, there is also opportunity and advantage when individuals with clinical and teaching expertise partner in less formal or "real-time" projects. Thus, CNE staff began to partner in new ways with clinicians to support unit-/service-based projects and BWH initiatives.

Key design principles have emerged that guide our approach to teaching interventions and program design:

- The clinical nurse as coach/mentor is central in learning and practice development
- Learning occurs best when it is contextual and socially based
- Learning is not an event, but an incremental process
- A partnership between expert clinicians and "teaching" and program development experts (CNE staff) often leads to the most effective interventions

These principles are synergistic with the DON vision of professional nursing, and have informed a set of guidelines used within the CNE for both "old" and new program/consultation and project development and evaluation.

CNE STAFF ROLE REDESIGN

In response to these changes, the practice of many CNE staff has shifted from teacher to coach, consultant, change agent, and project manager. As CNE staff redesigned their roles, the CNE was able to expand and diversify its central educational offerings to include programs beyond initial orientation (e.g., National League for Nursing (NLN) nurse practice development, palliative care programs, simulation and computer skill development for PCAs, and consultation and convening on projects). Typically, consult requests are synergistic with changes occurring in the BWH/DON clinical environment. We are able to offer expertise, customize a teaching/learning plan to the staff's particular needs and patient population, and assist in implementation as needed. For example, CNE staff partnered with nursing leaders and clinicians in oncology to develop several different strategies to support clinical practice development and new learning during the expansion of this service and the concomitant implementation of several new technologies. Onsite clinical support by CNE staff was provided in all phases of this project. In addition, the CNE staff has convened small groups of nurses to conduct evidence-based review of priority clinical practices. They have partnered with hospital-wide departments to implement new standards/technology and develop teaching strategies compatible with these changes.

The CNE staff also has begun to integrate scholarship into all programs. We have received more than $20,000 in grants that have supported the innovative area of designing and evaluating simulation learning strategies.

Change is best sustained when it becomes part of the norms and values of the department (Kotter, 1996). By carefully aligning the new work with the vision and goals of the DON, and by engaging the nursing community in creating the CNE, we were *able to create the organizational space for reflection and establish a new way of doing business*. Having taken care to set the table, we discovered that the BWH nurses could make their time at the table even more than we had imagined.

REFERENCES

Benner, P., Sutphen, M., Leonard, V., & Day, L. (2010). *Educating nurses: A call for radical transformation.* Stanford, CA: Carnegie Foundation for the Advancement of Teaching.

BWH Center for Nursing Excellence. (2008). *Future search final report and recommendations.* Boston, MA: Brigham and Women's Hospital.

Cooperrider, D., Whitney, D., & Stavros, J. (2008). *Appreciative inquiry handbook: For leaders of change* (2nd ed.). Brunswick, OH: Crown Custom Publishing.

Kotter, J. P. (1996). *Leading change.* Boston, MA: Harvard Business Press.

Kouzes, J., & Posner, B. (1995). *The leadership challenge* (4th ed.). San Francisco, CA: Jossey-Bass.

Weisbord, M., & Janoff, S. (2000). *The future search: An action guide to finding common ground in organizations and communities.* San Francisco, CA: Berrett-Koehler Publishers.

7

The Center for Nursing Excellence: Initiatives and Innovations

Patrice K. Nicholas, Laura Mylott, Katherine Gregory,
Mary Lou Etheredge, Angelleen Peters-Lewis, Leo Buckley, Jr.,
Ellen Bergeron, Julianne Nee, Janice Little, Laurie Cairns,
Ileana Jimenez-Garcia, Maria Teresa Panizales, and Dorothy Bradley

*T*he January 2008 Future Search process, sponsored by the Chief and Associate Chief Nursing Officers and described in Chapter 6, generated five priority areas to guide the Center for Nursing Excellence (CNE) in its work to create the future of nursing practice at BWH; the first priority was renewal. To achieve this, as staff of the CNE we realized that we would need to infuse our ongoing projects with an emphasis on renewal and create emerging initiatives in this spirit as we set out to achieve our goals. Throughout this book, numerous initiatives are described that demonstrate our capacity to renew. Innovations in technology (Chapter 13), in academic partnerships (Chapter 14), in integrative therapies (Chapter 15), in nurse transition programs (Chapter 19), and in global engagement (Chapter 23) all demonstrate the CNE commitment to meeting its goals and describe our outcomes. We also tell the story of our investment in evidence-based research in Chapters 11.2, 14.3, and 15.2.

These goal-driven initiatives all furthered the vision of the Department of Nursing (DON): *Excellent care to patients and families, with the best staff, in the safest environment.* In this chapter we describe the infrastructure and mechanisms created to make these initiatives and their embedded innovations possible, providing a roadmap to achievement of those goals that focused specifically on scholarship, recognition of achievement, cultural competence, and a global health agenda. All our efforts were grounded in our shared belief that scholarship, education, and diversity should be embedded in our understanding of professional practice and would encompass all role groups within the DON. One of our earliest realizations was that our goals would lead to an expansion of our partnerships, both present and possible.

Although the CNE had a tradition of partnering with a variety of stakeholders, we recognized that further expanding our partnerships would create new synergies. Some of these were internal, including the creation of funding mechanisms that would maximize the impact of our resources and manage them efficiently. Some involved external partners, such as the extensive collaborations we undertook with our academic partners in the Boston metropolitan area, our engagement in Partners Healthcare System (PHS) and its nongovernmental organization (NGO) initiatives, and our interface with the larger national nursing community through increased dissemination of our scholarly outcomes. Expanding our partnerships also unearthed new synergies through which we could meet two or more goals concurrently; for example, our goals to promote integrative care therapies into the practice of nurses, to support evidence-based practice, and to further nursing research converged in the awarding of a research grant for a group of nurses to study the impact of integrative therapies on stress reduction in nurses (Chapter 15.2).

RESEARCH AND SCHOLARSHIP

The CNE supports nursing research in a variety of venues. BWH has several signature programs that provide resources to nurse clinicians and investigators and ensure a pipeline of emergent initiatives, innovations, educational opportunities, and research projects. Concurrently, seeking additional external support has culminated in the establishment of a funded nurse-scientist position in collaboration with Boston College. Each of these furthers the CNE commitment to research and scholarship.

Lily Kravitz Nursing Studies Award

The Lily Kravitz Nursing Studies Award was established by Dr. Arthur Kravitz to honor his mother, Lily, whose life "exemplified the highest ideals of caring within the nursing profession." Since its inception in 1995, this award has financially supported more than 45 individuals and/or teams conducting nursing studies that contribute to the art and science of nursing practice. In 2002, the funds for this award were augmented from the estate of a former patient, Mr. David Coe, who wished to acknowledge the expert nursing care he received while a patient at BWH. In a health care environment challenged by increasing knowledge and advancing technology, the essential importance of compassionate, nurturing care warrants investigation. Nurses have their greatest opportunities to improve the health and wholeness of their patients when they practice in a professional environment where scholarly inquiry and innovation are encouraged and supported. BWH provides the environment and the Lily Kravitz Nursing Studies Award provides seed money and support that make it possible for the recipients to pursue excellence in nursing care. The following list of recent nurse recipients and their research focus demonstrates this commitment:

- *Implementing Alternative Complementary Therapies for the Purpose of Stress Reduction in Nurses While Improving the Quality and Care of Our Patients:*   Santina Wilson, Mary Absi, and Heather Hogan
- *Developing a Protocol of Care for the Prevention and Management of Pressure Ulcers in Cardiac Surgery:*   Maria Bentain-Melanson, Mary Aquilino, Trevor Herrin, Karen Politano, and Maryann Solari.
- *Central Venous Catheter Safety in the Emergency Department:*   Thomas Chafe

Past awards have focused on improving efficiency and quality of care; enhancing quality of life; increasing patient satisfaction; empowering patients, families, and caregivers; and increasing collaboration among caregivers.

The Mary Fay Enrichment Award

The Mary Fay Enrichment Award enables nurses to travel, observe, and learn in centers of excellence at other sites and to bring back to BWH the knowledge that they have gained as a result of their experiences. Initiated in 1999 and funded by Yousuf and Estrellita Karsh, Dr. Marshall Wolf, and the DON, this award gives BWH nurses an opportunity to explore innovative and evidence-based solutions to complex patient/clinical problems and implement those solutions in their clinical practice areas. The following list of recent nurse recipients and their focus of exploration shows the congruence of these initiatives with the goals of the CNE and the DON vision statement:

- *Palliative Care: Improving Our Delivery:*   Katie Fillipon and Eileen Molina
- *Nurse-Physician Communication and Collaboration: Improving Patient Outcomes:* Eileen Miller
- *Improving Discharge From the NICU:*   Jessica Marchetti and Jennifer Flückiger

Since its inception, the Mary Fay Enrichment Award has funded 34 projects involving 73 nurses who have explored best practices at other nationally recognized institutions and have implemented these practices in their own departments. Projects have had an impact on care in all nursing service areas of the DON. It is also noteworthy that the needs of our most vulnerable patient populations have been addressed through the funded projects.

The Karsh Visiting Scholar

In 2009, the DON received a very generous gift from Estrellita Karsh, a longtime benefactor and friend of BWH nursing: an endowment that funds the Estrellita and Yousuf Karsh Visiting Professor in Nursing, and an annual visiting scholar lectureship that coincides with Nurse Recognition Week and activities to celebrate nursing during the month of May. The endowment provides a yearly opportunity to invite a nationally or internationally known nursing leader to visit BWH and engage BWH nurses in conversations about excellent nursing care. The inaugural visiting scholar, Joanne Disch, a clinical professor, holder of the Lillehei Chair in Nursing Leadership, and director of the Katherine J. Densford International Center for Nursing Leadership at the University of Minnesota School of Nursing, presented on "How to Create an Expert Team From a Team of Experts."

The Genevieve Hope Blaney Scholarship Award

The Gretchen Stone Cook Foundation, inspired by its namesake's companion, Genevieve Hope Blaney, who was a registered nurse, donates money to support educational scholarships for nurses. These awards are given annually to BWH nurses who are pursuing baccalaureate and graduate education in nursing. The CNE also schedules a luncheon with the scholarship donor to highlight the award recipients and share their success with the donor.

The Steven and Kathleen Haley Nurse-Scientist Program

The Steven and Kathleen Haley Nurse-Scientist Program was created in 2009 through a $1 million gift from Steven and Kathleen (Powers) Haley, the creators of the Brain Science Foundation. It is the largest single gift ever awarded to the BWH DON and a significant achievement in meeting the CNE goal of establishing a center for evidence-based research so that our nursing practice might reflect the best science and clinical knowledge development. It also furthered our goal of enhancing our partnerships with academic institutions as we pursued our goals of research and scholarship. The program is designed to ensure that the nursing science generated by an academic nurse be "at the bedside" in collaboration with clinical nurses and that findings be integrated "at the bedside" by these same nurses.

In 2010, Kate Gregory, an assistant professor at Boston College's School of Nursing, was named the first Haley Nurse-Scientist to pursue a program of research in partnership with clinical nursing staff in the BWH Center for Women and Newborns. Using novel technologies and disease prediction strategies, Kate Gregory aims to better understand the pathogenesis of gastrointestinal disease in premature infants and develop new models of disease prediction, specifically for necrotizing enterocolitis (NEC). In turn, she aims to identify potential biomarkers for NEC that will provide neonatal clinicians with new tools for early identification and diagnosis of this disease in premature infants. She concurrently works directly with BWH nurses to further their research and scholarship and to advance the practice of nursing at BWH. To celebrate this successful collaborative achievement, our CNE sponsored an inaugural reception where Susan Gennaro, dean of the Boston College School of Nursing, and Mairead Hickey, BWH Chief Nursing Officer, served as co-hosts, introducing both the first Haley Nurse-Scientist and the Haley family.

CELEBRATING NURSING EXCELLENCE

The highest honor bestowed by the DON is the Mary S. Fay Essence of Nursing Award, presented annually to BWH nurses who best represent the highest ideals of the nursing profession. From the very best among our colleagues, we recognize those who step forward, placing patients first, day after day, and represent the true "essence of nursing." This award is the capstone recognition celebrated each May during National Nurses Week. The recipients who are nominated are singled out by those most capable of judging their excellence: the nurses who work with them daily.

ACKNOWLEDGING OUR PARTNERS IN CARE

The CNE, while furthering the scientific grounding of our nursing care, also turned to our partners in care, to support staff members and unlicensed staff who provide care to our patients and families and support our clinicians in their work. Because these essential resource persons evoked our utmost gratitude, we also wished to acknowledge their contribution through awards. We created two award categories to honor outstanding performance among these partners.

1. **Patient Care Assistant/Medical Assistant/Emergency Services Assistant Recognition.** This award recognizes a PCA, medical assistant, or emergency services assistant whose practice reflects compassionate care, customer service skills, a positive attitude, teamwork, effective communication with team members, and leadership skills. Recipients also must have demonstrated that they maintain standards of care by example and a commitment to learning. Recipients receive both a crystal award and a monetary award. In 2010, we initiated the inclusion of a video about the recipient that we play as part of the celebration of the award. This "Recognition Video" is designed to capture the recipient of the award "in action" to showcase the recipient's teamwork, customer service, and care.

2. **Administrative Support for Patient Care Services Award.** In 2010, we initiated the Administrative Support for Patient Care Services Award, designed to recognize staff in roles such as unit coordinator or business specialist who consistently demonstrate superior performance in their roles. Criteria for this award include strong customer service and communication skills, empathy toward patients and their families, professional demeanor, strong role model for others to follow, commitment to personal and professional growth, and an investment in the operation of the unit and safety and comfort of patients.

AFFIRMING CULTURAL COMPETENCE

The BWH patient population reflects the rich cultural diversity of the Boston metropolitan community, as does BWH staff. The CNE goal of developing a global health agenda was predicated on affirming and expanding the cultural competency of the DON. In addition, persistent disease and treatment disparities among minorities were of concern to the entire PHS, and the need for increased staff diversification as one way of addressing this concern was acknowledged. All these factors shaped the CNE's commitment to affirming cultural competence and investing in those best able to lead BWH in achieving this goal.

Three award programs were initiated in 2008 to honor representatives of three groups of nurses and staff who exemplify our cultural diversity. The criteria for all three awards are the same: The recipients must have demonstrated significant contributions in supporting our BWH diversity goals to improving culturally sensitive patient care within their unit; have served as active members of service/community and/or professional organizations; have been engaged in activities aimed at preparing the next generation of multicultural nurses/employees; and, for nurse applicants, have been involved in scholarly activities.

We recognized that the goal of advancing care to our multicultural patient populations can be supported through advancing our diverse workforce, including nurses, patient care assistants, administrative and support staff, pharmacy, interpreter services, and other departments. Supporting the goal of the very best staff includes those BWH employees who reflect the communities that we serve and are able to improve patient outcomes by advocating for the provision of culturally competent care.

The Ujima Award

The BWH Ujima Award was established to acknowledge, honor, and celebrate the contributions of BWH registered nurses of African descent. Ujima is one of the seven principles of Kwanzaa, a celebration of family, community, and culture: it describes the principle of collective work, culture, and responsibility. Under the leadership of Angelleen Peters-Lewis, Executive Director of the Connors Center for Women and Newborns, our inaugural celebration in 2008 honored Sondra Holland and included a lecture from our first Ujima Visiting Scholar, Deborah Washington, Director of Diversity for Patient Care Services at Massachusetts General Hospital and Nursing Spectrum Nurse of the Year awardee.

In 2009, our Ujima celebrations were broadened to include our BWH staff who are members of the Department of Patient Care Services. Sheila Jones Cannon, Assistant Professor at the College of Nursing and Health Sciences at the University of Massachusetts–Boston, served as our distinguished speaker and shared her expertise in advancing diversity in health care. In 2010, Rumay Alexander, Clinical Professor and Director of Multicultural Affairs at the University of North Carolina, Chapel Hill School of Nursing, spoke about diversity and learning how to better understand one another. Awardees included Nadia Raymond from the DON and Kerrie-Ann Jack and Michele Plaisiond.

The award ceremony and celebration are scheduled during Black History Month, a time to commemorate African Americans who have changed the world and to celebrate African American history and culture. Black History Month first began in 1926, when Carter G. Woodson, a Harvard PhD and historian, first initiated a celebration for African American history. He chose the second week in February because it included the birthdays of Frederick Douglass and Abraham Lincoln, the sixteenth president of the United States. Frederick Douglass was born a slave, yet was determined to be free: He escaped from slavery and became one of the most influential figures of the nineteenth century. He was a powerful speaker in the antislavery movement, an author, and an advocate for the rights of African Americans and women. In 1976, the bicentennial of the United States, the week-long observance was extended to the entire month of February to allow enough time for celebratory programs and activities. BWH is pleased to include its Ujima Award program among these national celebrations.

The Hispanic Heritage Award

The Hispanic Heritage Nursing and Patient Care Services Celebration and Awards ceremony were established to acknowledge and celebrate the contributions of BWH nurses and patient care services employees of Hispanic/Latino heritage; the celebration is held during the National Hispanic Heritage Month, September 15 to October 15. The DON and PCS at Brigham and Women's Hospital annually observe this month as a time to recognize, honor, and celebrate the contributions of our nurses and employees of Hispanic/Latino heritage who have made a positive impact on patient outcomes by advocating for the provision of culturally sensitive care and who have worked to enhance the competencies of the next generation of multicultural employees.

The observation of National Hispanic Heritage started in 1968 as Hispanic Heritage Week, under President Lyndon Johnson, and was expanded by President Ronald Reagan in 1988 to cover a 30-day period starting on September 15 and ending on October 15. It was enacted into law on August 17, 1988. This period celebrates the histories, cultures, and contributions of American citizens whose ancestors came from Spain, Mexico, the Caribbean, and Central and South America.

The population of the Boston metropolitan area has a rich representation of these varied Hispanic cultures, including those of Puerto Rico, Mexico, Chile, Colombia, Honduras, Guatemala, El Salvador, and Argentina. Our staffs are our most valuable resource in ensuring quality patient care to these communities.

The first two recipients of this award were Hilda Gallegos-Dargon and Marta Solis. Much as with the Ujima Award, the second year of celebration included a guest speaker, State Representative Jeffrey Sanchez. Mazie Anckle and Mishel Burgos were honored during this ceremony. Oswald Mondejar, Vice President of Human Resources at Partners Continuing Care, spoke at our third celebration, where the honorees were Ana Lora, Wanda Ocasio, and Lina Sanchez.

Asian-Pacific Islander Award

The BWH Asian-Pacific Islander Award was established to acknowledge and celebrate the contributions of Asian and Pacific Islands nurses. In pursuing the DON's vision to provide excellent care to patients and families with the very best staff in the safest environment, we realized that the very best staff includes those BWH employees who reflect the communities we serve and are able to improve patient outcomes by advocating for the provision of culturally competent care—in this case, care to our patients of Asian or Pacific Islander descent.

Asian Pacific American Heritage Month (APAHM) is celebrated in May to commemorate the contributions of people of Asian and Pacific Islander descent in the United States. Congress passed a joint congressional resolution in 1978 to commemorate Asian American Heritage Week during the first week of May. This date was chosen because two important anniversaries occurred during this time: the arrival of the first Japanese immigrants in America on May 7, 1843, and the completion of the transcontinental railroad (by many Chinese laborers) on May 10, 1869. In 1990, Congress voted to expand it from a week to a month-long celebration, and in May 1992, the month of May was permanently designated as "Asian/Pacific American Heritage Month."

The celebrations described here are also part of the recognition, in May, of nurses or staff of Asian/Pacific Islander heritage. Tess Panizales was the first recipient of this award in 2008, and Grace Mascarinas Huebsch was recognized in 2009. As with the other award celebrations, a guest lecturer became part of the celebration in 2009. Haeok Lee, an associate professor at the College of Nursing and Health Sciences at the University of Massachusetts–Boston, explored the question of "Health Disparities or Data Disparities."

We believe that these awards do much more than recognize nurse and staff leaders who are champions of our collective move toward cultural competence.

They also give heightened visibility to and awareness of the multicultural nature of our staff and patient populations, and acknowledge that affirming cultural competence is a choice and an area in which one can excel. As noted earlier, this focus on cultural competence was in part viewed as a precursor to the successful development and implementation of a global health agenda.

A GLOBAL HEALTH AGENDA

As we began to explore our role in our global nursing initiative, we realized that although nurses play a pivotal role in the delivery of health care in the United States and globally, they often go unrecognized for their contributions to the health care team and to the achievement of optimal patient outcomes. Despite growing interest in global health nursing in the United States, nurses are remarkably underrepresented in the field of global health delivery. Coupled with the nursing shortage in the world, these factors create an increasingly challenging situation. In resource-limited countries, complex issues (including a lack of educational and professional opportunities and migration of nurses to Western nations) contribute to the nursing shortage. We believed that the nursing profession could and must provide leadership to overcome the obstacles that contribute to the nursing shortage in the United States and abroad while providing opportunities for careers outside the typical. With the support of our DON and chief nurse, we developed the Global Health Nurse Fellowship Program (GNFP) as an initial contribution we could make, in partnership with our BWH and Partners In Health (PIH) colleagues to the development of a diverse, well-educated global nursing workforce. This first step set the stage for our emerging global health agenda.

The Global Health Nursing Fellowship

Our intent in creating the GNFP was to enhance the diversity of the nursing workforce and provide support to colleagues in the global nursing community. Our goals for the GNFP included providing opportunities for U.S.-based nurses to contribute to the efforts of caring for the world's populations by working shoulder-to-shoulder with nurses in resource-poor settings and, upon returning to the United States, to share their experiences with colleagues. The result of this professional exchange would be an expanded understanding and appreciation of the nursing profession by health professionals from all backgrounds. Our program was also aimed at attracting and retaining nurse leaders in the United States who could contribute to solving the problems of emigration and "brain drain" from resource-poor countries.

The role of nursing in global health is still developing, and strong clinicians are needed to advance that role. We believed that our GNFP could attract new clinicians to the nursing profession; a similar medical residency program at BWH, the Doris and Howard Hiatt Global Health Equity and Internal Medicine Residency, attracts applicants from around the world. We believed that our unique fellowship program would be attractive to young professionals considering careers in nursing. This emphasis in the CNE's investment in global health is well illustrated through our pioneering work in Rwanda.

Partners In Health Rwanda

In 2005, Partners In Health began working in two rural health districts in Rwanda as the implementing partner in the Clinton Foundation HIV/AIDS Initiative. The aim was to launch an integrated HIV treatment, care, and prevention program based on the model of care that PIH first developed in Haiti with its sister organization, Zanmi Lasante. Work in Rwanda was part of PIH's collaboration with the Rwandan Ministry of Health (MOH), and the Treatment and Research for AIDS Center (TRAC), the aim of which was to scale up HIV treatment and care and strengthen national training and evaluation programs in Rwanda. The intent was to develop a rural care model for HIV that could be adapted and replicated throughout Rwanda and in other African countries.

When the country director and project manager arrived in Rwanda's Rwinkwavu Hospital, it was supposed to be serving nearly half a million people—but lacked a single doctor to do so. Within the first 8 months, 30,000 people were tested for HIV (the first test for many), and hundreds were started on lifesaving drug and nutritional regimens. Since that time, the model has expanded to provide resources and infrastructure to seven health centers in Kayonza and Kirehe districts in the eastern province, as well as health centers in the northern province of Burera. Nurses play a significant role in the programs PIH provides, with more than 300 nurses involved, in contrast to only 20 physicians.

The nursing shortage is a challenge around the world. In the United States, there are approximately nine nurses for every thousand people. In Rwanda, there is less than one nurse for every thousand people. The burden of work on these nurses is enormous, especially in places where doctors are rare. At the District Hospital in Rwinkwavu, the first site for PIH in Rwanda, there are 81 nurses and 11 doctors for 80 patient beds. All too often, one bed holds more than one patient. Nurses fill roles of all kinds in the hospital, from bedside nursing to staffing the laboratory, providing strategic planning leadership, and dispensing medications in the pharmacy. In essence, nurses maintain these health care systems.

We realized that the minimal education and widely varying responsibilities among these nurses made this an ideal site for our fellowship program, where an experienced nurse clinician, through a 6-month fellowship, could help address the myriad of challenges these nurses faced. We believed that understanding the perspectives of Rwandan nurses and working in collaboration with them to establish goals for training and system improvements were two tenets of a fruitful fellowship. We initiated a call for applicants, with these tenets guiding our selection process.

In September 2008, our first nurse-fellow, Kate Sullivan, arrived in Rwanda and initiated the GNFP. She was able to make a substantive difference in maternity care through her training, role modeling, and advocacy for nurses. Her work and her success are described in more detail in Chapter 23.3. We continue to evaluate our BWH Global Nursing Program while seeking additional funding sources and developing a closer relationship with PIH.

The PIH global programs emerged more than 20 years ago after a devastating earthquake struck in the island nation of Haiti. When Haiti once more suffered a devastating earthquake on January 12, 2010, volunteer BWH clinical nurses were an essential resource in the relief efforts. Along with physician and nursing leadership, our clinical nursing staffs were deployed in the acute phase after the earthquake and in partnership with our colleagues at PIH. Their story is also told in Chapters 23.1 and 23.2.

CONCLUSION

This chapter has provided a roadmap for change when the goals of a center committed to nursing excellence, in a spirit of renewal, focuses its energies, creates appropriate initiatives, and embraces innovation. Because our work has a never-ending quality to it, we anticipate that our future will continue to be rich in initiatives and innovations.

8

Beyond Regulatory Compliance: Our Quality Journey

Diane R. Lancaster and Carolyn Hayes

I think one's feelings waste themselves in words; they ought all to be distilled into actions which bring results.

—Florence Nightingale

An oncology patient once told a gathering of patient and family advisors that he wanted to have t-shirts made up for all of them that said, "I survived cancer. Don't kill me with your dirty hands." This was said in the context of a discussion about the national "Speak Up" campaign encouraging hand hygiene among health professionals. His point was well taken. Evidence shows that hospital-acquired infections from inadequate hand hygiene is a known risk factor for patients. In fact, according to the World Health Organization (2009), each day 247 people die as a result of a health care associated infection. That is the equivalent of a Boeing 767 aircraft crashing every day (Blouin, 2010). Knowing this places patients in a vulnerable position. At this meeting, it was suggested to these patients that they be vigilant in prompting health care team members to maintain hand hygiene as needed.

ROLE OF LEADERSHIP IN QUALITY AND SAFETY

As nurses, we often pride ourselves on our role as the advocate or agent of safe passage through our systems. Excellent care to patients and families, the cornerstone of our vision within the Brigham and Women's Hospital (BWH) Department of Nursing (DON), mandates that we create an environment where outstanding hand hygiene is not only an expectation, but also a reality. Despite our belief that no health care team member ever intends to ignore hand hygiene or harm a patient, it still happens. Evidence also tells us that patients are more likely to be harmed by restraints than kept safe, but we still had more patients in restraints than evidence-based criteria would dictate (Gilbert & Counsell, 1999; Miles & Meyers, 1994). Falls with injuries continue to occur in academic medical centers (AMCs) (Dykes, Carroll, Hurley, Benoit, & Middleton, 2009; Dykes et al., 2010). Health care professionals know how these events affect patients and families all too well, and we were no exception. As leaders, we needed to keep our line of sight on patients and families, incorporating our worldview that they are the reason we exist and excellent care is our commitment to them. We believe we are obligated to lead from our awareness that evidence-based practice supports a culture of safety and that improved system and process reliability maintains a safe environment while it improves efficiency.

As leaders, we also know that the very best staff highly value and intend to deliver nothing short of excellent care, but the conditions for their success have to be present. For "the very best staff," it is not just a question of values: Clinical nurses can and will change practice when leaders provide them with the tools they need to do so. Clinical nurses need leaders to reinforce that the line of sight on patients and families is at the core of every decision. For DON leaders and clinical nurses, it is about patients and their families. The very best staff asks: "What actions influence patient and family care?" and "What do I need to know/have/do to provide that care?" To answer these questions, we set out to create the infrastructure, leadership roles, and processes to support their work.

INFRASTRUCTURE AND ROLE CREATION

In early 2005, health care agencies were barraged by an explosion of required external reporting criteria, the proliferation of National Patient Safety Goals by the Joint Commission (TJC), and, for us at BWH, a pending TJC hospital survey and the arrival of a new chief nursing officer (CNO), Mairead Hickey. In addition, I (DRL) was only a few months into the role of Executive Director for Quality Improvement and Measurement for the DON. After I completed a 3-month assessment, it was crystal clear to me that the DON needed more than a "party of one" to successfully create an infrastructure that would support the delivery of excellent care to our patients and families.

Thus, I envisioned a role that would serve as a catalyst at the unit level to stimulate activity around needed improvements in patient care through examination of current practices and/or work flow or system issues. Nurses in this role would have to be willing to acquire more than just clinical knowledge related to the discipline in order to improve and advance nursing practice: They would have to become change agents. It would require nurses with a strong clinical understanding of practice who could also diagnose system failures and apply quality improvement methodologies to the design, implementation, evaluation, and sustainability of innovative solutions that address systems problems and/or patient care issues. Ideally, they would work to eliminate unnecessary steps in key clinical processes, reduce and more effectively redeploy wasted resources, and enhance workflow. Their efforts would help to preserve and/or recapture time for value-added bedside nursing functions.

My 3-month assessment of the state of the quality program at BWH also revealed that the hematology/oncology service line had introduced two master's-prepared nurses in the role of nursing coordinators. They brought a specialized skill set and focus that would augment the work of the nurse director in relation to quality improvement, as well as support the work of the clinical nurse and the actualization of the department's vision. As members of the unit and service line leadership team, the work of these nurses was designed to influence patient care through deliberate and collaborative efforts. I had found my solution to moving beyond my "party of one" and initiated a collaborative partnership with the executive director of this service line, Carolyn Hayes, to make this template into a BWH model of quality improvement.

Leveraging the success of the innovative leadership role of the nursing coordinator within the hematology/oncology service line, we changed the role title to quality program director (QPD) and replicated it within each of the DON's service lines. These master's-prepared nurses, who bring at least 5 years of clinical experience to the role, fill a void in the required skill set that ensures a unit's success in designing, implementing, spreading, and sustaining quality programs relevant to the care of their patient population. The skills we required for this role included understanding of quality improvement theory, methodologies, statistics, principles of collaboration, and creation and translation of evidence-based practices to the bedside. Their work is multidisciplinary and cross-departmental. Thus, effective communication and team building/management skills are a must to establish effective collaborative relationships with a variety of disciplines and departments.

The QPD is accountable for programs related to patient safety, quality measurement and improvement, nurse-sensitive outcome measures, evidence-based practice, and regulatory compliance for units within a particular clinical service line, as well as a core set of measures that cut across the DON. She or he oversees and is accountable for ensuring collection, maintenance, analysis, interpretation, and dissemination of quality, safety, research, and compliance data findings. The QPD also hires, trains, supervises, and evaluates program staff associated with safety and quality initiatives as necessary to fulfill a project goal. Furthermore, QPDs provide leadership, management, and facilitation of related quality improvement teams and efforts within the nursing division and across related operational departments.

QPDs develop and lead their service line's quality improvement program to effect change and accomplish the established goals and objectives of the DON. They conduct needs assessments to identify practice/systems issues and create or enhance processes and systems for meeting program goals and objectives. Hence, they assume the role of project manager for specific projects that include overall accountability for operational outcomes and supervision of the project team, including feedback on work performance. They are accountable to the project sponsor. In addition, nurses in this role work with service line leaders, directors, and care improvement teams. They monitor and/or perform data collection and compilation and ensure entry of accurate and reliable clinical/compliance data into web-based or Access databases for all eligible patient cases. They also analyze, interpret, and present quality/safety program results to various audiences, including the CNO and Senior Vice President of Patient Care Services, chiefs of service, executive nursing directors, nursing directors, and educators, as well as frontline nursing and medical staff. Based on project findings, the QPD also leads the development and review of patient care policies and nursing standards associated with their projects for the service line and department. They may also facilitate and/or participate in nursing research and/or grant writing, as appropriate, to generate new evidence that meets program and departmental needs.

By 2007, each service line within the DON was able to create and hire into this role. The position enjoys a matrixed reporting structure. Each QPD has accountability for DON as well as unit-/service line-specific work. In such a structure, the QPDs have both the joy and challenge of clinical, operational, and quality improvement perspectives in the approach to and oversight of the work. As part of a large health care system, the focus of this role can be as broad as systemwide. However, to stay true to the vision of changing practice at the level of the nurse-patient dyad, accountability within the units of a service line and the DON grounds the work best.

METHODOLOGY

We believe that quality happens from the deliberate and intentional actions of individuals within an organization. It is *not* a single project, nor the responsibility of a single committee, role, or person. It *is* a way of thinking about our work in health care, keeping our eyes focused on patients and families, approaching its improvement, and getting everyone involved.

The entire DON leadership team contributes to the prioritization of project-based work that is built upon annual review of audit, patient satisfaction, and process improvement data as well as current research and regulatory standard requirements. The voice of the customer, our patients/families and/or clinical nurses, and the voice of the process carry equal weight in this prioritization process. A focus on risk reduction and prevention as intervention is a common thread in the work.

In creating and implementing the DON quality approach and methodologies, we have been highly influenced by the work of two key individuals at the Institute for Healthcare Improvement (IHI), Roger Resar and Robert Lloyd. Resar's (2006) work on high-reliability principles has provided us with excellent tools that are helping us achieve our vision of becoming a high-reliability DON. The premise behind health care becoming a "high-reliability" industry rests on our ability to identify the precise reasons for adverse events and find ways to keep them from happening in the first place, or at least to reduce them (Blouin, 2010). To that end, one QPD successfully used Resar's framework to reduce the spread of vancomycin-resistant enterococci (VRE), a hospital-acquired condition, on one patient care unit from a baseline rate of 4.7/1,000 patient days to 1.9/1,000 patient days.

Lloyd's (2004) work has provided the framework for how we approach continuous quality improvement (CQI) and its measurement in the DON. He identifies three foundational elements that are important components to any quality journey:

1. Listening to the voice of the customer (VOC); that is, the end user of a process
2. Listening to the voice of the process (VOP)
3. Using data to make decisions

Quality results when each of these activities is in effect simultaneously on a daily basis.

Voice of the Customer

As clinicians, we have a long history of being quick to prescribe or intervene and slow to listen—and yet we are perplexed when patients do not comply! Constant and deliberate listening to the VOC is a necessary but insufficient approach to achieving quality. Listening provides the context for responding (Lloyd, 2004). The next step is to turn what we hear into our tactics or strategies for action for the identified primary customer.

Key Quality Characteristics

Key quality characteristics (QCs) are what the customer cares most about (Lloyd, 2004). They will vary from customer to customer. For us, defining the key QCs of a process or product is an essential part of the VOC process. It prevents us from falling prey to thinking that we know what our customer wants, needs, or expects, much like the tool of a process map prevents us from thinking we know what the elements of an important process are.

Voice of the Process

After listening and hearing the VOC, our next step is to identify the processes that influence the customer's perspectives. Listening to the VOC without a plan for improving the process demonstrates "listening without responding." Listening to the VOP without connecting the process to the customer's expectations results in "responding without listening" (Lloyd, 2004). For us, successful CQI requires both, in addition to use of data for decision making.

What Should We Be Measuring? What Will Be Different?

The strongest business case for health care quality measures is the case for investment in the prevention of hospital-acquired conditions (e.g., infections, pressure ulcers, falls with injury, medication errors). The science of quality measurement within nursing is in its early developmental phase. Initial work focused on determining the relationship between RN staffing and patient outcomes (Aiken, Clarke, Sloane, Sochalski, & Silber, 2002; Burnes Bolton et al., 2007; Kane, Shamliyan, Mueller, Duval, & Wilt, 2007). Our attention now needs to shift toward the study of systems and processes in the RN work environment (Aiken, Clarke, Sloane, Lake, & Cheney, 2008). By way of example, we do not actually know if nurse-sensitive outcome measures are reflective of the process of nursing practice or of the degree of effectiveness of the hospital's documentation system. We keep focusing on outcomes when the payoff is in the study and standardization of the process. Useful examples of this include our studies on handoff communications and rapid response teams.

While these have been good starting points for sharpening our understanding of what our quality vision and skills should be, we need to begin to move toward developing metrics that matter: process and outcome indicators reflective of the VOC and VOP. For example, there is a clear need to reinvest nurses' time in direct care and other value-added activities that are meaningful to patients and families. "A 2008 study of 36 hospitals published in the summer 2008 issue of the *Permanente Journal* found that medical and surgical nurses spent only 15 percent of their time on patient care activities. The majority of their time was spent on documentation, care coordination, and medication administration" (Bisognano, 2010, p. 84). We believe the QPD role could help analyze and streamline sustainable changes to current nurse work flows in a manner that ensured that nurses' direct patient care time is improved.

How Will We Know That a Change Is an Improvement?

In analyzing our quality improvement data, we remind ourselves of what we consider one of the most helpful principles quality improvement practitioners can invoke before embarking on the data analysis phase of their work: "You and I do not see things as they are. We see things as we are." We are committed to using a rapid-cycle Plan, Do, Study, Act (PDSA) framework, as well as gaining skills to understand and accurately interpret variation in the performance improvement data. We believe that this is key to helping us filter out our own perceptions of the data story.

Rapid-cycle PDSA quality improvement allows us to analyze specific breakdowns in processes of care, determine their specific underlying cause(s) of failure, develop tailored solutions, and test those solutions in real time in actual patient care environments before spreading a practice change throughout our organization. We focus on speedy implementation of small tests of change in real time and under real conditions that produce new knowledge that is used to create the next test of change. Such changes are documented through a data collection process. To translate the data into meaningful actionable information requires understanding the data's variation through application of statistical process control theory and techniques.

Some precautions guide our process. First, we must understand the type of variation in our data: Is it special-cause or common-cause variation? We must further know how to interpret that variation. Special-cause variation does not mean "good" variation, just as common-cause variation does not mean "bad" variation. Finally, we realize that we must know how to depict variation in the process so that others will understand the story the data are telling. Understanding variation in quality improvement work is accomplished by using run and control charts. Run and control charts are plots of data over time that serve to identify and distinguish between special and common causes of variation. These are the best tools to determine if the improvement strategy had the desired effect.

In implementing our methodology, we became increasingly convinced that as leaders of a clinical discipline, we need to prepare current and future nurses with knowledge of and expertise in the application of quality improvement methodologies and concepts such as high-reliability processes, standardization, spread, sustainability, and statistical process control. This will create the conditions we need to develop and measure meaningful nurse-sensitive outcomes. It is from understanding and use of these methodologies and skills that a high-reliability DON, capable of creating and sustaining improvements in patient and family care, will be created.

REINFORCEMENT

Our DON quality program and the projects that support it are designed in partnership with staff at the local level. The QPDs lead or co-lead interprofessional or interdepartmental teams created to address a practice problem or change. The attention each QPD can bring to a specific patient population, geographical environment, and clinical team while applying the rigor of quality improvement methodologies learned not only fosters change, it sustains it. The infrastructure we created is in keeping with the DON goal of moving toward high reliability. We believe that goal is advanced considerably by the QPD's ability to assess, intervene, and evaluate at a local level while implementing initiatives from an integrated department-wide quality team. By design, the work product from this role is presented at unit-based project team meetings, department-wide leadership meetings, and interdisciplinary committee forums, all of which are attended by a variety of role groups to ensure the dissemination of best practices as well as learnings about what was tried and did not work.

At every opportunity, the QPDs reinforce the connection among evidence, change, and patient outcomes. Nurse directors, executive directors, and other clinical leaders conduct practice rounds routinely with clinical nurses. In addition, the nurse directors have made a commitment to assessing their patients at risk for skin issues, delirium (see Chapter 11), and falls (see Chapter 14.3) in their daily rounds with their clinical nurses. Nurse directors, executive directors, and the chief nurse send notes to clinical staff acknowledging work done, highlighting the project's contribution and connection to our vision. In these communications, we specifically articulate how a project improved safety, enhanced patient and family care, or developed staff.

We have created an infrastructure, role, and processes to maximize sharing best practices and sustaining change. The entire leadership team is accountable for prioritizing this work. The process is designed to stay true to our belief that clinical nurses are motivated by excellent patient care and our commitment to create the conditions for their success.

SUMMARY

Ever since the IOM's challenge posed in *Crossing the Quality Chasm* (2001), it has become commonly accepted that focused attention to quality is what clinical practice is about and what health care needs. We launched these personnel, in this new role, under this program based on the principle that if your line of sight is excellent patient and family care with the very best staff in the safest environment, then "Quality equals practice, there are zero degrees of separation." As we reflect on our successes, ever-mindful of the need to constantly introduce new evidence into practice and increase our reliability, our future is seen to be full of possibilities and ongoing challenges. And we are looking forward to them.

REFERENCES

Aiken, L. H., Clarke, S. P., Sloane, D. M., Lake, E. T., & Cheney, T. (2008). Effects of hospital care environments on patient mortality and nurse outcomes. *Journal of Nursing Administration, 38*(5), 223–229.

Aiken, L. H., Clarke, S. P., Sloane, D. M., Sochalski, J., & Silber, J. H. (2002). Hospital nurse staffing and patient mortality, nurse burnout, and job dissatisfaction. *Journal of the American Medical Association, 288*(16), 1987–1993.

Bisognano, M. (2010). Nursing's role in transforming healthcare. *Healthcare Executive, 2,* 84–87.

Blouin, A. S. (2010). Helping to solve healthcare's most critical safety and quality problems. *Journal of Nursing Care Quality, 25*(2), 95–99.

Burnes Bolton, L., Aydin, C. E., Donaldson, N., Brown, D. S., Sandhu, M., Fridman, M., & Aronow, H. U. (2007). Mandated nurse staffing ratios in California: A comparison of staffing and nurse-sensitive outcomes pre- and postregulation. *Policy, Politics, & Nursing Practice, 8,* 238–249.

Dykes, P. C., Carroll, D. L, Hurley, A. C., Benoit, A., & Middleton, B. (2009). Why do patients in acute care hospitals fall? Can falls be prevented? *Journal of Nursing Administration, 39*(6), 299–304.

Dykes, P. C., Carroll, D. L., Hurley, A., Lipsitz, S., Benoit, A., Chang, F., . . . Middleton, B. (2010). Fall prevention in acute care hospitals: A randomized trial. *Journal of the American Medical Association, 304*(17), 1912–1918.

Gilbert, M., & Counsell, C. (1999). Planned change to implement a restraint reduction program. *Journal of Nursing Care Quality, 13*(5), 57–64.

Institute of Medicine. (2001). *Crossing the quality chasm: A new health system for the 21st century.* Washington, DC: National Academy Press.

Kane, R. L., Shamliyan, T., Mueller, C., Duval, S., & Wilt, T. (2007). The association of registered nurse staffing levels and patient outcomes. *Medical Care, 45*(12), 1195–1204.

Lloyd, R. (2004). *Quality health care: A guide to developing and using indicators.* Sudbury, MA: Jones & Bartlett Publishers.

Miles, S. H., & Meyers, R. (1994). Untying the elderly: 1989–1993 update. *Clinics in Geriatric Medicine, 10*(3), 513–525.

Resar, R. K. (2006). Making noncatastrophic health care processes reliable: Learning to walk before running in creating high-reliability organizations. *Health Services Research, 41*(4), 1677–1689.

World Health Organization. (2009). *WHO guidelines on hand hygiene in healthcare.* Retrieved from http://whqlibdoc.who.int/hq/2009/WHO_IER_PSP_2009.07_eng.pdf

PART THREE

From Principles to Projects, Programs, and Practices

9

The Standards, Policies, and Procedures Steering Committee: Notes From the Field

Barbara Bauman, Cindy Jodoin, and Sharon Swan

The tradition of equating nursing standards, policies, and procedures with clinical nursing practice is a long and rich one throughout our profession. Evidence of it remains here at Brigham and Women's Hospital (BWH) in our online nursing policy and procedure manuals that are labeled "Clinical Practice Manuals." However, as we, the nursing leadership and staff, have worked to understand, define, and promote professional nursing practice, a new conceptualization of practice has emerged through our systematic process of change. We believe that characteristics of excellent nursing practice at BWH are:

- Knowing the patient and having the patient and family feel known and cared for
- Making clinical judgments specific to the individual patient
- Demonstrating caring practices, including interactions and interventions guided by strong notions of good care
- Staying attentive and in tune with patient responses and providing care in an individualized way
- Working with and leading others to act on the patient's and family's behalf

This description of excellent nursing practice emerged from a department-wide commitment to our vision statement: *Excellent care to patients and families by the very best staff in the safest environment.* As Mairead Hickey, our Chief Nursing Officer (CNO), regularly reminded us, in today's complex world, nursing practice is so much more than performing technical tasks. It requires a critical blend of knowledge, skill, and comportment that results in interventions that are specific to each patient and family.

Standards, policies, procedures, guidelines, and the like provide a strong foundation to support and guide practice. They are essential in ensuring patient care that is reliable and safe. However, they do not in and of themselves constitute practice. *Practice* is the nurse's use of skill, knowledge, and judgment in rendering care to a particular patient in a particular moment. It is contextual, not prescriptive.

We collectively realized that differentiating practice from standard processes of care requires constant vigilance. There is a natural tendency to want to develop policies, protocols, algorithms, decision trees, and comparable formulas that will cover every clinical scenario and tell every level of practitioner what to do in any situation. This, however, is not their function. Standards, policies, and procedures are among the tools in the clinical nurse's toolkit that can be used to carry out interventions guided by the nurse's clinical judgment and the patient's plan of care. They provide standardized methodologies to perform essential tasks and functions. This not only ensures safety and quality of care, but also allows the clinical nurse to focus more on the critical thinking and judgment required to provide excellent care to highly acute and complex patients.

STARTING UP: WHERE WE CAME FROM

By spring 2007, after months of discussion, reflection, and design, the nursing executive leadership at BWH was ready to implement our new committee structure (described in detail in Chapter 5). For the newly designed Standards, Policies, and Procedures (SPP) Steering Committee, this implementation would require restructuring, as an active model was already in place to do the work of developing, revising, and reviewing standards, guidelines, policies, and procedures. As part of my role, I had had responsibility for leading two large Department of Nursing (DON) committees that managed the policy and procedure review and approval process. The first, the Clinical Practice Committee, essentially covered all of medical surgical policies and procedures and had been established for several years. The second, the Clinical Practice Steering Committee, had been established only a few years earlier as a central forum through which the DON channeled all nursing policies and procedures from all the various practice sites (surgery, medicine/emergency, cardiovascular, peri-operative, women's health, oncology, and ambulatory).

These two committees were the primary elements of a rather loosely organized confederation of committees, task forces, and ad hoc interest groups and individuals that generated a variety of documents, policies, procedures, and guidelines to support the clinical practice of nurses. Other areas that had similar efforts included the Center for Women and Newborns (CWN), the Emergency Department (ED), and Peri-operative Nursing Services. The membership composition of these groups varied widely and consisted mostly of nurse educators and other persons with clinical leadership roles; few if any clinical nurses were represented. This model was to some degree able to do the job. It was also a somewhat traditional model that tended to equate policies and procedures with practice. We were ready to implement a change and the change had to begin at the top with our SPP Steering Committee.

The exceedingly broad scope of work to be done required a structure that drew on the expertise of a large number of nurses from every service. It also required a thorough yet efficient process to ensure that material brought forward and approved by the committee was evidence based, conceptually sound, relevant to and representative of current nursing practice at BWH, and consistent with larger organizational and regulatory requirements. We realized that we would be creating not only a new structure, but also a new way of doing our work. How our steering committee operated would be as important as what we did in engaging our nurse colleagues in our goals.

STARTING UP: DETERMINING GOALS AND RESTRUCTURING

As the conception of the new committee structure, its purpose, and its function became clearer to all of us, the initial charges of the newly named SPP Steering Committee also became clearer. They were to:

- Coordinate the review and approval of standards, policies, procedures (SPPs), and guidelines for all inpatient, peri-operative, and ambulatory areas
- Ensure consistency of SPPs and guidelines based on evidence/research, new technology, or practice changes
- Identify any need for new/revised SPPs based on new evidence, technology, or practice changes
- Develop communication and implementation plans
- Provide a forum for discussion of clinical issues and questions
- Create a network for experts on practice standards, policy, and procedure

As a means of ensuring the voice of the clinical nurse in decision making, the nursing executive leadership team had determined that all the committee memberships would be 50% clinical nurses and 50% nurses in leadership roles. We already had carefully detailed which units would designate clinical nurses and which would designate leadership nurses to participate on which specific committees. Our intent was to ensure an even distribution of clinical and leadership staff representation both across committees and across the various patient care units.

Membership of our prior committees did not follow this model. Therefore, it was necessary to restructure when starting up the SPP Steering Committee. This meant we had to make some painful decisions and conduct some difficult conversations, as we identified specific committee members who were no longer appropriate for the new committee. As advisor, I initiated conversations with these nurses, describing the change in membership as restructuring and not as a reflection on performance or contribution, and thanking them for their hard work to date. As the CNO, Mairead Hickey also sent formal letters thanking them for their contributions to the work of the department. This situation was unique to the SPP Steering Committee, as other new committees either had no prior existence or had an appropriate membership structure that was maintained.

We also restructured and refined the previously mentioned confederation of committees, task forces, and interest groups into five service line subcommittees that would regularly meet to do the preliminary development work on standards, policies, and procedures. These subcommittees are Medical-Surgical (includes oncology and cardiovascular), Women's and Newborn, Peri-operative, Emergency Department, and Ambulatory. Each subcommittee had two co-chairs who then became members of the SPP Steering Committee. The co-chairs and individual members of these five subcommittees do a tremendous amount of work in preparing standards, policies, and procedures for presentation and review for final approval by the SPP Steering Committee. Thus, the SPP Steering Committee benefits from the expertise of approximately 50 nurses who participate in the service line subcommittees, as well as of the numerous nurse experts and other expert clinicians they consult in the course of doing their work. The detailed work of the subcommittees is essential to ensuring that the 25 members of the SPP Steering Committee are able to focus on overall accuracy, relevance, and coherence of the material they are reviewing, rather than focusing on wordsmithing and typographical errors.

STARTING UP: SELECTION AND DEVELOPMENT OF CO-CHAIRS, STAFF SUPPORT, AND ADVISOR ROLES

As chairperson of the previous policy and procedure committees, I had observed several leadership and clinical nurses doing this work. Now, as advisor, I had the responsibility to recommend to the Chief Nurse who I thought would be appropriate as the first two *co-chairs* of the new SPP Steering Committee. Knowing that one co-chair had to be a nursing leader and one a clinical nurse, I was fortunate enough to be able to recruit a nurse director from the Hematology-Oncology nursing service and a seasoned critical care clinical nurse from the Surgical Intensive Care Unit. Both had demonstrated leadership and expert clinical knowledge in previous committee encounters, and I had developed a comfortable working relationship with both. For developing a start-up group, I had found that previous solid working relationships proved essential. The co-chairs lead the monthly committee meetings, help determine the agendas at our monthly planning meeting, and communicate the committee's work to the nursing community at large through formal and informal channels.

Because of the tremendous workload, dedicated administrative resources are essential to the successful functioning of the committee. A critical role is that of *staff support*, currently provided by a program director from the Center for Nursing Excellence. A master's-prepared nurse, she takes minutes at all meetings, assembles agendas for review, coordinates presentations for committee meetings, works with secretarial staff to finalize documents and get them online, and in general manages the flow of work. For this particular committee, it is essential that the staff support person has a clinical background in order to appropriately interpret and manage the work. Superior organizational skills, we quickly learned, are another must. The Center for Nursing Excellence proved to be an invaluable resource in our work.

As *advisor*, my role is to assure that the co-chairs have the resources to do their work of leading the committee. These resources are my time, energy, and focus on them and on the work at hand; my experience and organizational expertise in leading groups and committees; my overall perspective and insight; and sometimes the authority of my role for decision making or leveraging resources from elsewhere. My underlying conception here is that of the leader as teacher. That is, I believe that to lead is to foster the learning of others. My primary aim was that the co-chairs would learn to be effective leaders of the committee through their experience and through reflecting with me and each other on that experience. Additionally, I was quite intentional as a role model in demonstrating a thoughtful, direct, and consistent approach in my relationships with them.

GROWING: MANAGING THE MEETINGS

Before the first meeting of the new committees, all committee co-chairs and advisors attended a formal educational session on the overall committee structure and fundamentals of managing and leading a committee meeting. This included how to set an agenda and how to manage the group and the dynamics. This foundational work allowed us to move quickly to the specifics of managing this particular committee.

In the initial meetings of the SPP Steering Committee, a major focus was bringing the members together into a functioning group and establishing the co-chairs as the leaders. This was particularly important given the positional authority I have as an executive director. It needed to be clear from the beginning that this was not my committee or my meeting; rather, it belonged to the co-chairs and the membership. Fortunately, as I knew they would, the co-chairs stepped right up to the plate and took charge from the start, while I gratefully receded into the background.

The first meeting included light refreshments (now part of every meeting) and an ice-breaker exercise. We carefully considered the configuration of the room and the seating of the co-chairs, along with the staff support person and the advisor. From the beginning, the co-chairs sat together at the head of the table facing the screen (all material is electronically presented and edited in real time) with the membership to the side and in front of them. As advisor, I sit off to the side, or in some cases behind the co-chairs. The staff person takes minutes and manages the on-screen editing in real time at the computer, which is also off to the side.

The volume of work and nature of reviewing, revising, and developing approximately 160 standards, policies, and procedures a year requires that meetings be organized and efficient. As co-chairs, staff support, and advisor, we meet monthly for an hour, 2 weeks before the SPP Steering Committee meeting to review and plan the next meeting. We finalize the agenda that has been drafted by the staff support person. The SPP Steering Committee meets monthly on the third Wednesday; meetings typically last 2½ hours. The staff support person posts detailed agendas and all draft documents at least a week ahead, and members are expected to have reviewed all material before attending the meeting in order to facilitate comprehensive discussions. Clinical nurses are paid a total of 4 hours/month to support this commitment. Table 9.1 shows a typical agenda demonstrating the complexity of issues the committee addresses. It also validates the importance of time and process management.

The balance between allowing enough time for discussion and moving the group to consensus or decision is a constant dynamic. One of our strategies has been the development of a "Presenter Template," shown in Table 9.2, which uses a standardized format to facilitate and streamline the presentations of the material for review. All presenters complete the template before presenting to the committee and submit it to the staff support person, who then inserts portions of it into the agenda so the group can review essential content ahead of time. They also use it during the actual presentations. This resource not only enhances efficiency, but also signals the expectations of professionalism by the SPP Steering Committee.

Another strategy we have used is to ask guest speakers to present topics that contribute to the knowledge and development of the members so that they are better grounded in the topics under discussion. For example, the medical librarian presented on how to do a literature search; the director of risk management spoke on liability issues; and the advisor and co-chairs from the Patient Education Committee discussed the new patient education Website.

The two co-chairs have become quite skilled at managing complex and aggressive agendas. For example, sometimes a discussion goes on for some time with no sign of resolution, because of disagreement among members, because the presentation itself is unclear, or because the conversation uncovers gaps in information or knowledge. Strategies to manage these scenarios include asking the presenter to research further and return next month; determining that resolution will require an outside resource or decision maker, such as a regulatory agency or hospital or nursing executive leadership; or enlisting support for someone to work with the

TABLE 9.1 *Sample Agenda: Standards, Policies,*
and Procedures Steering Committee Meeting

Meeting date December 16, 2009		Time: 4:00–6:30 PM	Location: PCS-Tower 1
Time	**Topic**	**Who**	**Follow-up**

4:00–4:30 PM	Welcome/Introductions
	11-18-09 minutes review
	Identification of Nursing
	   Ops agenda items
	Equipment Committee
	   update
		Sharon Swan
		Cindy Jodoin
		
		L. Buckley	

4:30–4:35 PM	CWN	J. Daisy	

	DISCUSSION:
	WNH F.4 Formula Use and Storage
	WNH P.2 Post-Partum Check
	NICU T.2 Transfer/Transport of BWH NICU Infant to Children's Hospital Boston
	   (CHB)
	WNH M.4 Mumps, Measles, Rubella Immunization
	NICU E.2 Assisting With Partial Volume Exchange Transfusion Procedure
	   Archiving 3 pgs
	NICU I.1 Blood Glucose Confirmation Using I-Stat
	NICU F.1 Family Focused Care Guidelines
	WNH V.2 CWN Visitor Policy		

4:35–4:40 PM	AMB	M. Reynolds	
	DISCUSSION: **AMB-04** Monitoring Guideline Post-Endoscopic Procedures—S. Cialfi **Revised**		

4:45–6:00 PM	Med-Surg	M. Willis &
		   I. Fleischer ~4:40
		C. Daddio-Pierce
		   ~4:45
		A. Bane ~4:50
		L. Preston ~5:00
		J. Praetsch ~5:10
		A. Feinberg ~5:15
		V. Vacca ~5:20
		J. Beloff ~5:30
		D. Lancaster~5:40	

	DISCUSSION:
	GIT-15 Applying an Ostomy Pouch to a Stoma, Fistula, or Draining
	   Wound—M. Willis, D. Bryant and I. Fleischer **Revised**
	New products—one is cut to fit and the other is a moldable product. Use no
	   other skin products with moldable product. Positive response from
	   patients and nursing staff.
	
	CDV-05 Assisting With Cardioversion and Defibrillation Zoll M Series Biphasic
	   Automatic External Defibrillator (AED)—C. Daddio-Pierce **Final copy for**
	   review
	CDV-29 Assisting With External Transcutaneous Pacing—C. Daddio-Pierce
	   Final copy for review		

TABLE 9.1 *Sample Agenda: Standards, Policies,*
and Procedures Steering Committee Meeting (continued)

	ICU-14 Guidelines: Pulmonary Artery Pressure Monitoring—C. Daddio-Pierce **Final copy for review** **MED-01** Nursing Medication Administration—A. Bane **Revised** • Respiratory Therapists (RTs) employed by BWH may accept verbal or telephone orders. RTs may administer inhaled medications on ventilated patients. • Chemotherapy medications no longer documented on blue and green med sheets but documented in eMAR. • Lockable bedside Med Storage unit distribution continues. Added attachment 2: Bedside Medication Storage Containers: Instructions for Use. **CDV-28** Care of the Patient With a Temporary Transvenous Pacemaker— L. Preston **Revised** How to stabilize or properly secure. Two pacemaker generators have been retired. New battery must be replaced for each new patient. MD order for patient activity. **ICU-15** Cardiac Output Measurement Techniques—L. Preston **Revised** Title changed and other changes reflect the Vigilance II upgrade. The look is different; will provide pictures and the front buttons are not labeled. Policy #3 is new: MD order for Fick CO calculation with venous blood gases. Cardiac Output is from PA lines. Vigaleo is an art line-closed delivery. **EQU-26** Guidelines for the Completion of the Emergency Equipment Checklist—J. Praetsch **Reviewed** Removed green tube of gel called Signa gel due to minimal usage and safety concerns. **EQU-30** S-SORT Portable Suction Machine Policy—J. Praetsch **Reviewed** No changes **EQU-32** Continuous Passive Motion (CPM) Machine—A. Feinberg **Revised** Added details and embedded pictures within procedure for clarity and updated CCL. **MISC-02** Postmortem Care of the Adult Patient—A. Feinberg **Revised** Added Med-Legal information after consultation with Janet Barnes ("Other relevant resources" new section with links to Adm Med Staff Manual). Nursing gets direction from attending or from resident after resident discussion with attending. Committee: add death within 24 hours of admission. Discussion of present practice demonstrates variation in practice, leave everything in, remove ETT, variation between ICU and intermediate areas as well as variation among intermediate areas. Family visitation, palliative care, postmortem practice. • If unsure of requirements for tubes, lines, drains, may leave in but need to cap or tie off. • Sample pathology record book documentation **EQU-25** Intermittent Pneumatic Compression Boots—V. Vacca **Revised** Title changed to Use of Sequential Compression Device (SCD) SCD Express and Intermittent Compression Sleeves and Foot Cuffs

(*continued*)

TABLE 9.1 *Sample Agenda: Standards, Policies,*
and Procedures Steering Committee Meeting (continued)

	Conflicting information received by nurse educators and staff nurses between nurse educator presentation and unit presentations (prioritization of component effectiveness). Consulted with Dr Goldhaber to define sequence: **General Guidelines:** 1. Thigh-high sleeves are preferred 2. Knee-high sleeves if thigh-high contraindicated 3. Foot cuffs if clinically indicated and ordered by MD **NEU-03** Care of the Patient Requiring Cerebrospinal Fluid (CSF) Drainage With an External Ventricular Drain (EVD) System—V. Vacca and H. Doucette **Revised** NEU-04 embedded in NEU-03. Archive NEB-04. Reflects new equipment: Codman EDS-3 CSF Drainage System with pictures. Laser used for lining up anatomical landmarks. **Physician Approved Order and Screening Form for Inpatient Pneumococcal/ Influenza Immunization—**J. Beloff **Revised** Added to Influenza vaccine <u>not indicated</u> section; Influenza vaccine has been ordered but has not been received by hospital due to problems with vaccine production/distribution. Also stickers with same information available. **H1N1 update:** MD must screen for this vaccine and write order. Next year H1N1 will be a component of the annual flu vaccine. **Care of the Suicidal Patient—**D. Lancaster **Informational presentation** This suicide policy is a revision of a former policy and was reviewed and revised with input from the suicide committee members. It has been reviewed by the executive sponsors, legal, compliance, quality, and some others, and is now ready for final sign-off. Policy addressed requirements for JC NPSG-15 includes risk assessment of patient and environment, resources when patient discharged. High frequency in ED but patient may be admitted. Role of 1:1 sitter discussed (1 sitter may not be assigned to 2 suicidal patients). Policy located in Adm Med Staff Policy Manual. **STD-01** Documentation of Clinical Nursing Practice in the Patient Record—D. Lancaster **Revised** Date, Time Sign Nursing (Medical Records Policy): New JC signature policy (STD-01 updated to reflect changes). **FOR-08** Guidelines for Completion of Patient Assessment Form—B. Griffin **Archive**		
6:00–6:10 PM	PeriOP	C. Kubiak J. Walion	
6:10–6:30 PM	Practice changes for Nursing Ops agenda Open Agenda:	S. Swan C. Jodoin	

presenter to strengthen the original work. Knowing "when to hold 'em and when to fold 'em" requires that the co-chairs know and read the group well, so that members feel the amount of time spent on an issue was right, and that the decision to push for resolution or not was right.

TABLE 9.2 *Presenter Template: Standards, Policies, and Procedures Meeting*

PURPOSE:

Provide a standardized, comprehensive approach to presenting material at the Standards, Policies and Procedures Steering Committee meeting. Ensure that all substantive and salient issues are covered in a thorough and, to the degree possible, succinct fashion.

Date: _____

Title of standard/policy/procedure: _____

Who is affected (check all that apply)
❑ Intermediate RNs
❑ ICU RNs
❑ LPNs
❑ PCAs/MAs
❑ Unit coordinators/ops supervisor
❑ Other _____

Status of SPP
❑ new
❑ revised
❑ reviewed

Key points/substantive changes:
❑ _____
❑ _____

Departments/individuals involved in development/revision:
❑ _____
❑ _____

Who can act as a resource regarding this SPP?
❑ _____
❑ _____

For questions/support about your presentation, please contact:

Cindy Jodoin, RN, Heme-Onc/BMT *cjodoin@partners.org*
Sharon Swan, RN, Surgical ICU *sswan1@partners.org*

The co-chairs, the staff support person, and I always debrief for 15 to 20 minutes after each meeting. We discuss how the overall meeting went, particularly with regard to participation and group dynamics. We identify and clarify issues that were raised and determine what (if any) intervening actions or follow-up will be done and by whom before the next planning meeting.

SPPs that receive final approval from the committee move next to the Nurse Executive Board (NEB) for review, discussion, and approval. This is a standing monthly agenda item for NEB. Once approved at NEB, they are put on line.

GROWING: MANAGING THE WORK OUTSIDE THE MEETINGS

Like any other acute care hospital, our practice environment is complex, frequently intense, and always fast paced. Questions and challenges present daily when unforeseen clinical issues arise; new innovations, knowledge, or technology are introduced; or regulations change. There is constant e-mail communication and consultation among the co-chairs, the staff support person, and myself, as issues and questions can be and are brought to any one of us. Any issue not answered with a quick look-up in the online manual or redirection to an appropriate resource is taken to our planning meeting for potential inclusion on the next agenda. Occasionally, there is an urgency to quickly resolve or address an issue; for example, when a new product or piece of equipment has been implemented and the procedure must be updated to be available at the same time. In such cases, we use an expedited review and approval process, where the critical information is sent out by e-mail to the committee members with a response deadline.

SUSTAINING: COMMUNICATION AND FEEDBACK STRATEGIES

As we gained experience, we realized that we needed to develop a more robust communication process to ensure that all BWH nurses were appropriately informed about new or changed SPPs. Historically, e-mails to all staff had been used episodically, depending on the nature of the changes. We developed a template consisting of a grid that categorized the approved SPPs according to their content and practice areas affected, with bullet points that highlighted the important changes. This document was dubbed "New to You/Time to Review" and is distributed monthly to staff from the co-chairs. Staff can look at the category titles to determine which content has relevance to their practice without having to review everything. Table 9.3 shows an example from a recent "New to You/Time to Review" prepared by Brenda Griffin, the Center for Nursing Excellence Program Director who provides our staff support.

At the close of each SPP Steering Committee meeting, the committee reviews the approvals for that meeting and determines which ones are of particular importance or impact. The co-chairs then highlight these selected SPPs in the monthly committee update column of *BWH Nurse*, our in-house nursing newsletter.

Another important piece of feedback we depend upon is the "hit rate" for the SPPs, that is, which SPPs were most frequently accessed via the online manual. This information is collected annually and shared with the committee, so that we know where there may be areas of focus, potentially indicating a knowledge gap or a recent influx of nurses new to the department.

Midway through the second year of the new committee, we decided to survey our SPP Steering Committee members to assess how they felt they and the group were doing and to solicit ideas and feedback to guide the leaders in determining the future direction of the committee. Although this had been an area of discussion within the group during meetings, we wanted an anonymous survey as well to provide each member an opportunity to freely voice his or her thoughts and opinions. Seven survey items were developed and scored using a simple Likert scale. Results are presented in Table 9.4.

TABLE 9.3 *Sample Monthly Update E-mail Message to BWH Nurses*
From Standards, Policies, and Procedures Committee

A message from Standards, Policies, and Procedures Committee . . .

Please review the attached list of policies that have either been revised or are new. If the policy is pertinent to your practice, you will find all the updates here.

The Standards, Policies, and Procedures Committee wants to effectively communicate changes to you, the clinical nurse. If you have any questions or comments, please feel free to contact us.
Thank you,

Cindy Jodoin, RN, and Sharon Swan, RN
SPP Co-Chairs

New to You/Time to Review Policies and Procedures
Submitted by Brenda Griffin, RN, MBA

Chapter	Section/Title	Who Is Affected?	Key Points/Substantive Changes
CDV	**CDV-00** Guidelines for Nursing Roles/ Responsibilities in Adult Cardiopulmonary Resuscitation	Inpatient	• Added role of nurse educator during code, how to obtain a code summary.
	CDV-01 Tower Code Team Nurse Responsibilities	Inpatient	• Title changed to: Code Team Nurse Responsibilities. • Coverage provided by Tower, ED and Shapiro code teams with an attached appendix outlining the specific locations described in the policies. (Need further detail related to special circumstances; e.g., Adult code in NICU, visitor collapse in Tower room after unexpected death, L1 & L2 codes become confusing—Team called needs to be driven by location.) • Deleted all the code team equipment lists. • Added obtaining the Zoll Code Summary printout.
	CDV-17 Code Blue Obstetrics	Inpatient Outpatient	• Additional language re: OB emergency release blood and management of hemorrhage. • Additional information re: neonate separation from mother at any time during placement of proper ID bands. • Listing of OB hemorrhage meds and updated references.

(continued)

TABLE 9.3 *Sample Monthly Update E-mail Message to BWH Nurses*
From Standards, Policies, and Procedures Committee (continued)

Chapter	Section/Title	Who Is Affected?	Key Points/Substantive Changes
			• Information needed for Code Team members for tower pregnant inpatients. • Code OB for deliveries.
	CDV-26 Obtaining a 12-Lead Electrocardiogram (ECG) Utilizing a MAC 5000/5500	Inpatient Outpatient	• Added 5500 model to procedure which functions the same as the 5000 except that the 5000 has floppy disk the ECG techs take care of. • Scanner function for patient ID (5500 only comes out with 1st 5 letters of patient's last name, but all other demographics present). • Noted that in Shapiro there are 2 analog jack sites. • ED process added reflecting process for MUISE system when inaccurate information entered in error or patient subsequently identified by name.
DAG	**Amicar®**	Inpatient	• New
	Flolan-inhaled	Inpatient	• Flolan inhaled route only administered to ventilated patients in the ICUs by respiratory therapists with the nurse monitoring the patient.
GUIDE	**GUIDE-06** Guidelines for Timing Subcutaneous Insulin Administration	Inpatient	• To define appropriate clinical procedure for subcutaneous insulin administration related to POCT. • Nutritional Subcutaneous Insulin, Correctional Subcutaneous Insulin, and Basal Subcutaneous Insulin related to patient eating, delayed trays, NPO, tube feedings, and TPN.
S	Care of the Suicidal Patient	Inpatient ED	• Policy addressed requirements for JC NPSG-15 includes risk assessment of patient and environment, resources when patient discharged. High frequency in ED but patient may be admitted. Role of 1:1 sitter discussed (1 sitter may not be assigned to 2 suicidal patients). Policy also located in Adm Med Staff Policy Manual

TABLE 9.4 *Survey Responses From SPP Steering Committee Members: Evaluating Our Progress*

	Strongly Disagree %	Disagree %	Agree %	Strongly Agree %	Don't Know %
1. I have enough time to prepare for the meetings.	0	39	56	5	0
2. I have enough information in order to participate in the meetings.	5	6	61	28	0
3. The amount of material we cover in a typical meeting is about right.	0	6	72	22	0
4. The pace and length of the meeting are about right.	0	17	55	28	0
5. I think the work we do in the committee is important for the Department of Nursing.	0	0	22	78	0
6. I am seen as a resource by my colleagues because of my work on the committee.	0	6	61	22	11
7. I feel that I am an important member of the committee.	0	0	78	17	5

We also developed three open-ended questions with a large, free text box to allow our respondents to provide as much detail as they wished. We asked the following three questions:

1. What works best about the committee?
2. What one thing would you change about the committee or the way it functions?
3. Please make any other comments or suggestions for improvement

Responses to the open-ended questions included the following comments that provided guidance in planning changes and validated the processes we were using:

- Encourages all voices to be heard
- Allows time off from work at bedside to participate
- We receive feedback
- Although not as frequently as in the beginning, we still sometimes get bogged down in editorial work; would like to work toward decreasing that further
- The way the co-leaders are non-biased, and want everything to be done correctly. They equally give members and guest a chance to express their ideas.
- I feel my voice is heard by the nursing department when I raise a concern re: a policy.

SUSTAINING: REFINING AND REDEFINING GOALS

As our experience deepened and we entered the third year, we redefined the goals of the SPP Steering Committee as follows:

- Coordinate the review, consistency, and approval of standards, policies, and procedures.
- Identify any needs to develop or revise these documents.
- Ensure that language and content of standards, policies, and procedures meet regulatory requirements.
- Ensure homogeneity and congruity of language with other disciplines' standards, policies, and procedures.
- Promote evidence-based practice by providing education to membership on use of library resources.
- Refine and clarify process of development of standards, policies, procedures, and guidelines, ensuring consistency on how information is organized and presented.
- Develop strategies to improve accessibility for staff.

Now, as we approach the conclusion of the third year, more opportunities to grow and develop the SPP Steering Committee are emerging, as staff turnover has occurred, and planning begins for leadership transition. And we continue to evolve. Cindy and Sharon, the co-chairs of the SPP Steering Committee, complete this chapter with reflections on their experience and share their wisdom with the nursing community.

Co-Chairing SPP: A Narrative by Cindy Jodoin

When I was first approached regarding the role of co-chair for the SPP Steering Committee, I felt honored, apprehensive, and ambivalent—pretty much in that order. As a member of the previous steering committee that reviewed nursing policies and procedures for this large nursing department, I knew the volume of work this entailed each month. In addition, the sense of responsibility to provide evidence-based, useful work as a resource for the bedside nurse had always evoked a serious commitment of time and energy. The opportunity to provide leadership for this committee with a clinical nurse, though, was too compelling to not accept.

The past 3 years have been a wonderful challenge, including the opportunity to work as co-chair with the clinical nurse, executive director, and program director from the Center for Nursing Excellence, and all the members of the committee. My clinical nurse co-chair and I have established an environment where all feedback is welcome and valued, participation is encouraged, and evidence-based practice is the guiding principle for all decisions. Our initial meeting included establishing ground rules for all future meetings. These rules included starting and ending on time, only one person speaking at a time (avoid sidebars), attendance is expected, cell phones and pagers are on vibrate, and the commitment of the co-chairs to keeping the agenda items and discussion within the allotted time frames. These rules help to keep the agenda on target and show respect for members as well as guests.

This committee has brought the voice of the bedside nurse to each and every policy and procedure. The varied experience from so many specialties has contributed invaluable knowledge that is integrated into the Clinical Practice Manual, making it a useful tool. In addition, we have been able to improve the search engine and organization of the manual so that information is found with more ease. In a recent review of how often the top 10 policies/procedures in the manual are accessed, the percentage has almost doubled during the last 2 years. The manual has become a more user-friendly document that continuously evolves just as nursing care and practice continue to evolve.

I think our greatest accomplishment has been improving the accessibility of the policies and procedures. We routinely track the number of "hits" for the SPPs, including the "Top Ten SPPs," that is, the SPPs most frequently accessed via the online manual. In February 2009, there were 2148 hits for the Top Ten; in February 2010, there were 3918. Just one example is **IVT-21** (Guidelines for Flushing Central IV Catheters), which had 21 hits in June 2008, 166 hits in July 2009, and 629 hits in February 2010. This has become a useful and used manual, not just a resource in name only. Some next steps will be to streamline policies and develop a "Reader's Digest Condensed" summary for emergent situations. Of course, we are always searching for ways to improve communication to the staff.

The most important learning for me has been related to staying organized, keeping the members on track and within time constraints, and learning how very differently the various specialties may do the same procedure. I have a much broader perspective on the variety of ways each nurse functions at BWH.

My advice to those on this journey is to take it slow and bring the staff nurse into the process early. Education on committee structure and group dynamics may be helpful. It was for us.

Co-Chairing SPP: A Narrative by Sharon Swan

The strength of this committee is the feeling of safety within the group. Our committee had been recomposed with few original members. We were colleagues, but mostly strangers to one another. Clinical nurses had knowledge and skills to bring forth, but we were asked to utilize these in new ways, and how to do that created a large learning curve. I certainly experienced this as a novice co-chair who was humbled on more than one occasion. But it was okay; it was part of the process. The highest compliment we received, in my mind, was when a committee member told my co-chair: "It is safe to make a mistake here." Beyond the work, we had created an environment of trust, encouraging members to explore and expand. This allows individual members to grow and grows the committee as an entity.

The direction of this growth is outward. We must make relationships and communicate within nursing and the hospital organization at large. The work is interrelated, not isolated. Part of the committee growth is in seeing how our work fits in this bigger picture. This requires communication that reaches vertically and horizontally. Finding consistent and meaningful ways to communicate has been a challenge for individual committees as well for the department and the organization. To facilitate nurse-to-nurse and nurse-to-system communication, education and openness are key elements and must be incorporated into the work by the committee leadership. How to do this is an ongoing important learning experience.

As the committee reaches the ripe old age of two and a half years, the advice I would share with other nursing departments courageous enough to try this model is simple: Trust your nurses, both at the clinical and leadership levels. There is expansive knowledge and talent waiting to be tapped. The process elevates practice and the work environment. The end result is excellent patient care. The joy is in the journey and the love is in the details.

Change Through Narrative

10.1 *The Nurse Manager Narrative Project*

Eloise Balasco Cathcart, Miriam Greenspan, and Miriam Trainer

Creating a healthy environment for patients, families, and staff is a core responsibility of the nurse manager (Kramer, Schmalenberg, & Maguire, 2010). Knowing how to select and develop candidates for this central management role is necessary to achieve the Brigham and Women's Hospital (BWH) Department of Nursing's (DON) vision of providing *"excellent care to patients and families with the very best staff in the safest environment."* The literature is replete with studies describing traits of successful nurse managers, as well as factors that support engagement or create stress and challenge for frontline managers (Association of Perioperative Registered Nurses [APRN], 2004; Kramer, Schmalenberg, & Maguire, 2010; Mackoff & Triolo, 2008a, 2008b, 2008c; Shirey, 2006; Shirey, Ebright, & McDaniel, 2008). But in our work with nurse managers at BWH, we wanted to know something different: What did nurse managers experience in their day-to-day practice as they attempted to implement the DON's vision? How did they learn to do the situation-specific relational work that is germane to achieving good outcomes for patients and staff? How did they align staff to build nursing practice and improve patient care? How did ethical dilemmas show up for them? How was breakdown or failure in their practice manifested? How did they know what was good for patients, families, and staff? How did they learn how to make that happen?

As one of the first steps in a broader leadership development initiative within the DON, we undertook the Nurse Manager Narrative Project to illuminate our understanding of the lived experience of nurse managers at BWH. We utilized the methodology of practice articulation described by Patricia Benner in her corpus of research on clinical knowledge development. Benner used interpretive phenomenology to describe the lived experience, skilled practical knowledge, and ethical comportment embedded in the everyday practice of clinical nurses, and explicated the processes by which expert nursing practice develops (Benner, 1984; Benner, Hooper-Kyriakidis, & Stannard, 1999; Benner, Tanner, & Chesla, 2009; Benner, Sutphen, Leonard, & Day, 2010). At the time of this project, those who are in this book identified as nurse directors were designated as nurse managers, and it is therefore the designation we use in describing our project.

Based on our belief that nurse managers have a practice that is specific to their unique role, we sought to articulate in common language the specific knowledge and notions of good embedded in this central leadership practice. The use of narrative exemplars with guided interpretation made it possible for managers to describe what and how they knew about particular situations of their everyday practice in first-person experiential terms. We heard about the salient features of these situations that captured the managers' attention, and about the meanings and emotions that the situations engendered for them (Benner, 1994).

We divided 32 nurse managers into five groups based on their tenure in the nurse manager role. Participants' clinical services were mixed, so each group met with colleagues from groups led by directors other than their own. Each group attended 8 weekly seminars of 2 hours' duration over a 2-year period. Each participant wrote and read to the group a narrative exemplar of his or her best management practice or a story of a time of practice breakdown in which critical learning occurred for the manager. A consultant (Eloise Cathcart) and a program coordinator (Miriam Greenspan), a seasoned nurse executive and nurse manager, respectively, who have expertise in narrative interpretation, facilitated the seminars. In this chapter we describe our experiences and provide an exemplar from a nurse manager participant (Miriam Trainer).

The first group, the most experienced nurse managers, were comfortable inhabiting this pivotal leadership role and spoke from their perspectives as leaders. They talked of how knowing individual nurses and their practice was the basis for developing their staff and accomplishing programmatic goals. In their narratives, we heard stories of how they dealt with the challenges they faced as they worked to change the culture on their unit, how they coached staff to reinforce the value and worth of their clinical practice, and how they used finely honed skilled know-how to navigate the system for the good of patients and staff. This group was able to imagine how narrative could be useful to them in refining and extending the DON's vision on their respective units.

The second group had the shortest role tenure, and their narratives told of their experiences in transitioning into a new and unfamiliar role. Feelings of being alone, worries about being incompetent, and difficulties with time management and maintaining work-life balance were dominant themes in these narratives. The exemplars provided opportunities for situated learning. The facilitators coached participants to "see" these situations with the eyes of a manager, assisting them with their role transition from clinician to manager. Interpretation of the situations presented in the narratives helped these new managers develop a sense of salience and learn how to engage with staff, how to manage boundaries, and how to help staff develop as a team.

Subsequent groups, which met over the next 18 months, included managers whose tenure in their role was between 2 and 5 years. Their narratives often spoke of the relentless challenges inherent in the role. These challenges were experienced as administrative tasks that competed with the self-described "important work" of being with nurses around issues of patient care. Because these managers had not yet learned how to work through staff, they saw themselves as responsible for managing the breakdowns that occurred in the processes of patient care so that staff would be free to execute their daily assignments. Their experience of the role was shaped by the demands placed upon them by staff and senior nursing leaders to whom they reported, and they often spoke of the difficulty involved in managing these two forces they sometimes perceived as opposing. The facilitators coached these managers to "work through" rather than "do for" staff as a model of leadership practice, so that staff could learn to incorporate dimensions of clinical leadership into their own practice.

Our narrative work with these nurse managers and others has consistently shown that, in their best practice, nurse managers are able to engage in the demanding relational work which is at the core of this pivotal leadership practice, see what is at stake in particular open-ended situations, and intervene in ways that ensure good outcomes for patients and staff (Cathcart, Greenspan, & Quin, 2010). The following narrative by Miriam Trainer provides an exemplar of how this notion of good is lived out.

> A clinical alert was sent via e-mail that a patient who was 32 weeks' pregnant would be coming in to have a C-section birth before the due date. The baby had abnormalities that would be incompatible with life and the baby's head was three times the size of an average baby's head. The OB team decided that it was necessary to do this surgery early in order to get the baby's head out. The parents were well aware of the situation and wanted the baby not to go to the NICU but to stay in the room with them on the postpartum unit in order to spend as much time with the baby as possible. This was a practice that had not previously been done on the postpartum units. The nursing practice on these units has been limited to caring for postpartum patients and healthy babies. If a baby was going to die, that baby was in the NICU. These parents so very much wanted a baby and went through IVF [*in vitro* fertilization] in order to conceive. They were now planning for the birth and death of their baby and made a plan for their wishes to be carried out.
>
> During our daily staffing meeting, we were told that the patient would be coming in tomorrow and scheduled for surgery. We were asked to which unit the patient would be going. Since I was covering for another nurse manager and the other nurse manager was new in her position, I said that the patient would be going to my unit, CWN 9. Since this was a new practice for my staff, I thought, "Who was going to care for this family?" I wanted nurses who were comfortable with death and dying and remembered that I had sent an e-mail to staff regarding participation in a new palliative care program that we were going to develop. I had received several e-mails from staff stating they would love to be a part of this. I saw that three of these staff were on the next 2 days. I wanted staff to be prepared for this family, so I called each one at home and discussed the plan. I arranged to have extra staff in order to free the nurse for this family. We really did not have a practice in place and were just developing a bereavement book for the staff to use as a resource. I obtained the book and bereavement box and reviewed the policy.
>
> I thought all was set, but not so. The surgery had been rescheduled for the following day. I was thankful that the staff was still on. From the information given I thought that the baby would not live long. Wrong again. I came in at

7:00 AM and saw the night nurse starting to give report on this family to the day nurse. The day nurse had this look of horror on her face. I immediately went over and sat down and listened to report. The night nurse had bonded with this family and wanted the plan to go as the family wanted. I could see that the day nurse could not control her emotions regarding her assignment. I had not called this nurse and this was a surprise to her. I asked her if she was okay and she told me "No." She said that she had never cared for a dying patient and did not think she could handle this assignment.

I thought, "Oh, my God—what am I going to do?" I needed the patient and family to have a supportive, caring, and empathetic environment. I needed the program to go smoothly as an example for other families and I needed to have the nurse feel confident and comfortable caring for this family. I looked over the assignment sheet to see who was on and if I could make any changes.

I still thought that this nurse would have been the nurse I would have assigned to the patient. She is patient focused and always gives her all to her practice. I knew in that moment what I needed to do. I told her that I would be beside her all the way and that I would not leave her. I told her that I was very comfortable in caring for this family and I would be her support.

I knew that the staff was watching and I needed to be the leader. The nurse and I went into the patient's room and I talked with the patient about her being a new mother and we discussed who the baby looked like, what long fingers the baby had. The parents were talking with and reading to the baby. Mom put the baby to breast and kept touching the baby's face. The nurse started to engage in conversation and assisted the dad in holding the baby. I left the room to call the NICU for more morphine for the baby. The nurse came to me crying and said she thought the baby had died. She could not hear a heartbeat nor detect breathing. I went into the room, listened and told the parents that I could not hear a heartbeat but I was going to contact the physician to come and see the baby.

It was hard for these parents to know the end had come. They were crying and rocking with the baby. The nurse and I stayed in the room at the parents' request. The mother wanted to give the baby a bath and dress the baby. I offered to the nurse that I would do this. She declined the offer and wanted to be with the mom and assist. She let the family be with the baby for as long as they wanted. The nurse brought the baby to another room and I performed postmortem care as she watched. She carried the baby in her arms to the morgue with me by her side. We said goodbye to the baby and I put the baby in the drawer. She cried about how sad this was and what great parents these people were. She returned to care for the mother after we had a departmental debriefing.

This nurse e-mailed me several times that night about things that went on with the death certificate, funeral home, and told me how supported she felt. I knew that this experience had changed her personally. She had bonded with this family and still wanted to care for them.

Several weeks later we were asked to present rounds to the VP of Nursing. I was a bit surprised when the nurses involved in the care of this family came in on their day off. They had done the right work in the best supportive way possible. And when I heard the nurse say, "Before I didn't think I could care for this family and I now know that I can," I knew that I had made a difference in the practice of this nurse, the palliative care program, and for this baby and parents. Through my clinical skills of caring for dying patients throughout the continuum, I could demonstrate competence in practice, having family-centered care as our focus and that no nurse would be left alone; that support and anticipatory guidance would be there for the staff. My leadership skills in knowing practice and knowing the staff helped me help the nurse in developing the necessary skills to support this family. The nurses asked if they could present this case to the staff. Wow! I thought how great this is to share practice. Over lunch, the nurses told their story and the room was filled with unit assistants, unit coordinators, patient care assistants, and nurses and no one moved. Every person in the room was fixed on the narrative. On discharge to home, the patient and her husband thanked us for the kindness we showed and she held in her lap the precious footprints that we helped make.

This nurse manager tells of the challenges facing her when she learns that a baby with abnormalities incompatible with life would be admitted to her unit and that the parents of this baby had definite ideas about how they wanted things to go. Coincidentally, the nurse manager had been in the planning stages of developing a bereavement program for her unit, which had generated a good amount of interest on the part of the staff. The fact that she would have to deal with this devastating situation before the planning was complete and nurses were properly prepared demonstrates the nature of clinical work: It is unpredictable, unordered, and open-ended. This is the public stage on which nurse managers manage.

Despite this manager's preparatory work with selected nurses, whom she believed could provide good care for this family, she arrives one morning to find the patient's care being handed to a nurse with a "look of horror on her face." The nurse is clearly overwhelmed: "I asked her if she was okay and she told me 'No.' She said that she had never cared for a dying patient and did not think she could handle this assignment."

This is where the nurse manager eloquently gives voice to the ethical demand of her practice. She understands that she is there to ensure excellent care for this *particular* patient and family, to walk with the nurse through this rough terrain so that the nurse can come out safely on the other side, and to preserve this budding bereavement program so that families yet to come could have access to this kind of care. She did not need to go through a tedious list of alternative options to know what she needed to do. She was able, in an instant, to see the salient features of the situation and know immediately what was at stake. Her decision to reorder her agenda for the day and coach this frightened nurse is a superb example of an attuned response-based practice; she knew what to do and how to do it (Benner et al., 2010).

If this nurse manager were less skilled or less cognizant of what was at stake, she might well have diminished the significance of the look of horror on the nurse's face, or simply changed the assignment. But she knew this nurse and knew what this person was capable of, and realized what the benefit could be for her in persevering in this high-stakes learning situation. The nurse manager realized that only the experiential learning that could come to this nurse from remaining engaged in the care of this particular family would yield the complex skilled knowledge required to extend this nurse's practice (Benner et al., 2010). This situation reinforces the fundamental fact that our patients and our practice are our most important teachers.

The nurse manager engages with the nurse and coaches her through what Benner et al. describe as "clinical reasoning-in-transition" (Benner et al., 1999; Benner et al., 2010). The manager stands side by side with the nurse, teaching her how to think about what is unfolding before her and how to keep track of the changing situation while always paying attention to the meaning of the patient's responses. The manager models how to preserve the experience of parenting for this family, by "talking with the patient about being a new mother and who the baby looked like, what long fingers the baby had"—a vital gift for a family who will leave the hospital with memories rather than a newborn. This attunement, respect, curiosity, and willingness to be caught off-guard is all for the good of this family and illuminates the notion of good in clinical nursing practice (Benner et al., 2010).

When the baby dies, the nurse is distressed, but we see that she is beginning to claim the care of this family for herself. She declines the nurse manager's offer to bathe and dress the baby, saying that "she wanted to be with the mom and assist." The nurse manager skillfully modulates the boundary between herself and the nurse, giving the nurse more room but never leaving. We hear how the nurse reaches out to the nurse manager several times during the night, and finally the nurse says, "Before I didn't think I could care for this family and I now know that I can." This newfound competence and confidence make the transfer of accountability complete.

The nurse's practice has been transformed. She has acquired new learning, and she is reminded once again that she can make a difference in the lives of patients and families entrusted to her care. This situation taught this nurse important lessons about the value of care when cure is not possible (Cathcart, 2008). Along with this growth in her practice comes personal growth; the nurse manager tells us that she "knew this experience had changed her [the nurse] personally." The value and worth of her work with this particular family is recognized and reinforced as she proudly recounts the story for her coworkers and the chief nursing officer.

This narrative is an exemplar of highly skilled nurse leadership practice as well. The nurse manager walked into this emotionally charged situation and, with great care but no guarantee of success, helped both this family and this nurse to emerge intact. She is aware that this kind of risk-laden involvement always carries heavy scrutiny: "I knew the staff was watching and I needed to be the leader." She is authentic; what she does matches the values that shape her as a person and as a nurse (Shirey, 2006). We can hear her articulate her success in preserving those values that she identified early on as important to her: "competence in practice, family-centered care and that no nurse would be left alone" in the demanding but exquisite work of patient care. This nurse manager knows that her ultimate success depends on the competence of her staff (Hill, 2004). Her ability to improve practice on her unit and achieve programmatic goals is dependent on her staff's ability to live out a highly skilled practice, so walking into a quagmire like the one depicted in this narrative is usually worth the risk. She offers us a picture of leadership expertise that affects not only this particular family and nurse, but the entire nursing practice community and the organization as well.

The narratives presented as part of this initiative reinforced the essential role of the nurse manager in translating the DON's vision of providing *"excellent care to patients and families with the very best staff in the safest environment"* into reality. The nurse managers' narratives consistently illuminated what was at stake for patients and staff in the processes of patient care at BWH, how the managers' intents and goals were lived out, and how the managers' judgments determined strategies and actions. Being able to cull out and put language to the ways in which nurse managers work with staff to assure that patients and families receive the care they need in the safest environment provided an understanding of the complexity and undeniable importance of this frontline leadership practice (Cathcart et al., 2010).

REFERENCES

Association of Perioperative Registered Nurses. (2004). *Nurse manager skills inventory.* Denver, CO: Author.

Benner, P. (1984). *From novice to expert: Excellence and power in clinical nursing practice.* Menlo Park, CA: Addison-Wesley.

Benner, P. (1994). The role of articulation in understanding practice and experience as sources of knowledge in clinical nursing. In J. Tully & D. M. Weinstock (Eds.), *Philosophy in a time of pluralism: Perspectives on the philosophy of Charles Taylor* (pp. 136–155). Cambridge, UK: Cambridge University Press.

Benner, P., Hooper-Kyriakidis, P., & Stannard, D. (1999). *Clinical wisdom and interventions in critical care: A thinking-in-action approach.* Philadelphia, PA: W.B. Saunders.

Benner, P., Sutphen, M., Leonard, V., & Day, L. (2010). *Educating nurses: A call for radical transformation.* San Francisco, CA: Jossey-Bass.

Benner, P., Tanner, C., & Chesla, C. (2009). *Expertise in nursing practice* (2nd ed.). New York, NY: Springer Publishing.

Cathcart, E. (2008). The role of the chief nursing officer in leading the practice: Lessons from the Benner tradition. *Nursing Administration Quarterly, 32*(2), 87–91.

Cathcart, E., Greenspan, M., & Quin, M. (2010). The making of a nurse manager: The role of experiential learning in leadership development. *Journal of Nursing Management, 18*(4), 440–447.

Hill, L. (2004). New manager development for the 21st century. *Academy of Management Executives, 18*(3), 121–126.

Kramer, M., Schmalenberg, C., & Maguire, P. (2010). Nine structures and leadership practices essential for a magnetic (healthy) work environment. *Nursing Administration Quarterly, 34*(1), 4–17.

Mackoff, B., & Triolo, P. (2008a). Line of sight: The crucible in nurse manager engagement. *Nurse Leader, 6*(2), 21–28.

Mackoff, B., & Triolo, P. (2008b). Why do nurse managers stay? Building a model of engagement. Part 1, Dimensions of engagement. *Journal of Nursing Administration, 38*(3), 118–124.

Mackoff, B., & Triolo, P. (2008c). Why do nurse managers stay? Building a model of engagement. Part 2, Cultures of engagement. *Journal of Nursing Administration, 38*(4), 166–171.

Shirey, M. (2006). Authentic leaders creating healthy work environments for nursing practice. *American Journal of Critical Care, 15*(3), 256–267.

Shirey, M., Ebright, P., & McDaniel, A. (2008). Sleepless in America: Nurse managers cope with stress and complexity. *Journal of Nursing Administration, 38*(3), 125–131.

10.2 *Navigating Change Through a Narrative*

Pearl Cunningham and Phyllis Bailey

---

*I*n 2007, the Brigham and Women's Hospital (BWH) Department of Nursing (DON) began the journey of developing and implementing a vision: to provide *excellent care to patients and families, with the very best staff, in the safest environment.* I (Pearl) became the nurse director in the Operating Room (OR) department in May of 2008. As a new director, I believed it was important that I honor my commitment to staff to provide for them an environment where they could be examples of the vision we had developed. In late July 2008, we moved into the new Shapiro Cardiovascular building (see Chapter 17), which housed 16 additional operating rooms. Over the previous months, I had worked very hard to provide the staff with all of the resources they needed to care for our patients in their new environment. I felt that my responsibility was to provide the information and resources to make sure the staff could deliver the best care possible.

To say that it was a time of great change would be an understatement. Over the past 5 months, many hours had been spent orienting and integrating 30 new employees to the operating room. There was a massive educational program designed to orient more than 300 staff members to the newly constructed space and to the new equipment that was purchased. The physical plant grew by thousands of square feet. People had to reorient themselves to where supplies and equipment were stored. New locker rooms were necessary and the normalcy of the only personal space people could call their own was changed literally overnight.

The staff's work flow changed significantly. When staff voiced concerns about the perceived differences in the rooms, I reminded them that we were giving excellent care in all rooms. I made sure that we never talked about the "new ORs and the old ORs"; it was the "Tower or existing rooms and the Shapiro rooms." With our ORs spread between two separate buildings, many people thought that we now had two separate OR departments. To help people navigate the new traffic flow, we even had pocket maps printed!

I worked hard to try to sustain an environment where people would feel supported. This leadership core competency was an essential focus when we were developing the mission and vision for DON. It was within this context that I learned the value of narrative in addressing the challenges faced by the nurses who were dealing with these stressful work situations.

The first holiday in the new operating room was Labor Day weekend. When I returned on Monday, I assumed that all had gone well, because I had not heard otherwise. I was making rounds in the cardiac rooms. I approached Phyllis, one of the cardiac nurses with the most experience, to ask her about her day and the patient she was caring for.

She asked if I had a minute to talk to her about her patient from the previous Friday. She was very concerned about a series of experiences she had with a complex and challenging patient situation over the weekend. She wanted to know if she had "done the right thing" for her patient. She began to tell me what happened, described here in her narrative of the experience.

I was sitting in the media room in the cardiac area the Friday before the Labor Day weekend. We had recently moved into our new ORs in the Shapiro building, and we were getting used to the surroundings. I was reviewing my e-mail, when an anesthesiologist, with whom I had worked well, asked me to care for Mrs. A., a patient with a descending aortic aneurysm, which can be life-threatening. The repair is risky and complicated.

I enjoyed working with the anesthesiologist, so I asked the nurse-in-charge (NIC) if I could switch my assignment. The NIC looked at me in surprise when I asked for my assignment to be changed. I was assigned to the role of circulating nurse in a coronary artery bypass graft, commonly called by its acronym, CABG, a less complicated case than the one Mrs. A. was having.

As the circulator in the room, I was responsible for making sure that the scrub nurse, the team member who was sterile to assist the surgeon at the field, had everything needed. I was also responsible for providing care, monitoring the flow of the case, and assisting the team in maintaining the safety of the patient. When I went to meet Mrs. A., she was being transferred down the hall by the anesthesiologist. She was sitting straight up in the bed with her legs crossed. We had a brief meeting where I introduced myself; we talked about the new Shapiro building and her family. I asked her who was waiting for her. She said her husband would be in later. The anesthesiologist stopped outside the room to review her pain management. I returned to the room to help the scrub nurse.

Mrs. A. was brought into the room. I remained calm in my approach as I re-introduced the surgical technologist, the perfusionist, and myself. I gave explicit directions to the patient regarding the correct way to move from the stretcher to the OR table. I then performed the basic safety pause that included the patient's name, I.D. bracelet, date of birth, medical identification number, allergies, and I verified a signed consent form. No matter how much experience I have had caring for patients in the OR environment, the time constraints still cause me great stress.

The patient's primary concern was postoperative pain management. While the anesthesiologist reviewed her options, I was able to continue to open sterile supplies and instruments for the technologist. After reviewing her pain management choices, we made Mrs. A. comfortable on the table, provided a warm blanket, and a reassuring touch.

We then talked about her family. We talked about her husband and she mentioned her sisters. Mrs. A. was concerned about her husband, and she asked me to let him know how things were going. The anesthesiologist proceeded with the anesthetic induction.

The operation was long and complicated. Almost 8 hours into the case, multiple blood products were given and the procedure was going poorly. The surgeon asked me to get the husband on the telephone to let him know that things were not going well. I called patient liaison only to find out that Ms. A.'s husband had gone to move his car.

During that time, the patient went into cardiac arrest and they started CPR. I had multiple tasks to perform, such as ordering more blood supplies, administering medication, and asking for additional staff. In the chaos, the patient's husband returned the call to the OR. I asked the surgeon what I should tell the husband; he replied, "We need to prepare him." I felt a sense of panic knowing I had to tell him that we were performing CPR on his wife. He said, "What does that mean?" I told him that we were trying to save her life. He replied, "Is she going to die?" I said, "I don't know, sir. We are doing everything we can." I asked if he would like to see a pastor and he said, quite emphatically, "No!" Within 30 minutes it became obvious that we had done all we could, and that Mrs. A. was not going to survive. They called the code.

After the shock of her death, the surgeon, cardiac fellow, perfusionist, and anesthesiologist left the room, and I remained to clean Mrs. A. and make her as presentable as possible for her husband. Several nurses, who were unassigned, assisted with caring for her body, paying special attention to her hands, knowing her husband would want to hold them.

The unselfish actions of those nurses, who had forfeited their meal break to assist, moved me. Another nurse assisted me in moving Mrs. A. to the transfer room in the OR so that Mr. A. would be able to see her with some privacy. The nurse stayed with Mrs. A. while I went to get her husband.

Since moving to a new building, I was not sure of the location of the patient liaison waiting room. I called Patient Liaison for directions and then went to meet Mr. A., who was waiting by himself. After introducing myself, I asked him if I should call one of Mrs. A.'s sisters. He said, "No, I need to let my son know." Mrs. A. had never mentioned having children. I wondered where the son was, but felt it would not be appropriate to ask. Mr. A. attempted to make a call, but was so upset he could not operate his cell phone to find his son's telephone number. I asked the secretary in Patient Liaison to use directory assistance to find the son's number, but she had only recently started her position and she was unable to locate the number.

I took Mr. A. to view his wife. When we reached the transfer room, he broke down in anguish. I was devastated, as was the nurse waiting with Mrs. A. After viewing his wife, Mr. A. asked me what he should do. I called the NIC for assistance, but there was no response. Not knowing what to do, I took him to get his wife's belongings, including her cell phone. I hoped that the son's phone number would be in the phone. I called the front desk and asked for the NIC again, and waited for a while. When no one came to the phone, I thought of calling a social worker. I called a number on our directory and there was no response.

I felt that I was totally responsible for this man, who only wanted to go home. I did not know what to do so I walked him to his car, and since I had recently gone through the loss of my best friend's husband, I suggested that a funeral director would be able to help him. He thanked me and said, "Have a good life, Phyl." We both cried. I had never told him that people called me that.

I assured Phyllis that she had done the right thing, especially in transferring care of her patient to another nurse while attending to the husband. I was concerned that Phyllis felt that she had no support in helping Mr. A. navigate the environment. This was Phyllis's final act in caring for Mrs. A. I felt like I had let her down.

I coached Phyllis, giving her alternatives in how to find the resources she needed to provide care. She was not aware that there was a social worker in the Emergency Department. The OR had been fairly self-contained in the past, so we had always depended on our own resources, but the addition of the cardiovascular building and its infrastructure was the future.

The nurse administrator would have been a great resource to help with Mr. A., but not a resource we typically tapped into. I realized that we would need to do so in the future. I also reminded Phyllis that Mr. A. may not want a "pastor" as religious support if he was used to referring to a priest or another religious denomination. Even if he did not want clergy as religious support, the chaplaincy could help with escorting the family member down to the OR, or back to the waiting room. I assured her that she absolutely did the right thing in caring for Mr. A. as an extension of caring for his wife. I told her this embodied the mission and vision of the DON, the best care to patients and families. She had transferred the care of her patient to another expert caregiver in order to care for a family member.

Phyllis and I spoke about her being an experienced nurse with well-developed critical thinking skills. Phyllis still felt she provided care with an air of uncertainty. She prides herself on her ability to give care with ease. We spoke of our concern; if she had difficulty navigating the changes in the system, how could we support the newly licensed and inexperienced OR nurses, recently hired to accommodate our growth? We talked about the way that experienced nurses told their stories and how that was a way of transferring knowledge. We wanted to make sure that others learned from her experience. She said that she would talk about it to others and I promised to coach the NIC around ways to provide support to staff, how to utilize the resources that are readily available.

That fall, Phyllis entered the RN to BSN program offered by Emmanuel College onsite at BWH (see Chapter 14). Phyllis had asked if I would write a letter of recommendation to support her application to the program. I was very happy to hear that Phyllis had decided to enroll. She was apprehensive about going back to school after such a long period of time. We talked about it on multiple occasions, and I assured Phyllis that she was more than capable of successfully completing the program. I was proud of her decision to start the program.

During the first semester, Phyllis had to write a paper based on a nursing theory. She chose Katherine Kolcaba's Comfort Theory. She asked if it would be okay to write her narrative about Mrs. A.'s case. I assured her that it would not be a problem if she removed any identifying information. Phyllis worked hard on the paper, concerned about writing something that was, in her eyes, perfect. She brought it to me to look at and I assured her it was an excellent paper. She was uncertain, but resigned, about what would happen. When she received her grade, she brought the paper in to show me the "A" she had received on it. I knew that at that point, Phyllis realized for the first time that she really could meet the challenge of her decision to return to school.

At the end of the semester, Phyllis invited me to her final class to attend the presentation of the papers. As luck would have it, there were multiple crises in the OR, and I did not think I would make it to the class. Because of the work she had done and her commitment to growing as a practitioner and as a person, I did not want to let her down. Luckily, I managed to make it there just in time. When I walked into the room, I could see in her expression how much it meant to her that I had come. She made sure that her classmates knew that I was her director, and how much I had supported her.

The BWH DON encouraged the use of narratives as a way for nurses to reflect on their practice and to transfer knowledge. I asked Phyllis if she would present her paper as narrative to our executive director. The narrative would be a wonderful way to talk about the caring practice of the operating-room nurse: it embodied the voice of the OR nurse.

Phyllis was apprehensive but she said, "I will do it for you, because you believed in me." She was very nervous about presenting it and we got together to work on it and refine it. Our executive director was appreciative; she thought it spoke to nursing practice in the OR. She had been concerned that people did not know what occurred in the OR, so this was a way to express what OR nurses do. The chief nursing officer, Mairead Hickey, was attending staff meetings of individual units. I decided to ask Phyllis to present the narrative at the next staff meeting and explained that I would invite the chief nursing officer and the associate chief nurse officer, and others. This would be the first time that a staff member presented a narrative at a staff meeting.

During the months after the move, we worked through some of the "new house" issues, but it was definitely a stressful time. I felt it would be good for the staff to have the opportunity to reflect on their practice and this was the perfect format for that reflection. More than 100 members were expected to attend. Phyllis again said, "I really am nervous about this, but will you be there?" I told her I would absolutely be there. Again she said, "I will do it for you, I never thought I would be in a BSN program, but you believed in me and here I am." I explained that I appreciated that, and that this was for all nurses.

We asked a resource person in the Center for Nursing Excellence to help unbundle the narrative. She worked with Phyllis prior to the staff meeting and again during the meeting. This helped Phyllis to reflect on her practice.

The day of the presentation, Phyllis told me that she was so nervous that she was concerned that she would be ill. She wasn't sure that she was doing the right thing. She had encountered some staff members who expressed that they were not sure why Phyllis was going back to school and who made her doubt herself. I again assured her she *was* doing the right thing. She talked about how her approach to her practice had changed and of the growth she had experienced.

We walked in, I sat at the front of the room, and Phyllis began reading her narrative. For a second, her voice wavered, then we made eye contact and it was as if her voice took wings. She was strong and confident, and I was amazed that this was the same person who had been so apprehensive. You could hear a pin drop in the room as Phyllis read her last words:

> I later learned that the reason the son was not there was because he was with his fiancée who was with her mother who had died that day.
>
> My practice has been forever changed by this patient and her husband. I now ensure that I have proper contacts to assist patients and families who experience tragic loss, and I am not judgmental regarding family issues.
>
> I would like to acknowledge JL, the surgical technologist. Without his skill and spirit of teamwork, I could not have devoted as much attention to Mrs. A.

I would also like to acknowledge TR, who helped me care for Mrs. A., and prepare her for her husband. I transferred the care of Mrs. A. to her when I went to care for Mrs. A.'s husband.

There was a deep silence and then loud applause; many had tears in their eyes. Staff came up after and said it was the most profound presentation ever given by one of their peers. More than one person said they felt change in the air that day. They hoped that they could continue presenting their stories. As peri-operative leaders, we are committed to hearing those stories.

I was pleased to see the growth in Phyllis and really felt that this was the beginning of a culture change. I was really proud of the work that she had done and I looked forward to being there for the staff to help them develop and grow in their practice.

10.3 *Growing Up Brigham*

Katie Fillipon and Marsha Milone

As two relatively new nursing directors, we had learned that orientation to the hospital is critical to the socialization and successful integration of a new nurse into practice. We entered Brigham and Women's Hospital (BWH) as new graduate nurses 8 years ago and completed the original orientation process developed by the Center for Nursing Excellence (CNE). We were subsequently promoted to oncology nursing director roles as part of a rapid expansion of oncology services, and began planning to accommodate the influx of new staff. This provided us with a unique opportunity to review the orientation process currently used and adapt it, creating a new process based on lessons learned.

In this chapter, using narratives, we demonstrate these lessons learned through our lived experiences and through first-hand accounts provided by other nurses. Through the narrative work done here at BWH (see Chapter 10.1), we have learned that narratives provide a rich source of information in all areas of nursing. We chose to use narratives to better understand what was and was not working in the orientation process.

We first focused on the existing orientation process, the one we ourselves had completed. Using a fairly traditional model, it consisted of a week of classroom orientation to the hospital followed by 4 weeks of orientation on a medical/surgical unit under the guidance of the CNE, 2 weeks on days and 2 weeks on nights (see Chapter 19.1). Nurses transitioned to their designated specialty after this 5-week sequence. Our orientation experiences are described in the narratives that follow.

Narrative 1

As a nursing student I fell in love with oncology. Working as a patient care assistant (PCA) on a medical-surgical/oncology unit, I would watch the way the nurses would form lasting and sustaining relationships with these patients and their families, and think, "That is the kind of nurse I want to be."

In my last semester of nursing school, I had the opportunity to come to BWH and spend a semester doing a student practicum on one of the oncology units. It was the opportunity of a lifetime. My semester in oncology opened the door to a position as a new graduate nurse, and I couldn't wait to get back to Brigham and become a "real nurse." I spent a week in classroom orientation, met other new nurses who were sharing the same nervousness that I was, and prepared to head out onto the unit.

Our group of new-to-practice nurses were placed on 10ab and divided in half so there were five new nurses on each pod. In the first week on this unit, we worked with a faculty instructor, much like a nursing school instructor. This person was there to provide an assignment, answer questions, and serve as a resource. When she felt you were ready, you were assigned to two patients. The first week was great. I felt I had a safety net, a group of peers, and the comfort of a model I had come to know well in nursing school.

Week two brought a much different set of circumstances. We rotated to the evening shift, and that great faculty instructor was gone. We were paired with the nurse who was caring for our patients, and if you had two patients it would often be two different nurses. These nurses were also caring for three other patients; their patients were sick, the nurses were busy, and we were nervous wrecks. It was the first time I had ever provided unsupervised care, and I felt like I was doing the doggy-paddle in a tsunami. Having a group of other nurses who were new to practice and had the same deer-in-the-headlights look was the only comfort in what felt like the longest five days of my life.

At the end of this 2-week stretch I went down to the fifth floor, where I was to begin my oncology orientation. This was a comfort to me because I had been there before as a student, but in many ways it felt like starting over. I had to show my preceptor that I was able to do certain tasks, and I had a whole new group of staff to meet. I spent the next 6 weeks on this unit, with primarily one preceptor, but when he was not there, I would be placed with someone else, sometimes two people over the course of a 12-hour day. On days like this I would be told I was doing something wrong, when in reality I was only doing what I had been shown, what another nurse had done. It always felt like several steps backward; such a frustrating feeling.

At the end of my 6 weeks on 5, I was told it was time to move to yet another unit, and another preceptor. I arrived on the sixth floor feeling like I had on my first day on 10ab, and the fifth floor sent me with parting gifts of everything and everyone I should fear on the new unit. It felt like it took me about 2 weeks to earn the respect and trust of my preceptor and to adapt my practice to her preferred style.

Every nurse and every unit had a different practice. It felt so hard to build confidence, to get to know people and to form relationships. At the end of my orientation, there was no position available on any one unit, so I began to float to different units for about three months until a position opened up on the fifth floor, on another unit where I had not yet worked. It was here that I found a home and, in time, with that home I found my practice and my confidence.

Looking back at my orientation experience, I feel that it made me stronger, and more resilient, maybe better able to cope with change. It was the experience that didn't break me but certainly came close. This experience certainly made me who I am today, someone who knows that we can do better, that we should do better, and that I am creating better.

Narrative 2

I started at BWH in October 2003. It was a dream come true. After my cousin beat his battle with cancer, I knew cancer care was what I wanted to do. My first week of orientation was at the CNE where we reviewed benefits, did our medication test, watched videos, and decided what we would do if that were our patient. Once this week was over, it was time to go to the units. I went to the 15th floor, a medical/surgical unit, to begin my orientation. This part of my orientation was 4 weeks. I did 2 weeks of days and 2 weeks of evenings.

During this time, I felt like a student. We had a faculty advisor and we were given one patient with a staff nurse following us and being ultimately responsible for that patient. Although I was becoming increasingly comfortable with the systems, I was also developing relationships with the nurses on this unit and was becoming increasingly anxious about moving to the next unit. For my orientation, I was scheduled to spend 4 weeks on the 15th floor, and then move to the fifth floor (general hematology/oncology) for 6 weeks and then transition to the unit where I would work for the last 6 weeks to incorporate the bone marrow transplant piece of my orientation.

When I moved to the fifth floor, I felt like I was starting all over again. I did not know any of the nurses and I was scared of the oncology population because I had just spent the last 4 weeks learning about critical pathways for surgical patients. I never had a steady preceptor during this part of my orientation and I felt like I was given little guidance. By the time I got used to the nurses on this unit and the patient population, it was time to move again. My confidence was not where I wanted or needed it to be.

The last part of my orientation was on a hematology/oncology/bone marrow transplant unit where I would end up spending the first 4 years of my nursing career. These 6 weeks were the most structured of my orientation. I had one preceptor assigned to me on this unit, and I was able to develop a relationship and the skills that I would need to succeed. She helped me by pushing me and challenging me so that I would understand the oncology population and the complications that I needed to be aware of. I completed orientation after 16 weeks, and an overwhelming sense of responsibility came over me. I was on my own and responsible for four patients a night battling their cancer. I felt that my orientation was a whirlwind of activity, but I was able to learn what I needed and could provide safe care to my patients. I had an environment at the end where no question was a stupid question and I continuously learned as I went along. I spent the next 4 years loving every minute of my career, and knowing I was giving something to my patients everyday.

In reflecting on our narratives, we saw a fractured orientation process with a delayed socialization into practice. This awareness shaped our planning. We initiated our rapid expansion in the fall of 2008. To open the first of three units, we were going to hire 20 new nurses. Because we were new in our leadership roles, we partnered with the CNE to brainstorm the most effective way to transition these new nurses into practice. We knew we had an opportunity to improve the current process. In order to recruit and retain the very best staff, it was critical that we create a supportive environment, and help the new nurses establish relationships and partner with a nurse on their new unit.

Our first change brought the new nurse to the oncology specialty for the first 2 weeks, yet maintained a focus on learning systems. An expert nurse from within the oncology service rather than from the CNE filled the faculty member role. This change allowed for immediate socialization into our culture and our practice. After the initial 2 weeks, the new nurse transitioned to working with a preceptor. Our goal became consistency: We wanted as little change as possible. These new nurses were assigned 1 day and 1 night preceptor for the remaining 12 weeks of their orientation. Each week new nurses met with the nurse director, the nurse educator, and the preceptor, during which both the new nurse and the preceptor were asked to address three things that had gone well and three areas they were hoping to improve. This created real-time feedback and open communication, providing an opportunity for everyone to remain on the same page and ensure the successful progress of the new nurse. Attainable weekly goals were set at the conclusion of each meeting.

The following is the narrative of the nurse-in-charge on the first unit that was opened. She first describes her personal orientation, not unlike the ones just described, and then compares this to the new orientation, including her role in making it a reality.

Narrative 3

My dream had come true; I had been offered a job in oncology at BWH. I had just finished a 3-month senior clinical placement on 6b, one of the hematology/oncology/bone marrow transplant pods. I felt ready and versed in the basics of Brigham nursing and culture. The first week was tough, a new job in a big hospital, in a big city where I knew very few people. We started off with a week of classroom learning where all of the new nurses were grouped together. We quickly acknowledged each other's fears and became a support system for each other.

The next week we were placed in smaller groups. I was put in the "medical group" and the five of us went to a neurology floor. We had a wonderful instructor who supported us through the next 2 weeks. This was a very familiar feeling. It felt just like clinical in nursing school. What had I been so afraid of? We were limited in our responsibility for our patients' care. A "real" nurse from the floor still cared for the patient and we were just there to learn the systems. Things started to unravel a bit for me at this time. I noticed how different the care was here when I compared it to what I had seen with the oncology patients. When I asked my instructor about this, she confirmed my fears: Certain things are done very differently on the oncology service. Why was I on the neurology floor, then? I was here to be an oncology nurse. I conformed to how things were done and got through the next weeks with my new group of friends. Things were feeling better, I felt like I was supported.

After my month in this group, my world was rocked as I moved to my new home on 5a. The emotions all reappeared, all my security and confidence were lost. I was as nervous and anxious as my first day. Once again no one knew me, no one knew of my accomplishments the past month. My supportive group of friends had moved on to cardiology, thoracic, and medical floors. I was lucky to find myself with a great preceptor. She was a great nurse and good teacher. She eased me into the first week. Then, just as I started to feel secure again, she became ill and was out intermittently. I was passed from nurse to nurse on days she wasn't there. No one was truly assigned. Everyone was very informative on how they did things, so I quickly learned to do what was told to me on a day-by-day basis. No one communicated my progress to me or to each other. No one ever gave constructive criticism; it was always just "You're doing well." I felt overwhelmed.

The months flew by, and my orientation ended on Christmas Eve, 2 weeks ahead of schedule. I wasn't quite sure if it was because I was ready or because

I was a body to fill a hole in the schedule. I lucked out, though: All those nurses who shared the responsibility of teaching me continued to help me through the first year on my own. It truly had taken a village. I am still grateful to them for all they taught me. I gained a lot of confidence in this time, advanced my nursing practice, and decided to move to a new bone marrow transplant floor where I grew in my experience in the next 5 years.

When I heard there was a position for a nurse-in-charge available on a new hematology/oncology/bone marrow transplant pod that would be opening, I jumped at the opportunity. I was given the position and began to establish how we would orient our new nurses. There was a large influx coming to the new floor. Together with my director and the two new nurse educators, we started to discuss our experiences. The four of us had all started at the Brigham right around the same time. It was decided we would try something different, we would start our new oncology nurses on our floors. I was asked to precept the first 2 weeks of the "new" orientation. I would have two new nurses with me during those weeks so they would have the peer support we had in the old model. I was nervous; I had oriented, but never two people at the same time.

The experience for me ended up being a wonderful one. The lack of communication I felt during my own orientation had disappeared. I saw how supported the new nurses felt by the staff. It was the team they would be working with orienting them from the beginning. We had weekly meetings with the manager and educator to discuss each new nurse's progress. We began an open dialogue where we discussed progress, the things that were going well, and the things that needed to be worked on. As a preceptor I felt supported and that I was able to see progress week to week thanks to the open communication. As a nurse-in-charge, I was able to work with the majority of the new nurses during these orientations. I feel I was able to establish a mentor relationship with each of them. These relationships enable me to better support them as a nurse-in-charge. I know what their strengths and weaknesses are.

This experience has made me a better nurse and a better preceptor. I learned how to communicate more effectively, openly, and honestly with new nurses. I try to guide them in their practice, to support them rather than tell them how I do things. I try to instill confidence and a sense of team in them. I think my personal experiences as a new Brigham nurse shaped me into the nurse I am today. It taught me to be the take-charge person I am. I hope I affect the nurses I orient as positively as my preceptors affected me.

The following narrative was written by one of the new nurses who was in the first cohort implementing our new orientation program. From her narrative, we were able to begin to gather information about what was working with our new model and why.

Narrative 4

After a 6-month period following graduation spent applying to various positions at hospitals in Boston, I was ecstatic to accept an offer at BWH on an oncology unit. As I walked through the front entrance on my first day I was overwhelmed with both excitement and apprehension. I had spent most of my clinical rotations in school working at smaller community hospitals, so it was a shock to be at such a large institution. The first day was spent in a small room where we learned some of the basic skills of working with oncology patients. I was relieved to have another new nurse whom I had met in hospital orientation along with me. We listened to a recording of another nurse signing off her report. Immediately my stomach dropped to find out this was the way we gave report on the floor. I was already terrified of listening to myself on tape. As we continued to listen, the proficient nurse spoke in a foreign language with words like: "Hickman line," "AML," "7+3," "TBI," intertwined throughout. My stomach sank even further. I remember thinking to myself, "I will never understand this." Just as this thought crossed my mind, one of the nurse educators said, "I know you're both probably completely overwhelmed right now, but trust me, this will become like a second language to you sooner than you think." It was true. Within the first 2 weeks I was beginning to understand the vocabulary and even starting to tape reports on my own.

One of the experienced staff nurses on the unit guided me and another new nurse through the flow of a typical day of the unit. We each took only one patient. Although I was not completely responsible for my single patient yet, I still had a rush of accountability come over me. This feeling was something that I had never felt before in nursing school. Here I was, a licensed nurse accountable for the life of another individual. In report I learned this patient was a 30-year-old male with Hodgkin's lymphoma admitted for an autologous stem cell transplant. Instantly I was taken aback by how young he was. I wasn't expecting to have a cancer patient only 8 years older than me. I stalled for a while that morning, asking my clinical instructor questions, reading his chart, and researching more about his diagnosis on the computer. I was nervous about actually entering his room, fearing that he would ask me a question that I couldn't answer. I was no longer a student nurse, I was now working as a licensed nurse with a badge that said "RN" and I felt that I needed to have all the answers. Finally I put on my mask, gown, and gloves and walked into his room. I was surprised to see him sitting on the edge of his hospital bed, wearing pajama pants and a white t-shirt. I introduced myself and quickly added that it was my first day as a new nurse and that I was following a more senior nurse on the floor. We immediately bonded over the fact that we grew up just a few towns away from each other and my nerves over the situation seemed to dissipate. Throughout the rest of my first day, my patient gave me the history of his illness and explained everything that was expected from his stem cell transplant. I was lucky to have a patient who was so willing to talk about his illness. As most of the patients on the oncology units spend several weeks and sometimes months on the unit, they are understandably tired of telling the same story over and over again.

Through the next year, I continually followed this patient through a relapse, allogenic transplant, and several graft-versus-host complications that followed. It became evident how much this patient valued me and the other nurses on the unit. Each time he was admitted he would request to be put on our floor. He would always make sure to tell everyone that I was his nurse on my very first day of work. As I followed him through his therapy, he followed me through my first year of nursing. He would always laugh at how far I had come as a nurse from his first admission when he was teaching me about the treatment plan and the proper terminology.

People often ask me why I went into oncology, almost always leading into a question, "Isn't that so depressing?" I do find it depressing at times; however, despite the fact that the patients don't always have the best prognosis, the impact we are able to make to improve their quality of life throughout their treatment is the reason why I chose this field.

By the time we opened the second and third units, we had become more comfortable and competent with our new orientation model. This is evidenced by the following narrative from a nurse who was in the third cohort of nurses to go through this orientation.

Narrative 5

Having already worked here at BWH in a nonclinical capacity for several years, I knew as I was graduating from nursing school that there was nowhere else I would rather begin my professional nursing career. Fortunately, the opportunity arose for me to join a newly opening hematology/oncology/bone marrow transplant pod. I prepared myself to be overwhelmed by all the knowledge I would need to master about chemotherapy and stem cell transplants, in addition to simply learning how to be an independently practicing nurse! I didn't know what I didn't know, so I planned to ask many questions along the path. Fortunately, my initiation was quite smooth, thanks to the carefully constructed orientation process and my excellent mentors.

The first 2 weeks I was paired with another newly licensed nurse. Having someone at the same stage to share the experience was helpful. We each took just one patient and we worked closely with an experienced nurse to learn processes, documentation, and unit culture, helping me to develop a sense of work flow throughout the shift and become familiarized with everyday tasks like IV tubing, drawing labs, and changing central line dressings. Very quickly, it became apparent to me that nursing school had given me knowledge, but taught me very little to prepare me to actually work as a nurse. The thorough and focused on-the-job training I received in these first 2 weeks and beyond was essential for me to develop comfort and confidence in specific skills, problem solving, and multitasking.

Once the initial 2 weeks were complete, I was paired up with an experienced nurse preceptor to work with one-on-one for 5 weeks on night shift and subsequently, another preceptor on day shift for 5 weeks. These mentors were excellent resources, and willing and able to help me as much or as little as I felt I needed. As time progressed, I took on more and more independence and responsibility. I began to think for myself and answer my own questions. Or, at least, I knew where to go to find the answers! My preceptors were very supportive as I transitioned into more independent practice.

Perhaps the most instrumental element of my nursing orientation was my weekly progress meeting. My preceptor and I would sit down with my nurse director and nurse educator. I would prepare for the meeting by listing the three things I was feeling positive about and three things I wanted to improve. My preceptor, nurse director, and nurse educator also had the opportunity to give formal feedback and contribute to setting appropriate goals for the upcoming week. This meeting schedule and format provided a forum for open discussion and honest feedback and allowed me to track my progress over the course of the orientation period. When the end of the orientation period arrived, I felt more ready than I would have dared to hope. I knew my strengths and limits, my resources, and my challenges. My orientation yielded a strong basis in nursing practice, thanks to the challenging and inspiring Brigham patient population and my experienced nurse mentors. Now, almost eight months later, I continue to learn and develop on every shift I work, and I couldn't be happier or more proud to be a Brigham nurse.

After evaluating our own orientation experiences and understanding the value of socialization demonstrated in the literature, we created an orientation process whereby new nurses came directly into their designated specialty. Additional time spent on the unit and a supportive infrastructure ensured a more successful orientation process and earlier integration of the new nurse into the team. This increased comfort in their environment helped them develop critical thinking skills and form meaningful relationships with patients and families. As we have watched these new nurses develop over the past 2 years, we feel that they have the tools they need to provide excellent care to our patients and families.

The authors extend thanks to the following persons who provided input into our chapter: Caitlin Guerrero, BSN, RN, OCN; Laura Wesley Russell, BSN, RN; and Jenna Moran, BSN, RN.

Change Through Clinical Experts:
The APN Role and Impact

11.1 *The Psychiatric Nursing Resource Service:*
Building an Infrastructure for Practice and
Modeling the APN Role

Barbara E. Lakatos, Monique T. Mitchell, and Mary Lou Etheredge

On our journey to achieve the Department of Nursing (DON) vision—*excellent care to patients and families, with the best staff, in the safest environment*—a central focus and top priority for nurse leaders was building an infrastructure to support care and practice. To guide this work, the Nursing Executive Board (NEB) regularly reviewed patient quality and safety data, including data on restraint use, patient falls, and sitter utilization, as well as current care practices, such as nurses' use of security personnel to contain patients whose behavior was unmanageable. Board members determined they needed a more detailed assessment to understand factors underlying these practices and to guide improvements in the psychological care nurses provided to patients and families.

With the NEB's approval, we launched a process that ultimately led to the development of a program dedicated to supporting the psychological nursing care of patients and families. Mary Lou Etheredge, executive director for Nursing Practice Development, provided the executive leadership for this work and Barbara Lakatos performed the system assessment. Monique Mitchell joined Barbara, both advanced practice nurses (APN), and they became program directors of the Psychiatric Nursing Resource Service (PNRS), providing content and practice expertise. This is the story of how we developed and implemented the Psychiatric Nursing Resource Service.

Our work began in August 2006, with designing and conducting a system assessment (Lewandowski & Adamle, 2009). In this chapter, we describe the assessment process, how we used its findings to develop the PNRS, and how the PNRS assists nurses in providing psychologically based nursing care and serves as a model for the APN role.

ASSESSING PSYCHOLOGICAL NURSING CARE

The NEB specified five inpatient areas with high sitter utilization as target areas and allotted us 3 months to complete an assessment. From our previous APN experience, we knew there were likely a multitude of factors in different layers of the organization influencing the rate of sitter and security use by nurses. For this reason, we decided to use a systems approach to guide the assessment, obtain baseline data, and develop recommendations and a plan (Chaffee & McNeill, 2007; Clancy, Effken, & Pesut, 2008; Paley, 2007). A systems approach is comparable to the physical assessment conducted by clinical nurses when assessing patients, as it involves an organized process that considers the whole rather than separate disconnected parts and provides a foundation for action or intervention. We recognized that focusing on the whole rather than one part of the organization would help us understand the context of events and assess relationships among them, and provide a framework for designing an effective change process.

We were new to BWH, and entered the system without previous knowledge of any specific organizational issues. This gave us the freedom to explore multiple avenues and obtain a more comprehensive picture. As a first step, we outlined goals for the assessment process. First, we wanted to hear the perspective of nurses in many different roles and gain a deeper understanding about the status of psychological nursing practice at BWH. Second, we wanted to engender support for introducing change from nurses at every level and from other groups and departments involved in addressing behavioral and psychiatric issues in patients. We then mapped out a multistep assessment process. It included: (1) meeting with executive nurse leaders and nurse directors and educators of the five inpatient units identified by NEB; (2) obtaining input from clinical nurses on the five units through staff meetings and a clinical nurse survey; and (3) speaking with representatives from key departments (e.g., Security, Psychiatry, Social Services) involved in addressing behavioral and psychiatric concerns, and reviewing relevant policies and quality and safety data.

Input From Nursing Leaders

In discussions with executive nursing leaders, we heard about the culture of crisis that characterized nursing interactions with patients whose behavior they could not manage. As one executive director explained:

> We teach nurses what to do in a medical emergency—they call for the code team, and a group of expert professionals sprint to the medical emergency to assist them in assessment and safe treatment. There is a defined role for each staff member in providing care to the patient. During a behavioral emergency, we call for assistance and the only responders are the security team. Care stops and the nurse only returns to the bedside when the behavioral crisis is contained. There is no defined role for the nurse, and there are no experts who arrive to assist the nurses in their assessment and care.

Having nurses remove themselves from the care of patients was troubling to the executive directors. Also troubling was the rate of sitter usage and the dilemma confronting unit leaders each time a nurse ordered a sitter to watch an "out of control" patient. When asked whether the sitter was needed, nurses typically responded by sharing their worries and anxiety and their belief that a sitter was needed to keep the patient safe. The unit leaders generally supported nurses' requests for sitters, but struggled with how to provide the best care while keeping patients and staff safe and reducing or maintaining costs.

After speaking with the executive nurse leaders, we met with the nurse directors and educators on each of the five units. The unit leaders spoke candidly about their concerns regarding patient care, and shared their worries about the safety and quality of care for patients with psychological and behavioral issues and the safety and quality of life of the nurses who cared for them. They described clinical nurses' discomfort in caring for patients with unmanageable behavior, and were unfamiliar with the best approaches for meeting patient needs. They also shared their concerns about nursing practice involving patient restraints, and noted that restraint prevalence audits, in which nurses correctly identified the least-to-most restrictive measures utilized prior to introducing restraints, demonstrated their ability to identify these measures; however; it didn't change their practice. "We are compliant in checking off all the boxes but we don't seem to get out of the cycle," observed one nurse director. Importantly, the leadership teams on all five units agreed that change was needed, and our shared vision of how care could be different began to emerge. This was a critical step and marked the beginning of the change process.

Input From Clinical Nurses

Our next step involved hearing from clinical nurses. Nurse leaders on each unit invited us to staff meetings to explain the assessment process. Collaborating with us, they stressed the importance of hearing the "voice of the nurse" and encouraged nurses to share their worries, concerns, and stories about nursing care and challenging patient situations.

The nurses were very vocal during the meetings and readily discussed their fear of patients with behavioral problems, their belief that such behaviors were purposeful, and their worries about being hurt. They wanted to provide the safest and best care, but said they worried about their own safety and wanted help understanding why they felt frustrated and why caring for patients with behavior issues was so hard. The nurses also described "feeling sorry" for the pleasantly confused patients and "angry" at the agitated, not-so-pleasantly confused patients and their families. One nurse offered the following story as explanation: "If I see someone acting strangely while riding on the subway, I get up and move to the other side of the car because that person makes me anxious and scared for my safety. If the person continues to act crazy and talk to people who aren't there I usually leave the subway and inform security so they can deal with them. Public safety is important." The implication was that calling security made sense whenever one felt threatened.

To process this scenario, we asked the nurses to imagine what they would do if the threatening person was admitted to their unit. "Imagine you are now this person's nurse for the night," we suggested. "You cannot move away and you must provide care. How will you accomplish it?" The nurses described a process of "setting limits" on the patient's behavior and contacting security to "make them behave." When we pressed them further about their assessment, the nurses described how anxious they would feel, but could not describe how they would assess the patient and intervene to ensure safe and effective care. We then asked the nurses to imagine that the patient's behavior stemmed from a seizure or sepsis and asked how their assessment and interventions would be different. The nurses responded comfortably, because caring for patients with sepsis and seizures was familiar and the nurses had more confidence in their assessment and intervention skills. We identified that in the absence of a clinical framework for assessing patient behaviors, nurses adopted a social framework and used approaches they would utilize in social situations.

The nurses were also asked to complete a self-assessment of their comfort and competence in caring for patients with behavioral issues. Eighty-five of 250 nurses (34%) completed the survey. Among respondents, 47% identified "patients at risk for injury" (i.e., patients whose behaviors were unsafe or who were at increased risk for injuring themselves or others) as the most unmanageable patients. For 52% of respondents, this was the group they were least comfortable caring for, and for 54% this was the group for whom they felt the least competence. Respondents felt slightly more comfortable and competent caring for patients with changes in mental status or cognitive functioning. We found it striking that with both patient populations, nurses did not demonstrate an understanding of how to assess the patients or intervene appropriately.

Other Data Sources

We moved on with system assessment, speaking with representatives from other groups and departments involved in caring for patients with acute delirium and behavioral issues. Over several weeks, we met with nursing administrators and representatives from Psychiatry, the Division of Aging, Case Management, Security, Social Service, Pharmacy, Rehabilitation Services, and Patient and Family Services. We examined quality and safety data and policies and procedures related to security emergencies, restraint use, fall prevalence, staff injuries, sick calls, staff turnover, infection rates, and pressure ulcer prevalence; administrative and cost data related to sitter usage; and selected patients' medical records. Additionally, national quality and safety initiatives were reviewed to see where BWH fit within the larger framework (Armstrong, 2006; Hader, 2008; Institute of Medicine [IOM], 2000).

Analyzing the Data

In sifting through the data, we recognized that delirium was prevalent in many of the patients with behavioral disturbances, particularly in those for whom behavior containment interventions were utilized. This was not surprising: Delirium is one of the most prevalent cognitive syndromes in acute care settings. Delirium is caused by a medical condition and is characterized by an acute change in mental status and consciousness that fluctuates throughout the day (American Psychiatric Association [APA], 2000). Delirious patients are cognitively impaired and have difficulty following directions, remembering information, initiating self-care, and responding to cues. Despite its prevalence, delirium is not well understood or readily identified by nurses and physicians (Inouye, 2006; Steis & Fick, 2008). Adding to the challenge is the fact that delirium can present in different ways: as hyperactive delirium, in which patients become very agitated; hypoactive delirium, in which patients are somnolent and quiet; and a mixed presentation, which combines the hyperactive and hypoactive states.

Besides patients with delirium, nurses cared for two other groups of patients presenting behavioral challenges. One group consisted of patients with overt psychiatric diagnoses who were admitted to the hospital for medical or surgical care. The other group was smaller and consisted of psychiatric patients admitted while waiting for a bed in a psychiatric facility.

We realized that a lack of knowledge about how to assess and care for patients with behavioral issues was a major factor contributing to the high rate of sitter use and security emergencies. Because nurses did not understand the causes of acute delirium and other behavioral disturbances, or know appropriate assessment, prevention, and management techniques, they struggled to meet their goal of providing good, safe care. Nurses also lacked standard tools for performing mental status assessments and delirium screening, which further limited their ability to individualize and optimize patient care (Lakatos et al., 2009). In the absence of an evidence-based clinical framework for assessing and managing patient behaviors, nurses used a social framework and relied on containment strategies that, in some cases, exacerbated the behavior and increased a patient's risk for iatrogenic events such as pressure ulcers and falls.

We concluded that the nurses needed more training to meet the psychological needs of patients and families. Although most nurses working in medical/surgical specialties learn basic psychiatric nursing skills in nursing school, this training alone does not prepare them to provide the care required by patients with delirium and psychiatric conditions. At BWH, as in most acute care hospitals, nursing orientation and annual competency days focused on technological aspects of care and not on helping nurses acquire and refine skills needed to establish interpersonal connections with patients and families in emotionally charged situations. Additionally, nurses with expertise in psychologically based nursing were not available to coach nurses and model best practices. Given these factors, it was not surprising that nurses felt powerless in the face of a behavioral crisis and relied on sitters and security to maintain control.

Recommendations

We prepared a report for NEB summarizing the results of the assessment and outlining recommendations for improving the psychological care provided to patients and families. We emphasized nurses' knowledge deficit, noting that the results of the nursing needs assessment indicated that the majority of nurses were at a beginner level of psychological nursing practice and did not have the knowledge and skills required to recognize delirious patients or effectively intervene in their care. Without this knowledge base, nurses responded to patients using a social rather than clinical framework and turned for support to the resources that were available to them (i.e., sitters and Security).

We were convinced that a programmatic approach, blending education, evidence-based care guidelines, and expert resources, was needed. We proposed creating a Psychiatric Nursing Resource Service staffed by expert, advanced practice psychiatric nurses who had the knowledge and skill to help nurses develop the required nursing competencies. Our goal was to create a service that advanced the vision of the DON, was integrated into nursing practice, and modeled contextualized, engaged learning and unit-based practice change. The PNRS, the NEB believed, would also serve as a model for how to utilize and maximize the impact of advanced practice nurses, and agreed to its development in February 2007.

DEVELOPING AND IMPLEMENTING THE PSYCHIATRIC NURSING RESOURCE SERVICE

From the outset, we envisioned the PNRS as encompassing three components: consultation, coaching, and education. Numerous nursing experts and researchers have highlighted the importance of these components to developing and supporting psychological nursing practice (Benner, Sutphen, Leonard, & Day, 2010; Gilje, Klose, & Birger, 2007; Lewis & Levy, 1982; Karsten, Baggot, Brown, & Cahill, 2010; McAllister, 2008).

At the NEB's direction, we focused on supporting nurses on the five targeted nursing units. Our intent was to shift the culture surrounding psychological nursing practice from a culture of crisis to a culture of care. As a first step, and with collaboration as a guiding principle, we focused on engaging nurse leaders and clinical nurses in finding the good in nursing practice and building on that good to create sustainable change. This was an example where "walking the talk" was a challenge, requiring commitment, courage, and a belief that by working together we could improve current practice and engage nurses in shifting their thinking and habits of care.

Guided by input from nurse leaders and clinical nurses, we began work to design and implement the three components of the PNRS—an educational curriculum, expert consultation, and coaching resources—developing them concurrently and with the goal of enhancing the ability of clinical nurses to provide psychologically based care.

Educational Curriculum

Our objectives for the nursing education curriculum included helping nurses learn how to assess their patients' mental status and helping them understand the principles and practices underlying psychologically based nursing practice. We also dedicated a portion of the curriculum to explaining the PNRS, how it would work, and how we, as APNs, would serve as resources to nurses.

We developed two educational modules, with pre- and post-tests and evaluations, and obtained contact hours for continuing education credits for participants. Each module included a didactic component and case presentations that facilitated interactive discussion. Working with nurse leaders on the units, we identified opportunities to offer several programs daily. Our aim was to reach as many nurses as possible, and over a 5-week period we taught a total of 50 programs. Eighty-two percent of nurses on the five units attended at least one of the classes, and 60% attended both. For nurses unable to attend the face-to-face sessions, we provided online modules that contained the same content.

Through the pre- and post-tests, we measured nurses' perceptions of their knowledge, comfort, and competence in caring for patients with mental status changes and delirium, using four-point Likert scales where higher scores equaled more of each dimension. Both modules yielded an improvement in scores. Nurses' ratings of their comfort and competence in caring for patients with mental status changes and delirium rose from a score of 2 prior to the sessions, to 3 after the sessions. Nurses also demonstrated an overall increase in knowledge related to both areas. In written comments, nurses spoke positively about how the content would benefit their practice. Comments included, "This was the best in-service," "Most relevant [in-service]," and "It gave me tools I can use with my patient today." A majority of nurses said they had not received education on mental status assessment or delirium during their formal nursing education or hospital orientation. "Most of our patients have delirium," said one. "Why aren't we taught this in school?" Said another, "I've been labeling patients as noncompliant and now I can see they couldn't understand what I was teaching them." For nurses on all of the units, the education and introduction of the PNRS was energizing; everyone was excited about getting started and utilizing their new knowledge in practice.

Once the majority of nurses had attended the educational sessions, we had a basic foundation and common language with which to begin discussions about patient care. Therefore, we moved into phase two of PNRS implementation: introducing our consultation and coaching services.

Consultation and Coaching Services

Before setting up our consultation and coaching services, we had to attend to a multitude of details, from finding and setting up an office to creating processes for referral, assessment, follow-up, feedback, and outcomes measurement. Our charge was to provide coverage to five patient care units. This translated to 150 beds and 250 clinical nurses. With 1.4 full-time equivalents representing two APNs (both working part time), we determined that we could provide coverage 4 days a week, 12 hours each day. This ensured that we would be visible and available to nurses on all shifts. Also, because our schedules overlapped one day each week, we would be able to coordinate our work and ensure a consistent and unified approach.

To guide our efforts, we developed a service vision statement and goals, which highlighted our commitment to supporting nurses in providing excellent psychologically based care for BWH patients and their families. In addition, we adopted a service model for the PNRS, rather than an individual practice model. This meant that instead of assigning each APN to a specific unit, we committed to providing a seamless response to requests for assistance by having each of us get to know, support, and respond in the same way to all of the units, nurse leaders, and clinical nurses.

We also examined the consultation process at BWH to understand what nurses might expect from us and whether we needed to reframe their expectations. We learned that within BWH, nurses generally viewed consultants as expert clinicians who evaluated patients, entered expert recommendations into the medical record, and focused on "taking care of the problem." Nurses could not initiate requests for consultation and rarely participated in discussions with consultants about the plan of care. We committed to changing this consulting framework by emphasizing the primacy of the clinical nurse role and positioning the PNRS as a resource dedicated to helping nurses enhance their practice and improve the care they provided to patients and families. Our goal was to empower nurses with new skills and support them in developing the competencies needed to provide care regardless of their patients' behavioral presentations.

We designed our referral process to ensure a timely response to requests for assistance. Any nurse, on any shift, could complete our referral form and fax it to our service. The referral form asked nurses to identify the reason they were requesting support and to supply some basic patient demographic data. Nurses with an urgent need for assistance were encouraged to page the APN for more immediate assistance. We also asked nurses to inform their nursing directors whenever they faxed a referral. This would help nurse leaders remain aware of clinical issues and would facilitate collaboration between our service and the unit leadership team.

Launching the Service

Nurses began requesting PNRS consults immediately after the service was officially launched. Our daily routine included evaluating new consult referrals, following up on cases previously referred, and rounding with the nursing leadership, nurse-in-charge (NIC), and staff nurses on each unit. This routine ensured our availability and was fundamental to establishing a reliable presence. It also allowed us to get to know each nurse and for them to get to know us.

Initially, nurses viewed us within the same framework applied to other consultants—as a resource who would "deal with" challenging patient behaviors. We sometimes found it difficult to break out of this mold and, during a crisis, had to hold ourselves back from rescuing the nurse and usurping the nurse's role at the bedside. We had to continually remind ourselves to shift our focus from solving the identified "problem," to teaching and modeling a new and better way to provide care. During the first weeks, nurses also expressed fears about "getting dinged" for checking off the wrong box or filling out the wrong form and about being evaluated or "judged." Gradually, by focusing on helping nurses provide care and using a nonjudgmental approach, nurses began to understand our practice and the PNRS APN role.

Although we received a steady stream of referrals, we soon realized that some high-risk patients were not being referred. We recognized that addressing this issue required the support of nursing leadership and we proposed conducting 2-hour weekly rounds with nurse leaders on each unit. Nurse leaders embraced this suggestion and also agreed to meet weekly to discuss patient care, nursing practice, and quality and safety, recognizing that this would facilitate the change process and contribute to building mutual trust (Karsten et al., 2010).

As APNs, our role in developing and implementing a new service model was unique. We believed the PNRS offered a valuable learning experience for APN students. During the first year of the program's development, we reached out to schools of nursing that offered master's degrees in psychiatric and mental health nursing and hired Leslie DeLisle, RN, for a 3-month student internship. Leslie's exemplar follows our second chapter; it illustrates the numerous practice and safety concerns that nurses face while caring for delirious patients, and illustrates how APNs can play a role in facilitating psychologically based nursing practice.

Expanding Our Reach

Our work on the five patient care units allowed us to develop relationships with departments throughout the organization. Soon we were involved in launching multiple interdisciplinary projects and initiatives. In one project, we partnered with the Center for Nursing Excellence and Simmons College to build on our educational modules and develop a simulation scenario on caring for a delirious patient. Nurse educators using this scenario have consistently received positive feedback from clinical nurses. In another initiative, we helped introduce interdisciplinary patient care rounds. During our work on one of the units, we learned that interdisciplinary rounds did not occur on a regular basis. Nurses were frustrated by the lack of reliable communication with physicians, and physicians were frustrated about being paged frequently by nurses. Working with nursing leadership, we formulated a plan for scheduled interdisciplinary rounds and participated in those rounds once they began. Throughout our participation, we offered observations and suggestions regarding patient care and modeled for nursing leadership and staff nurses how to engage in interprofessional dialogue and make their voices heard.

We are also collaborating with physician colleagues in medicine and psychiatry to develop interdisciplinary evidence-based care guidelines for patients who present with delirium, alcohol withdrawal, suicide, and harm (DASH). A PNRS APN co-leads the DASH subcommittees with a physician colleague, and has co-led the overall steering committee within the organization. The DASH project represents a major initiative sponsored by hospital executive leadership, and an enormous advancement in interdisciplinary practice in the institution.

SUMMARY

Our experience during the first 6 months of the PNRS rollout highlights the value of blending formal education with "situated coaching" (Benner et al., 2010). We found that formal education was important in, though not sufficient for, establishing a common language and beginning the conversation of care. Bedside coaching allowed us to model psychologically based care, support nurses in practicing new skills, influence the care environment, and more effectively shift the culture from one of crisis to one of care. For nurses new to practice, who are typically anxious and focus on mastering technical skills, being present at the bedside was especially important (Burritt & Steckel, 2009). By working side-by-side with new nurses, we were able to alleviate their anxiety and encourage them to try new interventions.

Our experience also taught us the importance of collaborating with nurse leaders on the patient care units. The nurse leaders were instrumental in helping us influence the level of nurse engagement, guide resource allocation, and stimulate requests for care assistance. Their leadership, receptiveness to change, and willingness to ask for help also served as a model for staff nurses, prompting them to join in the process of changing and improving nursing practice.

Since introducing the PNRS in February 2007, we have provided expert consultation and coaching for more than 2,100 patient encounters and offered more than 170 hours of formal education to hundreds of nurses throughout the organization. We continue to evaluate our practice outcomes, introduce changes to reduce variability in practice, and adapt to the evolving needs of the organization, while remaining committed to our core service components of consultation, coaching, and education. We recently obtained funding to expand our service by hiring our former intern, Leslie DeLisle. Within the DON, the PNRS is identified as a model for the ways in which APNs can serve as resources to nurses while directly contributing to patient care.

BWH, like other acute care organizations, continues to grow more complex, but as one nurse said, "Knowing my patient helped me provide the best care, in the safest environment." We believe our service has positively impacted patient safety and nursing practice and has resulted in improved psychological care to patients and families and an improved nursing experience. In Chapter 11.2, we review the outcomes of this psychiatric nursing resource service.

REFERENCES

American Psychiatric Association (APA). 2000. *Diagnostic and statistical manual of mental disorders* (4th ed.). Washington, DC: Author.

Armstrong, F. (2006). Keeping nurses safe: An industry perspective. *Contemporary Nurse, 21,* 209–211.

Benner, P., Sutphen, M., Leonard, V., & Day, L. (2010). *Educating nurses: A call for radical transformation.* San Francisco, CA: Jossey-Bass.

Berman, A., Mezey, M., Kobayashi, M., Fulmer, T., Stanley, J., Thornlow, D., & Rosenfeld, P. (2005). Gerontological nursing content in baccalaureate nursing programs: Comparison of findings from 1997 and 2003. *Journal of Professional Nursing, 21*(5), 268–275.

Burrit, J., & Steckel, C. (2009). Supporting the learning curve for contemporary nursing practice. *Journal of Nursing Administration, 39*(11), 479–484.

Chaffee, M., & McNeill, M. (2007). A model of nursing as a complex adaptive system. *Nursing Outlook, 55,* 232–241.

Clancy, T., Effken, J., & Pesut, D. (2008). Applications of complex systems theory in nursing education, research, and practice. *Nursing Outlook, 56,* 248–256.

Gilje, F., Klose, P., & Birger, J. (2007). Critical clinical competencies in undergraduate psychiatric-mental health nursing. *Journal of Nursing Education, 46*(11), 522–526.

Hader, R. (2008). Workplace violence survey 2008: Unsettling findings. *Nursing Management, 39*(7), 13–19.

Inouye, S. K. (2006). Delirium in older persons. *New England Journal of Medicine, 354,* 1157–1164.

Institute of Medicine (IOM). (2000). *To err is human: Building a safer health system.* Washington, DC: National Academy Press.

Karsten, M., Baggot, D., Brown, A., & Cahill, M. (2010). Professional coaching as an effective strategy to retain frontline managers. *Journal of Nursing Administration, 40*(3), 140–144.

Lakatos, B., Capasso, V., Mitchell, M., Kilroy, S., Lussier-Cushing, M., Sumner, L., Repper-Delisis, J., Kelleher, D., DeLisle, L., Cruz, C., & Stern, T. (2009). Falls in the general hospital: An association with delirium, advanced age, and specific surgical procedures. *Psychosomatics, 50,* 218–216.

Lewandowski, W., & Adamle, K. (2009). Substantive areas of clinical nurse specialist practice. *Clinical Nurse Specialist, 23*(2), 73–90.

Lewis, A., & Levy, J. (1982). *Psychiatric liaison nursing: The theory & clinical practice.* Reston, VA: Reston Publishing.

McAllister, M. (2008). Educational innovations. Looking below the surface: Developing critical literacy skills to reduce the stigma of mental disorders. *Journal of Nursing Education, 47*(9), 426–430.

Paley, J. (2007). Complex adaptive systems and nursing. *Nursing Inquiry, 14*(3), 233–242.

Steis, M., & Fick, D. (2008). Are nurses recognizing delirium? *Journal of Gerontological Nursing, 35*(9), 40–45.

11.2 Shifting From Crisis to Care: Outcomes of a Psychiatric Nursing Resource Service

Barbara E. Lakatos, Amy L. Kenefick, Monique Mitchell, Mary Lou Etheredge, and Laura Mylott

The assessment that we of the Psychiatric Nursing Resource Service (PNRS) conducted of nurses on five inpatient units at BWH in 2006 revealed knowledge deficits in providing psychologically based nursing care, mental status assessment, delirium care, and safety management. The nurses acknowledged a general discomfort and a lack of confidence in these areas. System supports were absent in the inpatient health care setting to assist nursing staff in providing psychologically based care. Of the affective, behavioral, and cognitive mental status domains, it appeared that only the behavioral domain was recognized, and interventions were limited to containment through the use of sitters, security codes, and restraints. Nurses often feared for their safety and viewed a patient's behavior as intentional rather than a symptom of disease (i.e., delirium). We developed and implemented our service to incorporate the core components of education, consultation, and coaching.

For 2 years we provided coverage (1.4 full-time equivalents [FTEs]) on four 12-hour days to five inpatient units (155 beds), and 250 staff nurses. Patient populations on these units included bariatric, renal transplant, brain injured, orthopedic, pain and palliative care, general medical, cardiac, vascular, trauma, and others. Implementation strategies (detailed in Chapter 11.1) included educational sessions on delirium and mental status assessment, consultation for patients, and coaching of staff nurses focused on psychological care interventions to improve safety and quality of care.

We utilized Peplau's (1991/1952) and Benner's (1984) theoretical frameworks grounded within the interpersonal relationship between the nurse and patient to guide the PNRS program development. Peplau (1991/1952) asserts that although nursing is both interpersonal and technical, the nursing process cannot be technical. When patients are hospitalized, basic psychological needs emerge, creating tension and anxiety in the patients, which lead them to search for ways to relieve the anxiety. Once the nurse understands the anxiety and importance of establishing a relationship, care can be provided. If the nurse does not attend to this interpersonal connection, the patient's anxiety may increase and the nurse may feel more anxious and distant from the patient and family. The nurse's role in helping patients feel safe and less anxious cannot be underestimated. The nurse's engagement with the patient helps the nurse to "know" the patient as a human being (Benner, 1984), creating a connection that serves to guide judgment and nursing care.

Evaluation of identified outcomes is an essential process for the development of evidence-based practice (Fineout-Overholt & Johnston, 2007), psychiatric nursing practice (Yakimo, Jurlowica, & Murray, 2004), and quality improvement (Lilford, Brown, & Nicholl, 2007). In this chapter we review the outcomes of the

PNRS (Lakatos, 2009). We obtained IRB approval for our descriptive study and sent e-mails to all 250 nurses working on the five units, requesting their voluntary participation in our study. Over a 3-week period, we administered an online survey through Survey Monkey (2009) to collect nonidentifying data, and analyzed the data utilizing SPSS release 17.0.0 (SPSS Inc., Chicago, IL).

Our sample ($N = 51$) was primarily composed of baccalaureate-prepared nurses, with fewer associate-degree and master's-prepared nurses. Compared to the direct-care nurses working at BWH, there were more new-to-practice nurses in our study who had been in the organization 1–5 years (44%), with 14% having been there 6–10 years, 14% with 11–15 years, and 28% more than 15 years. We compared this to the 2913 direct-care nurses working at BWH with 1 to more than 35 years of experience. Of this number, 25% of all nurses had been in the organization for 1–5 years, 24% for 6–10 years, 13% for 11–15 years, 10% for 16–20 years, 11% for 21–25 years, 10% for 26–30 years, 5% for 31–35 years, and 2% for more than 35 years.

We had two different sections in the survey. In section one, we asked the nurses to rate their comfort and competence (using a 1–4 Likert scale) in providing psychologically based care for 19 variables; in section two, we asked each nurse to complete a 10-item knowledge questionnaire regarding delirium. We utilized Pearson's correlation and independent t-test to analyze the scores in section one, and utilized Bloom's and Krathwohl's taxonomies of cognitive, affective, and psychomotor domains (Bloom, Englhart, Furst, Hill, & Krathwohl, 1956; Krathwohl, Bloom, & Masia, 1973) to analyze scores in section two.

The results of the survey were striking (Table 11.1). For the sample ($N = 51$), the 2009 comfort and competence scores resulted in an overall Pearson correlation of $r = .987, p = 0.000$. This strong positive correlation suggests that a nurse's level of comfort is related to her/his perceived competence. The strong linear correlation reflects the intuitive relationship between the nurses' perceived skill level or competence and comfort in providing psychologically based care.

The independent t-test (Table 11.2) was used to compare the comfort and competence ratings from the assessment phase (2006) to the evaluation phase (2009) of an unmatched sample of nurses from the same five units. On average, comfort scores in 2009 were higher ($M = 2.95$) than the scores in 2006 ($M = 2.87$). In addition, average competence scores in 2009 were higher ($M = 3.10$) than the scores in 2006 ($M = 2.91$). There was a significant difference in the comfort and competence scores for four variables (delirium, demanding, impulsive, and manipulative) at the $p < .01$ level and for one variable (needy) at the $p < .05$ level. Although this was not a matched nurse-to-nurse assessment, this study demonstrates a difference in the scores of nurses practicing on the unit in 2006 and in 2009.

Furthermore, the delirium responses in 2009 (Table 11.3) revealed that participants were able to identify delirium as a syndrome, the antipsychotic medication used to treat the behavioral symptoms, nursing interventions aimed at early mobilization, and a daily schedule of care to facilitate baseline levels of function. The respondents were also able to recognize that impaired cognition, irritability, and agitation may require family involvement for discharge teaching, and that patient advocacy is required when delirium is present to ensure informed consent. The subtypes of delirium, however, were not as readily identified.

TABLE 11.1 Nurses' Comfort and Competence Scores Responding to Selected Patient Care Situations, 2009 (N = 51**)

	Comfort (Range 1–4)						Competence (Range 1–4)				
	r	n	Min	Max	M	SD	n	Min	Max	M	SD
Alcohol	.821*	41	2	4	3.22	.525	41	2	4	3.10	.496
Anxiety	.822*	39	2	3	3.21	.522	41	2	4	3.27	.549
At-risk injury	.764*	41	1	4	3.27	.633	39	2	4	3.26	.498
Confusion	.927*	40	0	4	3.05	.714	40	0	4	3.08	.730
Delirium	.830*	39	2	4	3.15	.469	39	2	4	3.13	.469
Demanding	.955*	39	2	4	3.23	.536	39	2	4	3.21	.522
Dementia	.791*	39	2	4	3.21	.469	39	2	4	3.21	.522
Depression	.943*	39	2	4	3.08	.480	39	2	4	3.10	.447
DC PCA	.852*	39	2	4	3.26	.595	37	2	4	3.22	.630
Drug seeking	.859*	39	1	4	2.97	.628	39	2	4	3.05	.510
Impulsive	.928*	39	2	4	3.13	.615	38	2	4	3.16	.547
Manipulative	.787*	39	2	4	3.03	.628	39	2	4	3.05	.605
Needy	.829*	38	2	4	3.24	.542	39	2	4	3.28	.560
Order PCA	.962*	39	2	4	3.38	.590	38	2	4	3.37	.589
Violent	.911*	39	1	4	2.76	.667	39	1	4	2.79	.656
Psychotic	.935*	39	1	4	2.69	.614	39	1	4	2.64	.628
Restraints	.884*	39	2	4	3.25	.595	39	2	4	3.28	.560
Sexualizing	.798*	39	1	4	2.46	.720	39	1	4	2.56	.680
Suicidal	.928*	39	1	4	3.00	.725	39	1	4	3.08	.664

Note. Pearson's correlation of comfort and competence is computed for each variable.

* Correlation is significant at the 0.01 level (2-tailed). $p = .000$ for all variables.

** Of the total sample $N = 51$, there were 41 responses to this item.

TABLE 11.2 *Comparison of Nurses' Comfort and Competence Scores in Providing Care in Various Clinical Situations: 2006 (n = 81) Compared to 2009 Respondents (n = 51)*

	Comfort					Competence				
	06/09 n	06/09 M	t	df	p	06/09 n	06/09 M	t	df	p
Alcohol	76/41	3.07/3.22	1.32	115	.190	76/41	3.11/3.10	.045	114	.964
Anxiety	78/39	33.2/1.24	.357	115	.722	80/41	3.20/3.27	.607	119	.545
At-risk injury	79/41	3.19/3.27	.637	118	.525	79/39	3.20/3.26	.468	116	.641
Confusion	79/40	3.20/3.05	1.22	117	.225	75/40	3.20/3.08	1.01	113	.313
Delirium	78/39	2.77/3.15	3.49	100.87	.001	76/39	2.78/3.13	3.34	99.88	+.001
Demand	81/39	2.79/3.23	3.67	101.18	+.000	72/39	2.85/3.21	2.67	109	+.009
Dementia	78/39	3.17/3.21	.377	115	.707	77/39	3.13/3.21	.654	114	.514
Depression	80/39	2.95/3.08	1.18	101.04	.241	77/39	2.95/3.10	1.27	114	.205
DC PCA	77/39	3.05/3.26	1.42	114	.158	75/37	3.13/3.22	.564	110	.574
Drug seeking	80/39	2.81/2.97	1.21	93.44	.231	75/39	2.76/3.05	2.36	107.39	+.020
Impulsive	75/39	2.69/3.13	3.31	91.74	+.001	76/38	2.78/3.16	3.14	94.41	+.002
Manipulative	80/39	2.54/3.03	3.58	96.23	+.001	76/39	2.58/3.05	3.53	97.57	+.001
Needy	78/38	2.94/3.24	2.31	114	+.023	78/39	2.99/3.28	2.36	115	+.020
Order PCA	76/39	3.37/3.38	.130	113	.896	76/38	2.28/3.37	7.27	112	+.000
Violent	75/39	2.52/2.76	1.69	96.89	.093	79/39	2.27/2.79	3.58	97.53	+.001
Psychotic	77/39	2.38/2.69	2.22	98.66	+.029	78/39	3.12/2.64	3.71	115	-.000
Restraints	74/39	3.05/3.25	1.51	111	.135	79/39	2.17/3.28	8.16	109.94	+.000
Sexualizing	77/39	2.44/2.46	.122	114	.903	79/39	2.77/2.56	1.37	100.59	.175
Suicidal	79/39	2.77/3.00	1.45	95.77	.152	78/39	2.74/3.07	2.26	99.01	+.026

Note. Sig. (2-tailed) $p = < .05$.
Note. Missing data in 7 of the 2006 and 14 of the 2009 responses.

TABLE 11.3 *Percent of Correct Responses to Knowledge of Delirium,*
2009 Survey Respondents (N = 51)

Knowledge Item	n	Percent Correct Responses
Question 1: Delirium as a syndrome	38	89.5%
Question 2: Etiologies of delirium	38	60.5%
Question 3: Hypoactive delirium	37	51.4%
Question 4: Haldol administration	36	86.1%
Question 5: Nursing care of delirium	37	97.0%
Question 6*: DC teaching for delirium	37	100%
Question 7: Medication administration for delirium	35	48.5%
Question 8: Ambulation intervention	35	97.1%
Question 9: Nursing intervention for delirium	37	67.6%
Question 10: Informed consent and delirium	35	92.4%

Note. Percentage of correct answers within each question.
* Of the total sample, $N = 51$, there were 38 responses to this item.

We were not surprised that knowledge deficits regarding hypodelirium, proper administration of as-needed (PRN) medication for behavioral symptoms, nursing interventions for delirium, and recognition of evolving etiologies required ongoing support to become embedded in the nurses' practice. The literature identifies delirium as one of the most prevalent and underrecognized conditions in the acute care setting, with hypoactive, hyperactive, and mixed activity presentations (Idemoto & Kresevic, 2007; Inouye, 2006). The nurses have become skillful at recognizing behavioral markers of hyperactive delirium, such as crawling out of bed, pulling at tubes, fall risk, and agitation. Hypoactive delirium presentations, such as not participating in care, withdrawal, and lethargy (Forrest, Willis, Holm, Kwon, Anderson, & Foreman, 2007), remain challenging and may require different targeted educational interventions.

We reviewed the nurses' knowledge of delirium based upon years of experience and divided their responses into two groups. Group one includes nurses with 0–6 years of experience and group two includes nurses with 7 or more years of experience who had exposure to the PNRS during its formation or implementation. The findings suggest that nurses with 10 or more years of experience were no more knowledgeable about delirium than the nurse with 1–3 years of experience. Moreover, the nurse with fewer years of experience was more knowledgeable about delirium. Benner suggests that years of experience are not equivalent to expertise unless there is active engagement, reflective practice, and ongoing learning that informs the practice development.

Consultation requests covering 2006 through August 2009 are reviewed in Table 11.4. Nurses' requests for assistance in providing psychological care fell into three main categories: delirium (60%), psychiatric acuity (25%) (with subsets of violent, sexualizing, psychotic, and suicidal), and response to illness (15%). The majority of patients were referred to the PNRS for delirium (60%), which is not surprising given the rates of delirium in hospitalized patients and the limited knowledge

TABLE 11.4 *Reason for Consultation Requests by Unit Nurses for PNRS 2007–2009 (31 months)*

PNRS Primary Diagnosis	Percentage
Delirium/Confusion	60.1%
Response to illness	14.5%
Substance abuse	4.9%
Suicidal/Homicidal	3.8%
Dementia	3.3%
Ethical/Family	3.3%
Schizophrenia/Psychosis	3.1%
Mood disorder	3.0%
Anxiety	1.9%
Personality disorder	1.9%
Head injury	1.8%

nurses have about providing care for the delirious patient (Maldonado, 2008; Rigney, 2006). It was also consistent with the targeted interventions established by the PNRS during the assessment phase.

Psychiatric acuity patients, the second largest referral category (25%), represented immediate safety concerns and are identified by the nurse to be "at risk" for unsafe behaviors. Violent, suicidal, and homicidal patients can increase nurses' anxiety level and fear for personal safety (Ballard, Pao, Henderson, Lee, Bostwick, & Rosenstein, 2008; Cutcliffe & Stevenson, 2008). In any setting, suicidal patients represent some of the most at-risk patients and require specialized care. The number of psychiatric beds has decreased (Brown, 2007), leading to increased numbers of psychiatric patients being admitted to general hospital beds and straining the capacity of large urban systems nationally. When the at-risk patients with primary psychiatric disorders are admitted to inpatient medical or surgical floors, the staff nurses are primarily responsible for managing the patients' safety. The competence required to safely manage this population of patients often exceeds the skill (Chan, Chien, & Tso, 2009; Gilje, Klose, & Birger, 2007) and comfort level of the staff nurse in the general health care setting. The nurse requires expert coaching to safely care for and manage these patients to remain engaged with the care.

The third category of patients referred to us for consultation was "response to illness," at 15 percent. *Response to illness* refers to a patient's expected and anticipated emotional response to being hospitalized or ill. There is an essential role for the nurse at the bedside to connect with the patient and family to decrease their anxiety and suffering. Nurses who are new to practice are focused on mastery of task and technology, and cannot appreciate that connecting with the patient facilitates the provision of nursing care. Establishing an interpersonal connection with the patient often competes with the demands of our fast-paced, technologically driven environment of care. Nurses felt uncomfortable and unprepared to address psychological care and sought assistance from us in developing interpersonal connections with the patients and their families. We guided them on how to talk with patients who were crying or sad as a response to a diagnosis, treatment, or long hospitalization. Through education and coaching, the nurses were able to identify their role in the patients' psychological care and what was a "normal" response to hospitalization for that particular patient. When nurses gain mastery of the psychological skills necessary to provide quality holistic care, their ability to engage the patient interpersonally is enhanced, thereby improving the overall care of their patients.

Security assistance requests from the five units, compared for two quarters of each year 2007–2009, decreased markedly. Calls from nurses for assistance in containing patient behaviors decreased. Security assistance requests [2007 (n = 157, M = 2.00, SD = 1.227), 2008 (n = 67, M = 2.34, SD = .980), 2009 (n = 82, M = 2.00, SD = .852)] decreased 57% from year 2007 to year 2008. Nurses requested security assistance for patients with traumatic brain injury (TBI), delirium, psychiatric symptoms (psychosis, schizophrenia, bipolar, depression, PTSD, anxiety, suicidal, homicidal), substance abuse, and dementia. Nursing requests for security assistance shifted from punitive—"I'm calling security to set limits on this patient"—to treatment and provision of safe care—"I need help to medicate my patient." There has been a shift from a crisis mode to one of assessment, intervention, and improved care. There was a slight increase in security assistance requests from 2008 to 2009 in the categories of TBI and psychiatric patients, which reflected an increase in these populations.

Reducing 1:1 "sitter" budgets has been the focus of acute care hospitals for many years, but multiple attempts to "reduce sitters" has not led to sustainable change. The results of our study show a decrease in sitter or one-to-one patient care assistants (PCA) utilization. The 2007/2008 average of one-to-one PCA requests for assistance on the five units for delirium averaged 9.74 FTEs. The average utilization for 2009 was 8.07 FTEs, resulting in an overall decrease of 1.67 FTEs. As understanding of the etiology of the behavior disturbance increased, nursing interventions focused more on identifying and alleviating the patient's risk for injury instead of containment.

Nursing leadership supported this shift with increased attention to the director's role in aligning resources based upon patient care needs. Intensive coaching by the nursing leadership (executive directors, directors, and nurses-in-charge) provided increased fiscal oversight management, shifting leadership's focus from containment to care. The directors engaged in "knowing" which patients were at high risk, at the unit level, provided budget and clinical oversight for resource allocation and clinical support. The modification in language from "sitter" (a passive, noninvolved role) to 1:1 PCA (a more active caregiver) was imperative in changing the culture of care and reflected the shift to identifying the patients' care needs. The 1:1 PCA participates in creating a quiet, restful, and safe environment, in which the PCA provides delegated care to patients such as walking, toileting, and feeding, instead of talking on the telephone, watching TV, or reading. Nurses have learned what to expect from patients at risk for delirium or injury. They can identify the behavioral disturbances, recognize the safety risks, identify etiologies, and develop individualized plans of care.

Subsequently, the practice has shifted from crisis-oriented intervention to preventive and care-based intervention, which enhances patient safety. The comfort and competence of nurses, knowledge of delirium, and quality of psychological nursing care improved. Five items (delirium, demanding, impulsive, manipulative, needy) are significantly higher in 2009 as compared with 2006 in both comfort and competence scores. The patient who was formally described as "acting out" or "needing limits" is now assessed by nursing as delirious and in need of care. Furthermore, the nurses' requests for security assistance fell by 57% and one-to-one PCA/sitter use declined by 17%. Nurses anticipate behavioral presentations from delirious patients and provide psychologically based care, no longer experiencing the behavior as a crisis requiring security or behavioral limit setting.

Practice change requires energy, support, and leadership commitment to effect that change over time. Our environments of care are technologically complex, but attention to the psychological health of patients facilitates safe, holistic care. Education, consultation, and coaching by expert nurses at the bedside address the source of nurses' anxiety and build nurses' skills for reflective practice. Their engagement in active, ongoing learning and inquiry is essential. The nurse who feels safe in providing care to a patient who is exhibiting behavioral manifestations of delirium can meet the increased care needs of these patients. Providing an opportunity for the nurse to reflect on what worked and what did not work, and to practice newly learned approaches to care, leads to enhanced interpersonal skills and improved psychological care of patients.

Knowing the patient requires the nurse to develop knowledge of the particular patient; consultation and coaching provide an approach that models and assists in psychological skill development in the nurse. The decreased requests for security assistance and one-to-one PCAs reflect the nurses' enhanced comfort with and competence in providing psychological care to their patients.

Without clinical and leadership support at the bedside, nurses have difficulty embedding new knowledge into their practice. Nurses build comfort and confidence and display ownership of psychological nursing care as an important part of their work. When leadership and support in the practice environment are absent, care may be superficially safe from a technology/compliance standpoint, but the patient remains at risk due to disengagement from the nurse-patient relationship. We are fortunate to work in an environment where this is recognized and engaged care is supported, and look forward to passing on this knowledge to others who commit to changing nursing practice.

REFERENCES

Ballard, E., Pao, M., Henderson, D., Lee, L., Bostwick, M., & Rosenstein, D. (2008). Suicide in the medical setting. *Joint Commission Journal on Quality & Patient Safety, 34*(8), 474–481.

Benner, P. (1984). *From novice to expert: Excellence and power in clinical nursing practice.* Menlo Park, CA: Addison-Wesley.

Bloom, B. S., Englhart, M. D., Furst, E. J., Hill, W. H., & Krathwohl, D. R. (Eds.). (1956). *Taxonomy of educational objectives, the classification of educational goals, Handbook I: Cognitive domain.* New York, NY: Longmans.

Brown, J. (2007). A survey of emergency department psychiatric services. *General Hospital Psychiatry, 29,* 475–480.

Chan, S., Chien, W., & Tso, S. (2009). Evaluating nurses' knowledge, attitude and competency after an education programme on suicide prevention. *Nurse Education Today, 29,* 763–769.

Cutcliffe, J. R., & Stevenson, C. (2008). Feeling our way in the dark: The psychiatric nursing care of suicidal people—A literature review. *International Journal of Nursing Studies, 45,* 942–953.

Fineout-Overholt, E., & Johnston, L. (2007). Evaluation: An essential step to the EBP process. *Worldviews on Evidence-Based Nursing, 4*(1), 54–59.

Forrest, J., Willis, L., Holm, K., Kwon, M., Anderson, M., & Foreman, M. (2007). Recognizing quiet delirium. *American Journal of Nursing, 107*(4), 35–39.

Gilje, F., Klose, P., & Birger, J. (2007). Critical clinical competencies in undergraduate psychiatric-mental health nursing. *Journal of Nursing Education, 46*(11), 522–526.

Idemoto, B., & Kresevic, D. (2007). Emerging nurse-sensitive outcomes and evidence-based practice in postoperative cardiac patients. *Critical Care Nursing Clinics of North America, 19,* 371–384.

Inouye, S. K. (2006). Delirium in older persons. *New England Journal of Medicine, 354,* 1157–1165.

Institute of Medicine (IOM). (2000). *To err is human.* Washington, DC: National Academy Press.

Krathwohl, D. R., Bloom, B. S., & Masia, B. B. (1973). *Taxonomy of educational objectives, the classification of educational goals. Handbook II: Affective domain.* New York, NY: David McKay.

Lakatos, B. (2009). *Outcomes of a psychiatric nursing resource service.* Retrieved from Proquest Dissertations and Theses. (Accession Order No. AAT 340200.)

Lilford, R., Brown, C., & Nicholl, J. (2007). Use of process measures to monitor the quality of clinical practice. *British Medical Journal, 335,* 648–650.

Maldonado, J. R. (2008). Delirium in the acute-care setting: Characteristics, diagnosis, and treatment. *Critical Care Clinics, 24,* 657–722.

Peplau, H. E. (1952, reissued 1991). *Interpersonal relations in nursing: A conceptual frame of reference for psychodynamic nursing.* New York, NY: Springer Publishing.

Rigney, T. S. (2006). Delirium in the hospitalized elder and recommendations for practice. *Geriatric Nursing, 27*(3), 151–156.

Survey Monkey. (2009). *Survey Monkey user's manual: Customer guide for account navigation, survey creation, survey distribution, & data analysis.* Retrieved May 8, 2009, from http://s3.amazonaws.com/SurveyMonkeyFiles/UserManual.pdf

Yakimo, R., Jurlowica, L., & Murray, R. (2004). Evaluation of outcomes in psychiatric consultation-liaison nursing practice. *Archives of Psychiatric Nursing, 17*(6), 215–227.

11.3 *Advanced Practice Nurse in Action*

Leslie DeLisle

In 2009, my final year of graduate school, I participated in an independent clinical experience with the support and collaboration of the BWH Psychiatric Nursing Resource Service (PNRS). I was working toward an advanced degree as an Adult Psychiatric Clinical Nurse Specialist (CNS), a role emphasizing clinical leadership, staff development, and education. This internship helped me develop my clinical skills in that role, one of many in nursing with a common designation: advanced practice nurse (APN). This story is for me an exemplar of how I learned to put the APN role into action. I have changed the names of both the patient and nurse to respect confidentiality.

I arrived at work on a Monday morning and headed to the PNRS office to organize my day. I prioritized the new referrals and noted that one nurse was requesting assistance with a patient, Mr. J., for "acute agitation, noncompliance, assaultive behavior, and a challenging family." When I arrived on the unit, several nurses commented, "You must be here for Mr. J." I found the nurse caring for him, whom I will call Meghan. She looked overwhelmed and in distress. I told her I was there to help and would be reading the patient chart until she was available to review his care with me.

Mr. J. was a 72-year-old male admitted a week prior for an upper gastrointestinal bleed. He had required more than 25 units of blood products over several days to stabilize him. He was transferred from the ICU the day before to this intermediate care unit. The nursing notes described many potential safety issues, including crawling out of bed, refusing care, and striking out at nursing staff. His agitation increased overnight, requiring several security emergencies to be called, and finally resulting in the use of restraints and a 1:1 observer.

When Meghan came out of his room she stated, "I'm so glad you are here; this guy is just awful. I feel so bad." She looked exhausted—and it was only 9:00 AM. I asked her to tell me about the nursing-specific challenges and the medical priorities. She described the patient as being at risk of falling or injuring himself and others. "He doesn't follow directions, keeps yelling at me, tried to punch me, and the nurse last night said he grabbed her stethoscope! Someone is going to get hurt; I don't know what to do." She said the family was asking questions frequently; she was unsure of how to respond, and the physician was in surgery, unavailable. She was concerned that she had little time for her other two patients because Mr. J. had been so "out of control."

We looked at the medical record together. I asked Meghan what she thought might be causing these symptoms and she wondered if he had an alcohol or dementia history. These were both good hypotheses, but I felt she was missing the overall diagnosis: delirium. I reviewed the hallmark characteristics of delirium. Meghan stated she thought he was delirious, but was unsure and didn't want to sound silly. I reassured her that delirium is complex, not well recognized, and that she was right on target.

We evaluated the patient together. Mr. J. was a frail man who looked terrified. He had his bed linens pushed off to the side and his hospital pajamas twisted up near his chest. He was oriented to self only and had difficulty responding to any questions. He asked if he was dying and if I would help him "escape this prison." He pointed to his arm with the IV and talked about the snakes crawling on his arm. He turned to talk with people he believed to be standing near the window (there was no one at the window), and stated that he was "being attacked" and needed to defend himself. I reassured the patient of his safety and used simple language to reorient him to his surroundings. "Mr. J., this is a safe place. You are at Brigham and Women's Hospital in Boston."

I had assured Meghan that I would assist her in finding the words to talk to the family. The wife and daughter were at the bedside and distressed. The daughter was talking to the patient in a loud voice—"Dad, it's me, Alice; don't you know who I am?"—while the wife sat quietly in the corner, crying. I asked them to come outside the room so Meghan and I could discuss his care with them. We reassured them that a patient care assistant would remain in the room, and they reluctantly left the bedside. They voiced concerns that Mr. J. was "going crazy" and stated, "This is not our Mike." I modeled how to respond to the family's questions for Meghan, demonstrating how to actively listen to their concerns and decrease their anxiety by providing education. We discussed delirium, possible etiologies based on his major medical problems, and treatment. I reassured them that his delirium would improve as the medical problems stabilized. I demonstrated what they could do to comfort him and provided them with an educational pamphlet on delirium. They were relieved to know what was happening to their loved one, what the treatment approach was, and what they could do to help in his recovery.

Before leaving the unit, I met with Meghan and discussed the interviews with the patient and the family, the multiple etiologies causing delirium, and specific interventions she could utilize to keep herself and Mr. J. safe. She could first begin by advocating that Mr. J. receive the appropriate medication to relieve the subjective distress he was in given his paranoia, anxiety, and hallucinations. She would then be able to focus on getting him mobilized and providing him with assistance for activities of daily living, including supervision with meals so that he would improve his nutritional status. Meghan could also tailor the immediate care environment to be less stimulating and work side-by-side with the support staff on the unit to ensure that everyone was aware of the care Mr. J. required. Meghan now appeared more relaxed and more comfortable providing care to Mr. J. I left a detailed note in the patient's chart reflecting my involvement with the patient and family and our recommendations.

My role as the CNS is to calm and influence a stressful situation by providing expert consultation to the patient, information and comfort to the family, coaching to nurses, and education and treatment planning for the patient's ongoing care. Once Meghan understood that Mr. J. was experiencing delirium, she was able to shift her thinking about him from a difficult patient who was trying to harm her to a patient with a diagnosis that required assessment and intervention. With coaching and support, Meghan was able to fill in the gaps in her knowledge, decrease her anxiety, and connect with this patient and his family to provide effective care.

For me, this exemplar illustrates only a few of the safety issues and concerns that nurses face daily. My work with Meghan improved her experience in caring for a delirious patient, gave her skills to utilize in future practice with delirious patients, and positively influenced Mr. J.'s care. In May 2010, I was fortunate to join the PNRS as a member of the service. I experience daily how APNs' support of staff nurses at the bedside is valued and essential to positive patient outcomes. I have learned through practice that for me to be effective, it takes patience, a supportive environment, and valuable supervision and support provided by my PNRS colleagues. As I work alongside nurses at the bedside to model new approaches of care for patients dealing with psychological health problems, I strive to be authentic as I inspire these nurses to think differently about their patients.

11.4 *A Leadership Perspective on Improving the Care of Delirious Patients in an Acute Care Setting*

Kimberly A. Ternavan and Margaret Higgins

Within Brigham and Women's Hospital's medical-surgical patient care services, there are two levels of care: intensive care and intermediate care. Our unit is a 31-bed intermediate care surgical unit that includes telemetry and general care patients. Our primary patient population includes the burn/trauma and renal transplant/renal medicine patients, though we also care for other surgical patients based on census demands. Our nursing team has adapted well to handling patient assignments involving diverse surgical and/or medical teams and patients with various needs. We have approximately 56 nurses, whose average age is 37 and average length of service at the hospital is 6.4 years.

LEADERSHIP MODEL AND GOALS: POISED FOR CHANGE

Kimberly Ternavan, our nurse director, and Margaret Higgins, our clinical nurse educator, led our leadership team. The team also includes seven nurses-in-charge (NICs), designated clinical leaders who work collaboratively with the leadership team in planning and implementing patient care. The NICs meet as a group monthly for 4 hours to discuss operations of the unit. A key aspect of their role is to translate the goals of the leadership group to the rest of the nursing team and to give the leadership team feedback about what is happening on our unit at the staff nurse level. During the monthly leadership meeting, we address operational decision making, improvement initiatives, competency/educational plans, and any other concerns that may arise. At our first meeting, we developed four main goals that would support our work each month:

1. Enhancement of communication among the patient care team
2. Development of a teamwork approach to patient care
3. Establishment of a strong, respected leadership core
4. Participation and development of educational initiatives to support professional development

We believed our goals reflected the vision of the Department of Nursing (DON): *Excellent care to patients and families, with the best staff, in the safest environment*. If we could implement our unit-based goals, we believed we would be in close alignment with the DON vision.

As the leadership team began to develop, we invited guests to join us. Basically, we wanted to partner with other departments as a way to improve the care of our patients. We had a monthly forum where we could invite them to participate, and conversely, when there was an issue, they had a place to talk to us about it. Using our monthly meetings to reach out to other roles and services, the NICs have been able to build relationships throughout the hospital. In addition, they have been able to acknowledge their own nursing practice and realize that they have "voice" in our leadership team.

Building on the newly minted DON vision and our unit-specific goals, the team wanted to create a deeper vision for our unit and wanted to share this with all staff. During a monthly leadership meeting, we created our statement of where we were headed as a team, unit, and humans and what it meant to be a part of the 8AB nursing team. We proudly hung the following statement on each of our two nursing units: *"8AB is committed to providing exceptional patient care in an environment of professionalism, integrity, respect, compassion and humor."*

FINDING A CHANGE FOCUS: DELIRIUM AND THE SURGICAL PATIENT

Having developed a well-functioning nursing staff through streamlined systems and concrete operations and resources, we realized that many challenges remained in the care of specific patient populations. An important one was the confused patient. Staff often described the confusion and challenging behaviors these patients manifested using terms a layperson might use, a more social than professional description. These patients might be admitted post-operatively, following a trauma, or withdrawing from alcohol or drugs. Staff often labeled them with terms such as "crazy," "weird," "challenging," "difficult," or "forgetful." Our first step toward practice improvement was actually putting challenging behaviors and signs of cognitive impairment into a clinical context. Most often we found that the patient we had difficulty describing clinically was actually experiencing delirium due to clinical factors, such as brain injury, infection, sleep deprivation, or pain.

According to a study by Pandharipande et al. reported in the *Journal of Trauma, Injury, Infection and Critical Care,* 70% of surgical and trauma patients experience delirium (Pandharipande et al., 2008). As this is one of the primary groups of patients we care for on our units, it became evident that staff needed more support in dealing with this secondary diagnosis. Although it was a secondary diagnosis, the challenges of maintaining safety for these patients often became the bedside nurse's primary focus.

Many of these patients were transferred from the intensive care unit. They often had a complex history that might include significant administration of sedative and analgesic medications, prior drug or alcohol abuse, or recent surgical interventions. In addition, they were often transferred to our unit during the busiest time, during the change of shift for the nursing team. The noise volume on the unit could be quite loud, further disturbing the delirious patient who is often easily or already overstimulated. The nurse-to-nurse handoff process was often disrupted when patients arrived shortly before the end or beginning of a shift, potentially leading to communication failures. Sometimes the patient's care was transferred to a night float medical resident who had not been involved with the case previously. This off-shift team would do their best to get the patient's care plan in place without the primary team available, but it would essentially be all new care providers for the patient, leading to difficulties in transitioning to a different level of care. Often the nursing staff felt they needed to physically restrain patients and use a sitter/

observer to maintain the patients' safety. These interventions were a response to behavior but not to the diagnosis of delirium, which we possibly could have identified earlier. Often staff nurses would leave their shift with strong feelings of powerlessness and defeat, feeling the lack of a solid, consistent care plan. Many of these feelings were due to frustration at not meeting the standard of care they believed the patient required or that they knew they were capable of providing to the patient and family.

BEGINNING THE CHANGE PROCESS:
THE PSYCHIATRIC NURSE CONSULT SERVICE

In early 2007, the Nursing Executive Board (NEB) established a Psychiatric Nursing Resource Service (PNRS) to improve the psychological nursing care provided to hospitalized patients and their families and access to psychiatric services for hospitalized patients. The PNRS was designed to improve the experience of nurses caring for patients with behavioral health issues and help create a safe environment of care (see Chapters 11.1 and 11.2 for further detailed information about the PNRS).

The PNRS would offer staff an opportunity to be coached at the bedside, in real time, on specific patient needs as related to mental health care and specifically delirium in the hospitalized patient. The service required a standardized referral form to be completed by the nurse; a physician order was not needed to request this consult. The resource would be available Monday through Friday. Initially, the service involved one-on-one consultation with the nursing staff at their request. This bedside meeting could include "informal and formal education, including current research, evidence-based practices, interventions and approaches to care." Among the potential issues appropriate for referral, the PNRS listed "delirium or a change in mental status" and "potential or actual safety concerns: use of restraints and sitters." We had found our resource.

As the PNRS initial pilot program began, we believed it was important that as nurse director and clinical educator, we encourage the staff to reach out to the consult service, continuing the practice of seeking help from clinical experts we had used in our leadership meetings. This could be something as simple as a verbal reminder that the service was in existence. We would often identify patient care opportunities—and there were many—that would benefit from the service. We believed that it was also important for both of us to access the resource in order to support our practice. To provide a foundation before the one-on-one bedside consultation on the unit, the PNRS provided two 1-hour classes on "Mental Status" and "Delirium." We made a commitment to have all staff attend this education, including both of us, and it was extremely well received.

Initially, the staff expressed mixed feelings about an "outsider"—the PNRS clinical nurse specialist (CNS)—coming to our unit and making suggestions about care improvement. It took our own acknowledgment that we certainly weren't perfect (not an easy acknowledgment in a large academic center) to encourage the staff. More important, our patients experiencing delirium were the ones paying the price for our lack of education and awareness. We also noted that in certain patient cases, even when we were aware of delirium, the situation was still complicated by a lack of knowledge about what intervention should be implemented. Thankfully, most staff welcomed the opportunity to share their practice and learn new skills in the management of these difficult and challenging patients. Initially, some staff were not as comfortable with their practice and were less likely to engage with the psychiatric CNS. As nurses began to see the value in the consult service through a noticeable improvement in a patient's behaviors, with fewer safety risks and less agitation, they were more receptive and began to seek out the resource service independently.

Interestingly, an unexpected finding arose. Many staff nurses realized that they had not had the opportunity to discuss practice outside of their immediate nursing team responsibilities. This increased awareness of how our nursing team often works in isolation even though we work beside (literally) several other disciplines. Too often, the voice of the nurse was missing. Knowing how to communicate a finding, such as an altered mental status, was a challenge, even though it was a finding nursing would be much more prone to recognize due to the amount of time spent with the patient and the fact that delirium symptoms often wax and wane. We knew that what the physician team saw on morning rounds provided an incomplete picture of the patient's mental status. Struggles in communication existed amongst our own nursing team; we then further struggled to communicate with other team members taking care of this patient.

TAKING CHANGE TO THE NEXT LEVEL

After about one year of PNRS referrals and consultations, our unit was ready to move our leadership in caring for this patient population to the next level. The CNS suggested that a more concentrated initiative might be helpful; we were still in the beginning stages of learning how to help our patients with delirium. The PNRS was interested in working more closely with one specific nursing team to truly elicit change in nursing practice. Since our nursing unit had the highest use of patient care assistants related to close observation of delirious patients, several challenging patient populations, and an engaged leadership team, we were the first area identified to work intensively with the PNRS as a pilot project.

As leaders on the unit, we looked at this pilot as a great opportunity to continue the growth and development of our team. Staff were interested in new opportunities for development and appreciated access to increased knowledge about delirium and its management. The advancement of clinical practice would provide support for this new partnership with program managers. These partnerships allowed further mentorship and coaching for our entire team. In the past, both the nurses and their management team had survived by working separately, even though we were all supposed to be working together. This had also been seen on a larger scale within the DON, the surgical nursing team separated from the medical nursing team. There was little sharing of leadership practices across the teams. The DON was reversing that pattern. The partnership with the PNRS would serve as an opportunity to share our story and hopefully share our development and outcomes with the rest of BWH. As leaders of the group, we were given an opportunity to test out a new model that was an important DON initiative supporting the new vision statement and the new emphasis on collaboration.

As we began to develop our plan for the intensive pilot, we learned more about the importance of the nurses' voice in improving practice. The PNRS team had been successful previously in working with a group of nurse "champions" and proposed using this approach with our unit. The *champion* is a clinician who is confident with his or her practice, well socialized among and respected by his or her peers, approachable and comfortable collaborating with staff about practice. Other common terms for champions are *experts* or *super users*. We knew that to elicit a change in practice, we would have to have buy-in from staff and have support available on all shifts. It was our expectation that this champion group be diverse and able to represent all three work shifts. This was a new process and it was important to have the right team members to make a smooth transition for successful practice change. Once we brainstormed and developed our ideal group, the list was presented and accepted by the leadership team, including, most importantly, the NIC group. We included two of the seven NICs who had requested to be involved in this group. We called the group our "Delirium Experts." This was an important step for us, since we had never utilized a champion model on this unit and did not want to create two separate groups within the nursing staff. We wanted a connection where feedback went from one group to the other in both directions.

To provide additional training, the psychiatric CNS led a full-day seminar for 10 staff members, inclusive of the two NICs. This time away from our unit allowed us to take a more in-depth look at what current practice was, and more importantly, some challenges nurses encountered every day in caring for the delirious patient. As the director and educator, we watched the CNS lead the class in a way that was new to us. She had knowledge, but also shared her many prior experiences. While the seminar had a didactic dimension, hearing the stories of our nurses' frustrations and barriers to providing care was what we ultimately needed to know to find the motivation to change and the commitment to remove our current barriers to quality care for our delirium patients.

During the morning, the CNS gave us information on behaviors that would help us identify delirium (it's not always obvious!) and reviewed the possible causes of behavioral disturbances, including infections, myocardial infarctions, sleep disturbances, and especially medications; quite commonly, the medications we give in a hospital to treat one problem then create a delirium. This gave us the clinical context to work within, replacing our inaccurate terms such as *strange* or *crazy*. Giving us language to use that focused on data rather than behavior was an important step in preparing us to communicate our findings appropriately.

The most important information we, as leaders, gathered during the day was the recurrent themes we heard by listening to the nurses. This time was also a chance for the director to honestly share her perspective about budgetary constraints and the pressure she felt to reduce the expenses of patient observers used with this patient group. The afternoon portion was then much more of an open forum. We had asked each of the 10 nurses to bring a narrative story with them. It did not take much for each nurse to recall a shift or experience caring for a delirious patient. Often, the story was from the shift the nurse had worked right before the class. It made us aware of the magnitude of the problem. In listening to the narrative stories of each nurse and identifying the recurrent themes, we were able to create five working subgroups to address the issues we faced on the unit. The five subgroups were sitter usage, education of co-workers, family education, patient care assistant (PCA) role and safety rounds, and physician/nurse communication. Each subgroup consisted of two nurses who were particularly interested in that aspect of our patients' care. With the guidance of the nurse director, educator, and program manager, they would follow the project to its completion. These became our nurse champion groups.

Sitter Usage

Sitter usage obviously strained our budget in a difficult economic time, but it also made staff planning a challenge. With the focus on excellent patient care, we needed responsible review and utilization of our resources. It was important to address why sitters were used and the steps taken to use an alternative solution prior to this resource being implemented. This would facilitate the implementation of better patient care plans and ensure appropriate allocation of resources for patient care.

Through our baseline research, we discovered that a significant number of patients were being transferred from intensive care with a sitter in place prior to being seen on our unit. Therefore, this subgroup of champions addressed the "transfer of ICU patients" by developing guidelines to support the transition of care with delirious patients. With the support of the leadership team, staff would evaluate the patient in the ICU prior to transfer. A conversation and assessment would take place at the patient bedside prior to arrival on our unit. We could then evaluate the need for a sitter. This direct communication with ICU staff, for something other than report, was new and some staff were skeptical about its effect. We listened intently to all feedback because it was a new practice.

The most important lesson learned was the need to evaluate and then reevaluate the patient before, during, and after transfer. It was not always appropriate to remove a sitter right before transferring a patient. We altered the guidelines many times as we received feedback from staff. We knew it was important to listen and respond to concerns to sustain staff buy-in. We initially felt that sitters were not always necessary for transferring ICU patients, but realizing that shift change is such a loud, stimulating time to a delirious patient, we reevaluated and determined it might be best to keep the sitter for several hours during the transition phase. The new environment, the lower intensity of care and observation, as well as shared rooms, can be quite stimulating to a patient who is already delirious. We also reviewed the timing of transfer to avoid shift changes. We realized that these could all be important practice changes that we could do differently once we realized the role they played in trying to keep the patient safe.

Education of Co-Workers

We knew we needed all nursing staff to receive the information we had learned in the one-day intensive class. This champion subgroup studied unit education options and worked with the program manager to develop 1-hour "Delirium Rounds," scheduled Thursday at lunchtime. One of the staff nurses would present his or her patient and the concerns related to behaviors exhibited during the patient's admission. Clinical information about the patient, such as history, labs, and so on, would be presented, including a medication review. We would then brainstorm about an alternative plan of care, if needed. Subsequently, the psychiatric CNS would role-model how she would complete her initial assessment and then work with the group on development of a plan. The nurses benefited from real-time discussions that gave them concrete examples about how to handle difficult decisions where the answer was not always black and white; we needed to grow comfortable with trial and error. Slowly, there were fewer cases to discuss on weekly rounds and we moved the Delirium Rounds to biweekly and then monthly. Staff were becoming more comfortable with making assessments, communicating with the teams, and forming clinical judgments. In addition, this subgroup also developed a resource book for staff to reference should the psychiatric CNS not be readily available, in the middle of the night or on weekends.

Family Education

A third subgroup of the delirium experts focused on family education. Ask any nurse and he or she knows how nervous and worried a family member can become when a loved one is experiencing a delirium. They wonder what is happening to their family member and whether the patient will ever return to "normal." To reassure the family member, and also give some advice on how to care for such a patient, with suggestions like keeping the room quiet and reminding the patient that he or she is safe, we developed a family education brochure. It explained not only interventions, but three different types of delirium as well. It is reassuring to have a tool that nursing staff can utilize to provide support to families. It also lets the family know that delirium is common and they are not the only persons who have seen this happen to a loved one. Just knowing there is a term for the behavior change sometimes provides comfort.

PCA Role and Safety Rounds

After the nurses received additional training, we wanted to extend it to all members of the nursing team, including our PCAs, who spend a significant amount of time with the patients on our unit. We realized we were not utilizing them as well as we could to further support safety measures for our delirious patients. Two of our delirium experts helped coordinate a "PCA Education Day." This was extremely well received by the PCA group. The entire delirium expert group, with the addition of the nurse director and educator, planned and delivered the day. Multiple topics were discussed, including our fall rate, safety devices such as lap belts or chair alarms, and also safety features on the beds. We also discussed a safety rounds program, as well as ways to improve shift report to be more inclusive of PCAs. The PCA group also brought forth one of their concerns: They were having difficulty in reporting to multiple nurses during a single shift. As a result, the delirium workgroup altered the staffing pattern of our unit to create a PCA/RN team for each patient. Ideally, a PCA only works with two nurses during the day shift and evening shift. (Each pod only has one PCA at night, so that is not an option.) Our goal was to facilitate accountability for the PCA, improve communication, and make accessing the nurse a bit easier, rather than asking the PCAs to try to coordinate patient care they provided with four or five different nurses.

Physician/Nurse Communication

The last subgroup addressed physician/nurse communication, one of the most difficult challenges we faced. There are several reasons for this difficulty. We are a large, busy academic medical center and there are many competing demands on physicians. It also can be hard for nurses to demonstrate to other disciplines the importance of the work they do. One of the themes discovered from the narrative work was that often the nurses would be trying to share the picture they were seeing in the behavior of their patient and it was not well understood by our physician counterparts. Also, the physician team had not received the same level of education and support for care of delirium as the nursing team. The nursing group had been educated while we had inadvertently left the physician teams out of the work we were doing. Much of the communication between nurses and physicians is through text-message paging. Again, nursing often is in the best position to identify the delirious patient based on the amount of time spent with the patient. Nurses felt the concerns they brought forth were often ignored or that physicians were not responsive to what the nurses were telling them. Admittedly, in the past, the concerns had been presented in descriptions that lacked the clinical clarity of our new understanding of delirium.

One of our primary services, the trauma patient population, was an area we chose to focus on since we often had patients with brain injuries, alcohol/drug withdrawal, or delirium, and often all three. This particular patient group presented unique challenges to the nursing staff. We surveyed staff and found that the communication process with the physician teams was ineffective. In September of that same year, we began twice-a-week multidisciplinary trauma rounds which included not just the nurses and physicians, but the entire team, including physical therapy, care coordination, trauma CNS, social work, the director, the educator, and the psychiatric CNS, along with other disciplines as needed.

OUR CULTURE CHANGE

The engagement of staff in this performance improvement initiative increased awareness of safety concerns existing in our unit. Oftentimes, just as staff nurses can work separately even though they are right alongside one another, so too can the director and educator work separately from staff. This type of initiative took our entire staff coming together, facing the reality of the situation and having the energy to try another way—and it wasn't easy at times. We needed to be honest about our areas of deficiency and we needed to be willing to go back to a topic over and over until we got it right. We realized that our leadership team could increase their data sharing and give feedback not only to the NIC group, but also to every staff nurse on our unit. We succeeded in decreasing our fall rate by 35%, reducing employee turnover by 9%, and calling 50% fewer "code grays" or requests for security support on the unit. We needed to be willing to part with the illusion of perfection we wanted to believe existed. It was be painful at times, but in the end we gained so much more.

The second lesson learned was that peer-led practice changes could be very successful. This was our unit's first real attempt at having staff model the new way of approaching a patient population. Watching the group coming together was one of the best parts of the experience. Having a nurse assist another nurse who was struggling with providing care to a delirious patient is not only rewarding to the staff involved, but also rewarding for the director and educator. Most important, the patient and family, who might not even notice the difference, received better care. It seemed that when given more information on delirium and a basic focus on communication skills, staff nurses developed the voice that had been missing. Watching the relationships among all team members develop in a positive manner was rewarding.

Giving staff nurses a chance to practice their new knowledge in a safe setting was essential. We have had experiences where nurses are taught in a classroom setting but then never have the chance to actually implement the changes they have learned. In the change process we used, our nurses formulated plans for the patient and revisited the plans repeatedly, often involving the director and educator as sounding boards. Change can be challenging, but luckily we chose the right people for the "delirium expert" role, who took the knowledge from the class and put it into practice the very next day. It was also nice to see one nurse helping out another nurse. It created a team environment rather than a "my patient" and "your patient" mentality. The delirious patient became "our patient."

REFERENCE

Pandharipande, P., et al. (2008). Prevalence and risk factors for development of delirium in surgical and trauma intensive care unit patients. *Journal of Trauma, Injury, Infection & Critical Care, 65*(1), 34–41.

The Ethics of Caring

12.1 Ethics Conversations in Real Time: The Clinical Ethics Program at BWH

Martha Jurchak

*I*n 1996, BWH created the Ethics Service, a 24/7 consultation service staffed by a physician-director and nurse assistant director and supported by a full-time administrative assistant. I came to the Brigham and Women's Hospital (BWH) in 1999 as the assistant director. In the following 3 years, we worked to increase BWH's knowledge of and access to ethics consultation, which was available to anyone in the hospital who wanted help addressing the ethical aspects of clinical care. Patients, family members, nurses, and physicians called in increasing numbers. In our effort to "get the word out" and increase knowledge about and access to the service, I offered the nursing executive directors and directors the opportunity to work with them to address issues of ethics on their units. Some I never heard from. Some called me to ask about education programs or "talk sessions"; some invited me to conduct rounds.

I was appointed director of the Ethics Service in 2004 after the retirement of the physician-director. Collaborating with the co-chairs of the ethics committee, we expanded the group of clinicians providing ethics consultation, maintaining our commitment to multidisciplinary participation and colleagueship. Our model of ethics consultation was consistent with the recommendation of the national organization, the American Society for Bioethics and Humanities (Ausilio, Arnold, & Youngner, 2000). Called *ethics facilitation*, it reflects the focus of interpersonal conflict resolution and philosophical case analysis needed for concurrent ethics consultation. The ethics committee and the consultation service aimed to build and foster a vibrant moral community at BWH, where difference was expected and dialogue encouraged. In the words of M. U. Walker (1993), we sought to keep "moral spaces open" in the organization for conversation about differences in ethical values. This aim was consistent with the mission of the organization and vision of the nursing department— *excellence in patient care, with the best staff, in the safest environment*. It also contributed to the evolution of the nursing practice model at BWH that was being developed.

Ethics is essentially about the questions "What is good?" and "What is the right thing to do?" These questions are elemental in clinical practice. All health care professionals entertain an essential question when caring for a patient: "What is good for this patient?" Most of the time, this question is quickly answered without conflict: clarity about practice guidelines, the patient's diagnosis, and interests of the patient all align to move care along a clear and unconflicted course. This does not mean that the questions of ethics are not present, only that they are easily addressed. We tend to notice ethical issues when there is ambiguity, uncertainty, or conflict. Having affirmed that ethics is a fundamental aspect of nursing practice, how can we engage nurses in these questions, help develop the skills necessary for discernment of options, and then encourage the agency and, sometimes, the moral courage to act on the identified choice?

I addressed this question organically in my role as nurse-ethicist at BWH. I worked to be responsive to the questions of ethics wherever they arose. I applied this "wide-angle" view to ethics consultation requests. In nursing development forums, when I talked about the 24/7 availability of the ethics consultation beeper, I encouraged, "Don't just call when you *know* you want an ethics consultation. Call us when you're wondering 'Is this the right thing to do? I'm not sure this is best for the patient.' Don't worry alone! Call us!" And nurses did!

Because the offer was taken up, we can share the stories in this book that make specific what might have only been imagined. What do these stories reflect? They represent an interest in meeting nurses where they are. Following a fundamental tenet of adult learning, we build on our learners' acquired knowledge and skills that brought them to this point on their journey. The stories reflect the lived experiences of moral courage, moral uncertainty, and moral distress. Ethics conversations give voice to the challenges of "pushing back" against the assumptions that can or have kept nurses "in the middle," "powerless," and as "victims" of the perceived institutional power structures.

My aim is to stay in the conversation about ethics—with nurses, physicians, and other health care colleagues, and with patients and their families. Staying in the conversation means helping nurses develop the language of ethics that allows them to clarify their viewpoint and discuss issues of concern. It means creating the opportunities for inquiry and discourse in rounds. It means encouraging reflections on practice that acknowledge "the good" and encourage "the better." This work enacts the Department of Nursing mission: *excellence in patient care, with the best staff, in the safest environment.*

REFERENCES

Ausilio, M. P., Arnold, R. M., & Youngner, S. J. (2000). Health care ethics consultation: Nature, goals, and competencies. *Annals of Internal Medicine, 133,* 59–69.

Walker, M. U. (1993). Keeping moral spaces open. *Hastings Center Report, 23*(2), 33–40.

12.2 *Strengthening Moral Agency in New ICU Nurses*

Martha Jurchak and Mary Pennington

The Brigham and Women's Hospital (BWH) has more than 110 adult critical care beds staffed by more than 600 nurses. On an annual basis, 40 to 60 new nurses are hired into open positions in the intensive care unit (ICU) and participate in a critical care nurse-intern program, the gateway to ICU practice at BWH. New nurses are recruited from the medical-surgical intermediate units or directly out of school for the program, which has a robust curriculum prioritizing knowledge of fundamental pathophysiologic processes and interventions sequenced with clinical experiences through a dedicated preceptorship model. It is evidence based, consistent with American Association of Critical Care Nurses (AACN) professional guidelines and standards, and is benchmarked against other academic centers' programs.

Early qualitative program evaluation data were positive on all program aspects—with *one* exception. The critical care nurse-interns reported feeling unprepared, confused, conflicted, and upset in response to ethical issues they observed or experienced in the ICU. Some were shocked by the regularity with which life-and-death decisions were made by the interdisciplinary teams. Often the new nurses felt angry when they perceived that families were offered "false hope" with aggressive therapies that appeared only to prolong death and suffering.

> Although SK could not communicate any type of pain or suffering to us, I did feel that our treatment measures were prolonging her overall physiological distress, rather than improving it, which to me translates into suffering. As a caregiver, I felt as though I was doing things "to" the patient, rather than "for" the patient.

It is well known that ethical problems and worries are commonly encountered in critical care practices. This expectation occurs, however, in the context of substantive expectations placed on the nurse within the American Nurses Association Nursing Code of Ethics (2008):

- ■ "Nurses must bring forward difficult issues related to patient care and/or institutional constraints upon ethical practice for discussion and review" (p. 13).
- ■ "The nurse has a responsibility to express moral perspectives, even when they differ from those of others and even when they might not prevail" (p. 19).

Critical care nursing practice is fast paced, with continuous data coming to the nurse and with minute-to-minute decisions being made about treatment. Nurses often do not reflect on or process the emotions generated by the life-changing events in the ICU. How are these experiences processed? How do we teach and support the ethical skill of advocacy? Education for nurses on strategies for intentionally reflecting on moral perspectives is rarely offered in orientation programs. Nurses are expected to learn the skill of ethical reasoning through observation of peers, seemingly through osmosis. This approach tends to be inconsistent and unreliable.

Historically, critical care orientation programs prioritize the acquisition of technical skills, clinical knowledge, surveillance, efficiency, and organization. Yet, the profession of nursing is grounded in an ethical model. How are moral agency and ethical comportment developed, strengthened, and sustained for nurses?

We wanted to do something about these unmet and often unacknowledged needs of new critical care nurses. Each of us could bring our personal expertise to a shared concern. The critical care expertise of the intern program director (Mary Pennington) and the ethics expertise of the ethics director (Martha Jurchak) combined to create a program that not only addressed these needs but also made a direct impact on the quality of care the nurses were prepared to deliver. We achieved this through a targeted educational intervention. Our first step was to better understand the problem we were addressing. For us, this intervention was a very specific way to implement the BWH Department of Nursing (DON) vision.

NEW NURSES AND THE RISK OF DISENGAGEMENT

Benner, Tanner and Chesla (2009) have described new nurses as advanced beginners who commonly experience pervasive anxiety. These nurses regularly articulate their fear of harming a patient due to their lack of experience, driving them to rely on experienced nurses, protocols, guidelines, rules, and standards to guide clinical decision making. In the technical jungle of critical care, advanced beginners manage anxiety by viewing their patient as a list of tasks. Once the new nurses master the technical skills and tasks, they begin to see and connect with the patient as a person who has a family, a life, hopes, and dreams. This connection facilitates the development of caring practices and ethical comportment. Benner names this phenomenon "engagement" and defines it as the "emotional involvement or connection with a person and/or the situation", Hooper-Kyriakidis & Stannard, (Benner, 1999, p. 567).

As nurses move from advanced beginner to competent clinician, they begin to stand on their own two feet. Sometimes, because the new nurse "looks good" and appears independent, the manager, educator, or preceptor will begin to withdraw support and let them "fly on their own." It is during this transition that the new nurse may begin to wonder: "Why are we aggressively treating this patient when we know she will die?" "Why are we pressuring the family to donate their son's organs?" "Is terminal extubation ethical?" During this time of budding awareness, new nurses begin to notice things that create discomfort for them. Despite "looking good", new nurses may feel confused about the complex ethical issues that regularly bubble up in the ICU. They may wonder how to be a patient advocate.

This external appearance of clinical competency, coupled with the less visible inner dialogue of uncertainty and questioning, may lead preceptors to miss this teaching opportunity. To anchor these clinical experiences with caring practices, advanced beginners need a safe space to reflect on their nursing practice. The cost of not providing time and space to reflect on these issues is high: for the nurse, the patient, and the profession. It is also essential that the new nurse be guided and mentored through these vulnerable times. We believed that critical care orientation must include a model that creates space for new nurses to tell the story of their angst. We were convinced that when reflection is not part of orientation, the stage is set for disengagement.

Our direct experiences with our nurse-interns validated our convictions further. Many BWH nurse-interns were distraught and discouraged by the frequency of conflicting opinions between physicians and nurses or between clinicians and family members and the ambiguity of identifying the "right" thing to do. Some of the nurse-interns remained outside the situation, not seeing themselves as having the power to influence how a situation unfolded, but experiencing it as observers. Silence when confronted with perceived wrongs sets the stage for disengagement by damaging ethical values and self-esteem (Kelly, 1998). The research of Patricia Benner and colleagues (Benner, Hooper-Kyriakidis, & Stannard, 1999) finds that engaged ethical reasoning necessitates the nurse's involvement in the situation. Detachment from the clinical situation obstructs the development of the skill of ethical reasoning. As one intern noted:

> Although Mr. M.'s family knew of his very poor prognosis, they were not proactive in making decisions regarding Mr. M.'s care. I feel that this is because the doctors told them that they would not have to make any decisions for nearly 2 weeks after his admission. By delaying decisions regarding treatment, the staff put him at risk for not only further neurologic decline, but nosocomial infections, skin breakdown, DVTs, PEs, malnutrition and sepsis, just to name a few. I felt that Mr. M. was not being advocated for efficiently. His family should have been given options as soon as possible and been informed about the benefits of making decisions early in critical care.

When faced with ethical problems and worries, the critical care nurse-interns experienced moral distress, and some began to distance themselves from the ethical issues. When new nurses fail to engage, they don't necessarily leave the job. They come to work and competently perform the technical and clinical portions of their role. Yet they have no authentic patient connection, no story, and really no nursing practice, as there is no caring nurse-patient relationship. Symptoms of disengagement include not being in a relationship with the patient, viewing the patient as a diagnosis or outside one's own community, and approaching the patient as a list of tasks to be completed. This phenomenon prevents the nurse from acknowledging and responding to the patient's suffering (Benner et al., 1999). It also creates the conditions for moral distress.

MORAL DISTRESS

Moral distress is defined as a situation that occurs when a person knows (or perceives that he or she knows) the right course of action but cannot act upon it (Jameton, 1984). The result is psychological disequilibrium, painful emotions, and feelings of low professional self-esteem. When nurses experience moral distress, they may feel like they are acting against their personal and/or professional values.

Unresolved ethical problems that cause moral distress for critical care nurses may lead to disengagement if they passively accept or compromise at the expense of doing what they know to be the right action. Research shows that significant changes in ethical and professional values can occur when new nurses transition into practice, and are predicated on the extent to which new nurses incorporate the norms and values of the hospital culture as their own (Kelly, 1998). For new nurses, entry into practice is the time to develop and strengthen moral agency as they find their voice. Although nursing schools include ethics education for students, it has not been demonstrated to decrease the difficulty new nurses have in articulating their concerns. For new nurses to become self-determining, independent thinkers, and move into their role of patient advocacy, we concluded that deliberate and targeted education was needed. This specific educational intervention was consistent with the goal of transforming nursing practice at the bedside and actualizing the BWH DON vision.

Narratives

Toward the end of ICU orientation, each nurse-intern is asked to write a narrative describing an ethical problem that he or she experienced or witnessed during orientation. The narrative story provides a window into exploring the moral experiences of the nurse.

We ask them to consider the following questions:

- What were your concerns?
- How did you understand this ethical problem?
- How did you feel about the decisions made?
- Who was available to help you think about this?

The nurses come back as a group and share their experiences with each other, the nurse ethicist, and the critical care program director. We use the narrative as a tool to stimulate a conversation about an ethical framework, moral agency, and nursing practice.

Creating an Intervention

In designing this intervention, we had several goals. We wanted to introduce a framework for ethical analysis. We wanted to use the problems the ICU nurse-interns themselves identified as problematic as case examples that would be the focus of our intervention; we would apply our framework to the nurse-interns' narratives. The narrative provides an opportunity for the nurse-interns to think about their thinking, reflect on what was done, and uncover assumptions made. We also wanted to help them identify the resources in the institution that are available for addressing ethical issues.

We believe that the identification of ethical problems is inherently complex. Like much of clinical practice, the challenge is in finding patterns, identifying the issues from a sea of information and data. In clinical ethics, the questions of ethics—"What is right?" or "What is good?"—often first arise in nurses as a feeling of discomfort or anxiety (Alderson, 1991). Nurses often express their initial concerns about the ethical aspects of care in terms of feeling: "I just don't feel like we are doing the right thing. My gut told me this wasn't a good thing to be doing." The feeling of something being wrong or "off" initiates the identification of a potential ethical problem.

The challenge for clinicians is to move from their affective connection to the problem to an intellectual engagement with understanding and resolving it. Put another way, ethical problem identification is driven by affect and feeling while the work of ethical problem solving is driven by cognitive, intellectual processing. One almost always has a "gut reaction," an immediate response. But these unreflective, off-the-cuff initial answers to "What's the right thing to do?" do not reflect our best thinking. By systematically working through the elements of a framework for ethical problems in clinical care, new possibilities emerge; different perspectives can be considered, often leading to new insights about the problem at hand. The new awareness, often expressed as genuinely as, "Oh, I never thought of it *that* way," emerges out of the systematic application of a framework.

Many authors and clinical ethicists have suggested frameworks, and they contain several similar elements: attending to the factual information from which decisions about what to do must be made, identification of the persons who have moral authority or a stake in the decisional outcome, and a clear identification of the ethical problem or ethical issues. We elected to use the framework developed and tested by Jurchak (McCormick & Jurchak, 2006) over several years of work in clinical ethics, the FESOR framework. The acronym captures the essential elements of an ethical case analysis framework:

F—Facts
E—Ethical question or problem
S—Stakeholders
O—Options for addressing the ethical problem
R—Reevaluation of choice of option made

In our work with the interns, we briefly review this model, and also review the principles of bioethics and their meaning—autonomy, beneficence, nonmaleficence, and justice (Beauchamp & Childress, 1994). We then use narratives to apply the framework. The narratives that the nurse-interns write are stories about an ethical problem that they either experienced or observed during their critical care orientation. Some of the themes from the narratives have included:

- Differing opinions about choice for care among physicians, nurses, and families, particularly when the nurses who are telling the story believe they know what the patient wanted
- Responding to families when they are "hoping for a miracle" or have decided to "leave the decision in God's hands"
- Dealing with families that "want everything done"
- Limiting or withdrawing treatment when it is perceived as "giving up" on the patient
- Dealing with families or patients who request treatment that the nurses involved would not choose or do not think is best
- Providing support and care to patients when nurses believe that the medical team has disengaged from the patient who transitions from an acute unstable ICU patient to "chronic ICU patient"; noting that the emotional and ongoing treatment care of the chronic patient seems to fall primarily on the nurse and wondering how to reengage the medical team

EVALUATION

Because we were interested in measuring the impact of this work, we developed an evaluation survey and sent it to those who had completed the program. The evaluation was sent 6 to 12 months after completion of the program and the results confirmed that many of our goals were achieved. The goals were to provide a framework for thinking through ethical problems and to identify the institutional resources available that support ethical problem solving at the bedside. Survey responses further amplified these findings.

Feedback has been positive. The following are excerpts from survey evaluations:

> I feel that after the ethics program, I was able to better understand some things, know and learn that so much of what I was feeling was ok and not wrong. The ability to express how difficult these ethical situations can be. I felt supported. It was at that moment that I started to feel, though this was going to be a very big challenge in my life: I came to the ICU to make a difference and this is what I was going to do.

CONCLUSION

Excellence in modern critical care nursing demands nursing practice that is psychologically engaged, technically expert, and intellectually astute. In preparing new ICU nurses to meet these multiple demands, our initial program focus on the technical skill sets was revealed to be inadequate regarding ethical skill development. Our response was to create a program that addressed professional development, disengagement risk, and moral distress through the use of narratives. Identifying an ethical problem and writing about it in a narrative requires ICU nurse-interns to locate themselves in the context of the new ICU environment and culture and to find their voice in expressing their views. Discussing the narratives provides the opportunity to use a framework for ethical problem solving and to familiarize new staff with the nurse-ethicist, as well as providing a link to the 24-hour consult service available for addressing ethical problems and an invitation to use it in the future. The act of discussing the narratives with peers as well as clinical experts fosters an environment for reflection and critical thinking that acknowledges current problems, as well as sowing seeds of reminder of future supports.

This program has been ongoing for the past 5 years, with 181 nurse graduates from it. The narratives that the nurse-interns write have become richer over time. We believe this is due to shifting the culture through reflective practice: Now, nurse-interns are precepted by nurses who have been through the critical care nurse-intern program. The current BWH ICU preceptors coach and mentor the new nurses as they write about their ethical problems. Our critical care nurse-intern program provides support for the DON vision of excellence in nursing practice by creating a reflective practice model based on ethical comportment and agency.

REFERENCES

Alderson, P. (1991). Bioethics ignores human emotions [abstract]. *Bulletin of Medical Ethics, 68,* 13–21.

American Nurses Association. (2008). *Code of ethics for nurses with interpretative statements.* Silver Spring, MD: Nursingbooks.

Beauchamp, T., & Childress, J. (1994). *Principles of biomedical ethics.* New York, NY: Oxford University Press.

Benner, P., Tanner, C., & Chesla, C. (2009). *Expertise in nursing practice: Caring, clinical judgment, and ethics* (2nd ed.). New York, NY: Springer Publishing.

Benner, P., Hooper-Kyriakidis, P., & Stannard, D. (1999). *Clinical wisdom and interventions in critical care: A thinking-in-action approach.* Philadelphia, PA: Saunders.

Jameton, A. (1984). *Nursing practice: The ethical issues.* Englewood, NJ: Prentice Hall.

Kelly, B. (1998). Preserving moral integrity: A follow-up study with new graduate nurses. *Journal of Advanced Nursing, 28*(5), 1134–1145.

McCormick, M., & Jurchak, M. (2006). A pathway for moral reasoning in home healthcare. *Home Healthcare Nurse, 24*(10), 654–661.

12.3 *The Inquiry of Ethics Rounds*

Martha Jurchak and Elizabeth Eagan-Bengston

Nurses who practice in any acute care setting must not only be expert clinicians. They are equally challenged by a myriad of complex moral situations: end-of-life decision making, the use of technology that prolongs death, patient autonomy, and the many clinical decisions that require consensus among a diverse number of stakeholders. The ethical practice of nurses is put to the test every day, and even highly experienced nurses struggle with these challenging ethical dilemmas. The complex challenges of ethical responsibility are increasingly the focus of the nurse's framework of patient management in the ICUs and other patient care areas. At Brigham and Women's Hospital (BWH), the focus on ethics has been heightened as we have worked to enact the Department of Nursing (DON) vision statement: *"Excellent care to patients and families with the very best staff in the safest environment."* The ethical challenges the BWH nurse faces are shaped by all three dimensions of nursing articulated in this statement: care, staff, and safety.

In this chapter we tell our shared story of addressing those ethical challenges by initiating ethics rounds: Elizabeth as an assistant nurse director in the Coronary Care Unit (CCU) and the intermediate medical cardiology unit, and Martha in her role as BWH's nurse-ethicist. The nursing staff includes a blend of high-level expert nurses and moderately experienced to novice nurses. Over the past few decades, we have witnessed the evolution of new and advanced drug therapies, devices, and life-sustaining interventions that have counteracted diseases and prolonged life. While we can be quick to marvel and feel excitement about how these resources have changed the course of many illnesses, they have also ushered in ethically perplexing questions about patient/family situations. These new technologies have not only prompted new choices for patients, but also raised many questions for nurses at the bedside. Whether the patient concern is about continuing life support or initiating lifesaving actions that prolong death, these complex situations make it difficult to know what the right thing is for any given patient who is acutely ill.

Before we started ethics rounds, the CCU nursing staff had some prior experience with participating in informal ethics discussions, led by Martha as the hospital's nurse-ethicist. The discussions were held at a time when the word *ethics* elicited a "last resort" response from many of the unit's attending physicians. Nurses felt that if they requested an ethics consult, the physicians would see the nurse as questioning their clinical judgment. What the nurses really sought was the ability to speak honestly about their concerns or ethical uncertainties.

Often the nursing staff encountered physicians who were reluctant to discuss issues of redirecting a patient's care, withdrawing treatment, or even considering choices that would limit available treatment. When the nurses were able to initiate these conversations, they often felt they had unproductive, negative exchanges yielding few solutions. The contrast between the physicians' perspectives and the nurses' perspectives created a communication gap about the right thing to do for any given patient. It was this lack of understanding of each other's views that was impeding an open exchange about what was best for the patient, seeming to focus instead on what felt better for the individual caregiver.

These early conversations between the nursing staff and the nurse-ethicist began to give voice and credibility to the nurses' feelings and perspectives about their patient experiences. The discussions gave nurses the courage to share their "worries" in an open and safe forum and gave rise to a sense of "freedom without judgment," along with new confidence in their nursing practice and voice as patient advocates. The nurses felt that having the expertise of a nurse-ethicist provided "in the moment" guidance for identifying ethical dilemmas and facilitating tough discussions. These early discussions set the stage for what in time emerged as "ethics rounds." We had begun a tenuous program.

THE MOVE MOVED US

The cardiovascular service was moving to a new building (Chapter 17). The nursing management team began the work and planning for what promised to be a challenging process. Priorities shifted; so did our effort in creating ethics rounds, which got shunted to a back burner until the move was complete. The new building, which offered a unique environment for the patient/family care experience, also allowed family members to stay overnight with patients in the room, thus adding valuable dimensions of interaction with families, nurses, and the rest of the team. Our treatment philosophy, while always espousing concern for the family, now embraced their concerns, interests, and presence "front and center."

As the nursing staff assimilated into this new patient/family-centered care environment, they began to raise questions and engage in discussions about support, not only in managing their patient's medical care, but also dealing with the sometimes constant physical presence of family members in the room. There was much anticipation and some anxiety among the nurses prior to the move about the presence of family members in a patient's room. Many expressed a concern that such intense family presence might impede care. Interestingly, many of the more senior nurses had concerns about how it would feel to have family members right in the room while giving care.

These concerns opened the door again for us to refocus on ethics rounds. We realized that we could explore these issues through collaboration with the Ethics Service, which could thereby support our nurses and enhance their practice by giving them a chance to explore their concerns. We believed that if we provided a safe, nonconfrontational forum for discussion, our nurses could learn to work through routine concerns that appeared as barriers and ethical uncertainties.

So it was that the nurse director, assistant nurse director, and nurse-ethicist met to revisit their delayed implementation of formal weekly ethics rounds in both our CCU and our intermediate medical cardiology unit. It was agreed that the need for a regular forum existed. Indeed, the move had unveiled additional new dilemmas that warranted our attention. Our intent was to further cultivate the relationship between the nursing staff and the Ethics Service through our partnership with the nurse-ethicist. The CCU nursing leadership's decision to implement ethics rounds demonstrated a commitment to honestly address a salient need: nurses needing a space to share their often unspoken thoughts of distress on how to manage tough discussions with patients or family members as well as physician colleagues. We all concurred: nurses needed help with working through ethical worries or uncertainties.

RESPONDING TO THE NEED

The nurse director, assistant nurse director, and nurse-ethicist meetings led to a plan for addressing ethical concerns that nursing staff identified. We recognized that the ethics-rounds intervention had been successful in other units and could be replicated here. Ethics rounds are based on the assumption that "ethics" is a fundamental aspect of patient care. This is because ethics is about determining what is the right action to take or what constitutes "doing good" in a situation. Patient care requires that clinicians consider, in an ongoing manner, what are the right actions or good care. The questions of what is right or good may be quickly and easily answered—practice standards or the weight of evidence may point clearly to a good intervention to a clinical problem, so that the questions of ethics float below the plane of consciousness—until there is a conflict. Reflecting on clinical practice, thinking about what "good care" for a patient looks like, or giving voice to a nurse's internal musings about what is the right thing to do is at the heart of ethics rounds. They are a regularly scheduled opportunity to discuss the ethics of clinical practice with colleagues and an ethicist facilitator.

The format we agreed to was a weekly rounds led by the assistant nurse director and nurse-ethicist while engaging the nurse-in-charge (NIC) and the nurse caring for the patient, as well as other nursing or multidisciplinary staff as available. Each week we would start rounds by approaching the NIC, asking if there were any ethical questions, issues, or worries with any patients or families on the unit. Other questions followed, such as: "Who is the patient who worries you the most?" "Which patient is taking the most time in the unit?" "Of the patients here today, who would you say is the most 'problematic'?" After we had identified a patient and a worry, we included the nurse caring for the patient in the now-widening discussion. Our aim was clear: to engage the nurses in reflection on their practice.

The general structure of an inquiry-based ethics rounds begins with a brief summary of the clinical situation by the nurse. This is followed by an exploration of the ethical worry or concern by the nurse-ethicist, description of options for understanding or managing, and a plan for "next steps." For example, after hearing from the NIC that a particular patient had a vague history of drug abuse and had been refusing some medications and testing and demanding others, we moved the conversation of ethics rounds to the nurse, who was frustrated with the patient's lack of cooperativeness. We framed the issue as one of unmet trust expectations, and asked: "Do you know what he hoped or expected from the hospital admission?" She didn't, and agreed that it was a good question. From here, the team happened to come by on rounds and we engaged them as well in the question: "What do you think 'good care' for this patient looks like?" Options were considered and a tentative plan was formulated.

It was our belief that this format of inquiry supported our project goals to:

1. Provide a structured time and setting for nursing staff to have an "at-the-moment" opportunity to speak openly and comfortably about ethical concerns as they arose for "just-in-time" problem solving.

2. Use the resource of the nurse-ethicist for "just-in-time" teaching, problem solving, and triage of ethical problems.
3. Reinforce the message that institutional resources were available to address ethical issues in patient care.
4. Reinforce nursing leaderships' recognition and support of identifying and addressing ethical aspects of patient care.

These goals supported the DON vision of providing excellent patient care by helping the nurse to identify ethical problems and engage in problem solving about them before they became conflicts. It also supported the leadership group in their development of nursing practice through reflection.

To introduce ethics rounds and build support, we held three informational lunch sessions for the nurses-in-charge and the staff nurses over a 2-week period. These sessions gave the CCU nursing leadership and the nurse-ethicist an opportunity to introduce the idea to the staff, explain the goals, describe the format, and answer questions. We considered the response to be "cautiously accepting," with few questions asked. We did notice, however, that the discussion focused on one of two consistent topics. The first was about a current patient who was challenging, problematic, or "ethically worrisome." The second focused on a challenging but long-since-discharged patient: The nurses recalled gathering together to talk about the questions or issues this patient had generated. These themes were very helpful to us. We took them as endorsements for the program and a strong indication of the need for the rounds.

We also met with the NIC group at one of their regularly scheduled monthly meetings. Though the presentation was the same as it had been to the staff nurses, the response from this group was more lukewarm. There was little discussion and few questions, although when asked, they endorsed our plan and (cautiously) agreed to participate. One imagined they were thinking, "What are we getting into?" Indeed, a question we might all be asking!

With the goals identified and the introduction accomplished, we launched into implementing the rounds. Each week, the nurse director, assistant nurse director, and the nurse-ethicist would meet in a different unit of the CCU and intermediate care units.

The nurse-ethicist developed a standard opening statement she used in approaching the NIC: "We are doing ethics rounds, which is an opportunity on a weekly basis to touch base about the patients and families who are here currently, and to find out if there are any ethical questions or worries with them. The issues don't have to be an ethical dilemma, but can just be questions that have come up related to ethics—about what's right or good to do. Anything come up with these patients?"

Responses have been highly variable. They run the gamut from "Quiet; no problems" and "Oh, I forgot we had these rounds" to "It's so lucky you are here today! We were just talking in report about what are we going to do with this patient!" and "You have got to go and talk to Joan—she is having a really hard time with that patient!" Sometimes, in conversation with the NIC, we will engage in a shared discovery about a patient situation that warrants our attention. The conversation will start out with a look down the list of current patients, with a two- or three-word commentary on each one as the NIC scans the list, identifying each patient: "no problem," "going home," "delirious, but under control," "problems with wife, but social work is on it" . . . until we hit a worry:

"Now this one may be one you want to talk about. The patient has been admitted four times in the past 3 months. His heart failure is really in the final stages. The docs have said to us they've run out of options for how to manage his failure. And yet he comes in . . . again. He's been here 3 days now, and there's no code status! No one seems to have had the discussion with him about what he wants us to do if he codes . . . and he will! The docs just seem afraid to have that conversation with him . . . and you know what happens: The nurse is left holding the bag. That is just not fair! Now that's something you could do something about!"

In this specific situation, the nurse-ethicist engaged the nurse in inquiry. The dialogue that follows demonstrates how ethics rounds as inquiry might proceed. The nurse-ethicist starts the conversation.

"Yes, that sounds like a really worrisome situation! I wonder what the patient is thinking about all this—four hospitalizations so close together. He must be scared or worried, or who knows what. Do you know what he thinks of this? What meaning do all these admissions have for him? And I wonder what he thinks about resuscitation? Do you know?"

The nurse replies "No," but speculates: "I bet he thinks it's like what happens on TV. Most patients do. You know, you suddenly go, and the code team rushes in and works on you, and you are fine and walk out the next day! It sure doesn't happen like that!"

The nurse-ethicist probes: "Do you think the nurse might start that conversation?"

The reply: "I don't think so! We can get our heads chopped off [by the doctors] for telling the patients what we think, especially when it's different from whatever they [the doctors] were going to tell them."

The nurse-ethicist persists: "I wasn't thinking so much about the nurse telling the patient what the code status should be. I was thinking more about trying to find out what the patient thinks about it, just trying to get a read on where he is."

The nurse asks, "What do you mean?"

The nurse-ethicist continues: "I was imagining something like the nurse, while making the bed or maybe even finishing the nursing assessment, saying to the patient something like 'I know you've had to come into the hospital a lot in the past few months and I was wondering what you thought about that.' It would be an opening to find out where the patient is about the progression of his heart failure. Does he not have a clue about what it means? Is he scared or worried, and hasn't talked to anybody about that yet? Is he more worried about his wife? Who knows! But it would be an entry into finding out. Related to that, you could ask the question, 'Have you thought about what you wanted to do if you had a cardiac arrest?' So, it's really about asking questions; about inquiry. It's not about telling the patient anything, really. It's about listening and providing the space for them to talk about where they are. Do you see the difference?"

This nurse did.

We thanked the nurse, reminded her that we'd be back next week, and moved onto the next unit. As we were making rounds, the nurse director and assistant began to talk about how universal the themes we were discovering were across the units. They also noted that they saw differences in practice among the nurses and wondered how to engage the staff in the reflections and conversation that would encourage exploration of these recurrent themes. We stopped to discuss this more carefully. We determined that the difference in nursing practice that we were concerned about could be described in different ways:

■ The difference between "telling" patients and "asking" them
■ The difference between a checklist approach to patient interactions and an inquiry approach
■ The difference between seeing patient care as a series of tasks to be done versus engaging and "knowing" the patient

As we reflected on what themes we were discovering in ethics rounds, we observed that they gave the CCU nursing leadership an opportunity to better understand their staff and the nursing practice they provided. Leadership and staff were also seeing both from a different angle: Inquiry of rounds was opening a window into nursing practice issues as well as becoming an avenue for problem solving for particular patients. Some of the themes we noted and discussed included:

■ What are the obligations we have to the family of an international patient, when he or she arrives with little money, no place to stay, an inability to speak English, and no experience ever having been outside their native country?
■ What does advocacy for patients look like when they have lost decisional capacity and their spouses or health care proxies seem to the nurse to not be making decisions based on the patients' best interests but their own?
■ How do we address the needs and complications after a patient has accused a nurse of abusive care while hospitalized, when investigation reveals that the patient's response seems to be related to posttraumatic stress disorder unrecognized by the patient?
■ How do we manage the feelings that are activated in staff when they react to a patient who makes choices staff believe do not promote well-being and health?
■ How do we address the issues that arise when a staff person's family member becomes a patient?
■ How do we address the challenges to our commitment to family-centered care when we assess the family as one with poor boundaries, who have difficulty respecting the privacy of other patients, or whose requests, demands, and attention take an "unfair" amount of staff time?
■ How can we address the structure of nursing work and how it promotes or impedes good care for a particular patient (e.g., "The night shift always does this!")?
■ How can nurses better understand and work with religious and cultural influences that lead to what is seen as controversial health care choices?

From our discussions and our emerging list of themes, we determined that it would be useful to keep a feedback stream open with the NICs, and so met with them 3 months into the start of ethics rounds to check in. Their feedback was useful and informative. The NICs observed that the focus of the discussion in ethics rounds had shifted from talk about tasks and "nurse-centered concerns" (the work the nurse felt burdened by) to more patient-centered discussions. It was their view that the rounds had evolved, with more engagement in questions such as:

- What does good nursing care for this patient look like?
- What is impeding good care for this patient?
- What does it mean to be accountable for nursing care for this patient?
- What are our habits of practice that foster—or inhibit—care of this patient?
- How do our handoffs/continuity-of-care practices impact on patient care?

Using the narrative process that has guided much of the work of vision implementation at BWH in the DON, we were able to further articulate this change as seen through the eyes of the assistant nurse director. The following narrative by her captures our awareness of change and progress.

We were rounding on the last unit that day. We checked in with the charge nurse and asked if there were any issues that we could help with. The charge RN directed us to the nurse caring for Mr. S. Mr. S. was a 50-year-old male who had arrested, went on to have a very complicated medical course, and was now at the end of his life. His family held a constant vigil at his bedside. We approached the nurse and asked if there was any issue we could assist with.

It was obvious to us that the nurse was having a hard time or was in conflict. He immediately launched into the fact that his patient was CMO (Comfort Measures Only) and he was giving care that to him did not make sense. He posed the questions in succession to us: "Why are they ordering tests on this patient? Why am I replacing labs when this patient is a CMO? Why are we doing so much? It makes no sense!" It was clear the nurse did not understand the difference between CMO status and the withdrawal of care. The distress he was experiencing was palpable.

We listened while he vented his frustration. I remember the look of struggle on his face. It was in this moment when the nurse-ethicist brings such clarity to a challenging situation. She quietly walked to the computer and brought back a copy of the BWH's CMO Policy to share with the nurse. With much sensitivity toward the nurse, she directed him to specific areas of the policy to review with him and redirect his angst. She engaged the nurse in a conversation that emphasized the idea that certain interventions at end of life are regularly included in CMO care of the patient to ensure patient comfort and dignity. His struggle was driven by a lack of understanding.

The conversation that ensued between the nurse-ethicist and the nurse was done with gentle respect but to the point. The nurse appeared somewhat embarrassed but definitely well served by this exchange. I think our intervention at that moment created opportunity. First and foremost, it interrupted the nurse's cycle of distress that had created a barrier for him. His focus was driven by a cascade of negative thinking driven by a lack of understanding rather than what was best care for this patient. Second, he was given critical information that enabled him to refocus his attention and be empowered by next steps rather than being annoyed and distrusting. I knew we had made a difference in the direction of that patient's care and the nurse's ability to manage it in the best interest of the patient and family members. It was also an eye-opener for the leadership team that a senior clinician had such a misunderstanding of this policy. It highlighted and confirmed the knowledge that nurses perform at varied levels of capacity despite standardized practice policies.

As we have reflected back on the work accomplished since initiating weekly rounds, we identified several insights (that emerged from the intervention); insights that have helped both the staff nurse at the bedside and the unit leadership team. We have found that ethics rounds provide a forum for staff to reflect openly about any inner struggle or conflict that bothers them about a particular patient situation. They can ask for guidance: "What is the right thing to do with this situation?" Many times we have started our conversations with a nurse or charge nurses and find that they appear perplexed about a patient but are not readily able to form their question or present their concern, simply because they are uncertain. The nurse-ethicist's role is multilayered during these rounds: The nurse-ethicist offers nurses not only an expert opinion about an ethical worry or problem, but through questions also catalyzes insights that require nurses to think through their own questions and discover ways to form their questions! The nurse-ethicist facilitates our nurses' understanding of their worry and helps them to clarify their values. Ethical case analysis and exploration of their interpersonal conflicts guide them toward problem solving and resolution.

We have learned that the inquiry of ethics rounds, supported by nursing leadership, promotes respectful, open dialogue that acknowledges the differences in values among the nursing staff. Through inquiry of rounds, nurses are able to better understand their own questions or conflicts. It empowers our nurses to take action in the next step of their patient care. The outcome of each rounding varies. Often there is not an immediate answer and we agree that more involved follow-up is necessary. The nurse is guided toward potential options to consider and to pursue either with the team or the team working with the patient and family. Sometimes we come up with a plan in collaboration with the nurse about possible next steps to take. On occasion, the nurse-ethicist may recommend an ethics consult to facilitate a dialogue and, it is hoped, reach consensus amongst all parties.

We have also learned that ethics rounds give our nurse leaders an opportunity to participate on an active-listening basis. This makes it possible for them to stand back and observe: to hear the stories, the questions, the worries, and the exchange between the nurse-ethicist and the staff nurse. The role of nursing leadership is to listen to our nurses' experiences through their stories and learn about their individual practice. From this active listening we try to better identify what we can do to support our nurses' development and their clinical care at the bedside.

For our leadership team, the true value gained in participating in weekly ethics rounds is multilayered: There is a significant benefit to being able to observe individual behaviors and responses and thus identify things we might do as leaders both to support individual nurses and to develop nursing practice. This includes both development focused on ethical issues and other, more comprehensive, practice development concerns. An even better value for our team is that by listening to the path of inquiry and observing the nurse-ethicist's approach, our own skill set is enhanced. The concept of promoting ethical resolution through respectful communication has become a focus for the work in front of us. We too have become empowered by the need to engage in respectful but critical conversations with our nurses to support best practice.

CONCLUSION

Our journey with ethics rounds in the CCU and intermediate care units has been much like the journey of discovery of the DON. We identified a need, then developed a shared idea of how we might address it within the vision of the DON: providing *excellent care to patients and families with the best staff in the safest environment*. Our collaborations among the unit leadership team and the nurse-ethicist and with the NICs and staff nurses led us to an unexpected place of practice development and care improvement through inquiry on the fundamental question of our work: "What does good care look like for this patient and family?" Providing the conversation space for reflecting together has led to opportunities for teaching, support of the nursing staff, and intervention with problems, all of which support our aim of excellence and growth.

12.4 *Alleviating Moral Distress: A Journey to Create the Most Supportive Environment*

Cynthia Jodoin, Eileen Molina, and Katie Fillipon

We currently serve as nursing directors for the Hematology/Oncology/Hematopoietic Stem Cell Transplant Service (Heme/Onc/HSCT). Our Service also contains a palliative care population. This service consists of eleven separate units: three focus on solid tumor and pain/palliative care, one on high-risk HSCT patients, and seven are a mix of hematology/solid tumor and HSCT patients.

As the vision of the BWH Department of Nursing (DON) unfolded, we, as nursing directors of the oncology service, reflected upon how we could help nurses to feel supported and not alone. As a nurse, you face the loss of a life, the crisis of the grieving family, and the call from admitting asking when the bed will be available for the next patient—sometimes in a matter of moments. Having lived this experience ourselves and then observed it from a director role, the burden is truly palpable. In a busy work environment, it is a challenge to take time out to acknowledge these losses and cope with these difficult experiences. In order for our staff to make it through a day and be able to walk into the room next door with a smile after leaving a bedside vigil, it is critical to be able to create an environment that is supportive for them.

How do we create an environment that is healthy and allows nurses to reflect, process, and return to the bedside refreshed and ready to connect with the next patient and family? We had done some research and discussion around the moral distress that is inherent in witnessing human suffering and being part of difficult ethical decisions (Zuzelo, 2007; Shepard, 2010). In addition, the experience of assisting patients and families with death and dying profoundly affects nurses and continues to affect them years later (Gunther & Thomas, 2006). Moral distress also can adversely affect nurses' ability to care for their patients. Using methodologies that allow for discussion and communication around issues and expression of emotions can assist staff to deal with these traumatic patient events (Zuzelo, 2007).

The oncology service has 110 beds with more than 300 nurses. The day-to-day responsibilities encompassed by this patient population go far beyond their physical needs. Our nurses often struggle with the stress and emotional distress this specialty can evoke, including end-of-life issues, patients refusing care, and existential suffering. In addition, staff often voice feelings of grief and loss when a patient they have known for a long time passes away. When we couple this with the normal stress level of any busy academic medical center, it is clear that the staff need support in order to be able to care well for the next patient. Simply put, nurses cannot provide excellent care unless they have a safe place to discuss their thoughts and feelings in a way that helps them to process events that have affected them. Reflecting on the events and individual responses helps staff to learn from their experiences and continually grow and develop their practice.

To address these concerns, our leadership team developed several practices, each designed to bring difficult ethical and emotional issues to the surface for reflection, discussion, and processing. Only in this way can our staff continue to grow in their nursing practice, giving each new patient and family the same commitment of excellence. We thus describe four practices and their impact on staff and the care we provide: morbidity/morality rounds/case studies, spirituality rounds, ethics rounds, and memorial services.

MORBIDITY/MORTALITY ROUNDS/CASE STUDIES

To help our nurses deal with moral distress, we instituted a modified morbidity and mortality rounds/case study review in the Hematopoietic Stem Cell Transplant (HSCT) intensive care unit (ICU), inviting multiple members of the patient care team to participate: the attending physician, primary nurse, nurse-ethicist if appropriate, care coordinator, and a representative from pharmacy. The nursing director facilitates the discussion, keeping it on track, maintaining ground rules, and summarizing. We use a relaxed, conversational format. The ground rules are simple: Each member communicates respectfully, no one interrupts when someone is speaking, our discussion is confidential, and we will all work to avoid blame or disparaging comments.

Either the attending physician or the primary nurse begins with a brief overview of the patient/family, including why this case has been chosen for this review. Our conversation may focus more on the physiological care, including why certain treatment plans were used. Other times we review our experiences with a challenging patient/family, identifying what we did well and what we could do better next time. We conclude with a summary of lessons learned, what the staff did well, and why this case demonstrates the challenges of this patient population.

The staff report that they find these rounds very helpful. Each member of the team has a better understanding of the perspective of other members, including the shared responsibility and caring of all participants.

The program accommodates a variety of topics. At recent rounds, the attending physician discussed the cause of death of a young patient recently discharged; he spoke in a way that helped staff realize that they had not contributed to the unfortunate course of events that led to his death. On another unit, our staff were very distressed by the death of a patient who had experienced severe existential suffering during a protracted illness that included difficult social issues. In this case we invited the attending physician, nurse-ethicist, social worker, primary nurse, and other staff on our service. We wanted to give all the Heme/Onc/HSCT staff who work with pain and palliative care patients an opportunity to learn from one unit's experience. This patient was for us symbolic of our increasing focus on relieving existential as well as physical suffering (Rousseau, 2001).

As sometimes happens at these rounds, there were no black-and-white answers about how we can best deal with a patient/family who are suffering in so many ways. We do provide a forum, however, for a rich discussion of shared experiences and perspectives. The benefit is twofold. It provides us with an opportunity to understand how the different members of the team lived the experience with this patient/family. It also creates a confidential and safe environment in which to express the angst and moral distress that come with a career in nursing practice that often includes such emotional experiences.

SPIRITUALITY AND ETHICS ROUNDS

Spirituality and ethics rounds provide a safe setting for staff to openly discuss issues and concerns related to their practice as nursing staff that affect their spiritual, emotional, ethical, and physical well-being, and their ability to provide the best possible care for patients/families while also taking care of themselves.

Nursing staff give more than physical comfort to their patients by frequently "giving" themselves emotionally and spiritually in the process of providing care. They are constantly challenged regarding their own ethical belief systems. The daily work involved gives them little time to reflect on their practice or to share events that they encounter. The emotional cost of giving can also lead to compassion fatigue and burnout, leading staff to turn to self-destructive ways of coping when they are off duty and do have time to reflect (Keidel, 2002).

Spirituality and ethics rounds give staff a visible and powerful means of support and care that directly influences and affects the care provided to patients and families while maintaining the emotional well-being of the care provider. Staff can support each other, share learning experiences, debrief difficult situations, and acknowledge shared experiences that might otherwise be thought of as isolated events. Rounds also allow the director to identify areas where staff might need education or improvement in existing practices. We have also discovered that these rounds strengthen nurses' collaboration with the various departments that make up the multidisciplinary team (e.g., the Ethics Department or Chaplaincy). This is also an opportunity for nurses and patient care assistants (PCAs) to bond and support each other through challenging situations in a relaxed manner.

Spirituality and ethics rounds are conducted on consecutive days (spirituality rounds on the second Wednesday, ethics rounds on the second Thursday of each month). They are held for 1 hour in a conference room, in a round-table manner with lunch provided. Staff are asked if they want to bring up a specific case, though often the case is decided in advance. Often the same subject is discussed, but with different approaches or emphases. We send an e-mail to staff the day before and the day of the meeting, with the subject included (if appropriate). Basic ground rules regarding confidentiality of the subjects discussed are referenced at the beginning of each meeting.

Spirituality Rounds

Both a chaplain and a nursing director chair spirituality rounds, which are otherwise voluntary for staff. We often discuss case presentations that have been of interest to staff on one of the units. We usually prepare in advance by selecting some useful journal articles that the participants in the rounds can read following our discussion.

We have learned that various chaplains differ in their approach to conducting spirituality rounds. We believe this gives staff diversity of perspectives and makes the rounds more valuable. Chaplains may or may not emphasize a specifically spiritual focus. Some chaplains sometimes start off with a prayer, handholding, or meditation. Others do not bring religion into the conversation unless the subject is associated with religion.

Some of the subjects we have covered include existential suffering, bloodless bone marrow transplants (transplant done without the support of blood-product transfusions), end-of-life suffering, end-of-life viewpoints of specific families, humor in the workplace, and complementary therapies. Both RNs and PCAs are invited and urged to participate.

Our PCAs are most often the people who show the greatest comfort with spirituality. One such PCA was very comfortable with spiritual discussions with patients/families, but never imposing. When she came to spirituality rounds, we asked how she knows which patients/families to talk with about religion. She said that while making beds, she would quietly hum a piece of religious music. If the patient mentioned something to her about what she was humming, it would open up a conversation between them, and she would let the patient take the lead. Everyone learned that day that something introduced so subtly could make patients decide whether they wanted to talk about spirituality or religion. Discovering whether a patient wants to talk about religion often can be an awkward subject, but this PCA had handled it well.

Ethics Rounds

Ethics rounds (held on the second Thursday of every month) are conducted with the nurse-ethicist and nursing director. Because most of our staff works less than 40 hours a week, they do not get to both meetings, and we find a completely different group attending each day. Very often, the same subject is carried over from spirituality rounds into ethics rounds, although the conversation usually takes a different course. Again, this is usually guided by case presentations that are occurring in the moment or have recently occurred.

THE DEVELOPMENT OF A MEMORIAL SERVICE

The concept of a memorial service for our staff was created as a way to help with caregiver burnout. Because we were once the staff nurses and nurse educators whom we now direct in their work, we understand the toll it takes to care for critically ill patients at the end of life. We will hold our third Heme/Onc/HSCT Memorial Service this fall. We created this so that our staff could have a safe, designated place where they could focus on themselves and their loss. This service allows staff to take time away from the unit to connect with one another and in some cases to reconnect with the families who mean so much to them.

A multidisciplinary committee comprised of social workers, care coordinators, chaplains, physicians, nurses, patient care assistants, unit coordinators, educators, and managers created and developed the memorial service. There has been great value in making this work a collaborative effort. Representation from such varied groups has promoted greater staff involvement and participation.

The families of those patients we have lost are invited back to celebrate the life of their loved ones and to acknowledge the impact that this loss has had on our community. It is moving to see staff reconnecting with families and families connecting with one another. The service includes shared readings and songs by many different staff members. Perhaps the most meaningful part of the service is a ceremony where each family submits a picture of their loved one; the picture is then displayed on a screen with the name, which is read aloud. The family members are invited to hang an ornament on a tree to acknowledge their loss. Time is also included for staff to hang additional ornaments for patients they have lost who are not represented by family that day. The development of this service has been an excellent opportunity to share in the amazing impact each life has on every member of the health care team.

No program can eliminate moral distress, an experience inherent to the work we do. However, we can, and believe we have, alleviated some of that moral distress with our programs, and made it possible for our nurses to give the kind of exceptional care that they want to give and are most capable of giving.

REFERENCES

Gunther, M., & Thomas, S. P. (2006). Nurses' narratives of unforgettable patient care events. *Journal of Nursing Scholarship, 38*(4), 370–377.

Keidel, G. C. (2002, May/June). Burnout and compassion fatigue among hospice caregivers. *American Journal of Hospice & Palliative Care, 19*(3), 200–205.

Rousseau, P. (2001). Existential suffering and palliative sedation. *American Journal of Hospice & Palliative Care, 18*(3), 151–153.

Shepard, A. (2010). Moral distress: A consequence of caring. *Clinical Journal of Oncology Nursing, 14*(1), 25–28.

Zuzelo, P. R. (2007). Exploring the moral distress of registered nurses. *Nursing Ethics, 14*(3), 344–360.

Technological Change

13.1 *Clinical Practice as a Context for Developing Technological Competency*

Ann Furey, Cheryl Avitabile, Anne Bane,
Carol J. Luppi, Denise Goldsmith, and Laura Mylott

O ver the years, Brigham and Women's Hospital (BWH), like other acute care settings, has introduced numerous innovative technologies designed to support new treatment options and improve patient safety. While many of the early technologies targeted the administrative mechanisms that support workflow process, those introduced later often targeted aspects of patient care and had a direct impact on nursing workflow and practice. Although clinical nurses were often the primary users of these technologies, they typically were not involved in technology development or implementation planning.

As the Department of Nursing (DON) embarked on its vision-driven change process, we, as nurse educators and informatics specialists in the Center for Nursing Excellence (CNE), set out to change this approach to technology introduction. In particular, we aimed to ensure that nurses, as key end users of many technologies, contributed to technology development and implementation by serving on design teams, participating in testing, and leading training and implementation efforts on the clinical units. Our efforts were guided by an essential principle: Technologies used in the clinical care setting must *support* nursing practice and patient care rather than *define* it, and must not compromise nurses' efforts to know their patients and ensure that their patients feel known by them. This chapter tells our story of making this principle the touchstone for our decisions and outcomes.

CLINICAL PRACTICE AS A CONTEXT FOR TEACHING AND LEARNING

We believe that practice provides a useful and important context for helping nurses learn to use a new technology and integrate it into patient care. This is supported by adult learning theories suggesting that most adults find it easier to learn a new skill or acquire new knowledge when the teaching and learning process builds on prior knowledge and previous experiences and incorporates situations that resemble real-life events and problems. By using "contextual" teaching strategies, teachers expose learners to situations as a whole. Learners begin to recognize and understand what is most and least important as they assimilate the new knowledge and determine how to apply it in their practice and work environment (Baker, 2001). When augmented by coaching, supportive critique, and opportunities for discussion with peers, a contextual approach to teaching and learning becomes a powerful strategy for helping nurses attain technological competency (Benner, Sutphen, Leonard, & Day, 2010).

In changing our approach to technology adoption, we ensured that practice provided a context each step of the way. When planning implementation, we began engaging unit-based leaders and staff in discussions in which they anticipated how the technology would affect nursing practice and help them achieve desired outcomes. When training staff to use the technology, we taught nurses the necessary technical steps, and also used scenarios and examples from practice to help them anticipate how the technology would affect the patient and develop the critical thinking skills needed to resolve problems. We also provided feedback and coaching as nurses began using the technology in the clinical setting and created opportunities for nurses to share their experiences with one another. Our experiences taught us that using practice as a context for instruction synergizes the technology with patient care and promotes the harmonious coexistence of technology and caring practice. By helping nurses understand the nuances of using the technology while providing patient care, we reinforced technology's role as a tool for nurses.

In addition to using practice as a context for technology adoption, we also began engaging end users—nurse leaders and staff nurses from the clinical setting in which the technology will be used—in each step of the technology adoption process. This was an important change, as it advanced the DON's goal of ensuring that the voice of the clinical nurse helped drive decisions affecting the practice environment. In addition, clinical nurses have a unique and important perspective on how a technology will affect the patient, nursing workflow, and patient safety. Working with colleagues in Information Technology and nurse leaders on the clinical units, we arranged to have clinical nurses participate on teams that were engaged in technology design and began to involve them in implementation planning. We also began training clinical nurses as "super users" to provide real-time support to staff. Clinical nurse super users have a deep appreciation for the difficulties of incorporating a new technology into patient care and nursing practice. Because of this, they have a high degree of credibility among their peers. In addition to being change champions, the clinical nurse super users helped us sustain change by providing an infrastructure for continued learning and support.

LESSONS LEARNED AND RECOMMENDATIONS

We have used the principles and practices described here to help nurses in every clinical setting attain competency in many different technologies and computer applications while also supporting the DON change process. Based on our experience, we have developed the following recommendations for helping nurses attain technological competency.

1. *Use a project leadership model that blends clinical practice and informatics expertise.* Nurses leading technology initiatives must have a sound understanding of both technology and practice in order to help staff attain technological competency and master the critical thinking skills necessary for using the technology in patient care. We have found that a co-leadership model, involving a nurse educator/clinical specialist and a nurse informatics specialist, is an effective way to help nurses attain technical competence that is grounded in practice.

2. *Partner with unit-based leaders.* Technology implementation efforts are most successful when unit-based leaders are fully engaged in the process and partner with nurse educators and nurse informatics specialists to guide the initiative. Unit-based leaders can assure that the implementation process respects the unit's culture as well as nursing workflow and practices. They should take the lead in setting expectations for staff performance and overseeing communication efforts and surveillance. As project coordinators, nurse educators and informatics specialists can support unit leaders' efforts by providing appropriate language and informational materials to facilitate communication, developing training and other resources for clinical nurses, and implementing mechanisms to ensure real-time support and obtain feedback.

3. *Involve end users.* Clinical nurses and other end users have a unique appreciation for how a technology affects workflow. During the design phase, they can spot potential problems that might otherwise be missed; when planning for implementation, they can provide insights that help educators frame the technology within a practice context and develop appropriate usage guidelines; during evaluation, they can provide vital feedback on the technology's performance and needed changes.

4. *Use an incremental approach to teaching/learning and real-life problem solving.* Using an incremental approach to teaching allows learners to build on what has already been presented and assimilate information before moving on to new content. An incremental approach works well when introducing new technologies, which often require nurses to master multiple sequential steps. Instructional programs used to introduce new technologies should also engage nurses as active participants in their own learning by using experiential teaching methods, such as real-life scenarios. These help nurses anticipate issues that might arise when using the technology in practice, and help nurses develop the technological and clinical reasoning skills they need for problem solving.

5. *Have extra support available during implementation.* During the early phases of implementation, users face a steep learning curve and need to have ready access to expert, real-time support. Super users, or unit-based staff who receive special training in using the technology, are vital to implementation efforts. By providing one-on-one, real-time support and assistance with troubleshooting, super users help nurses master the mechanics of the technology and incorporate it into practice. Super users also play a key role in championing the technology and facilitating unit-level change. Additional support from technology experts, clinical experts, and online resources should also be available. Project

and unit-based leaders must continuously evaluate users' needs to determine how long round-the-clock super users and other special supports should be available.

6. *Provide opportunities for feedback.*   During the go-live period, users inevitably discover problems with the technology. Identifying and resolving these glitches is a critical part of the implementation process. Mechanisms to obtain user feedback should be introduced as go-live begins and continue throughout the implementation period. Identification of the problem should be followed up with expedient resolutions. Timely responses to the nurses' feedback sends the message that the nursing perspective is valued and encourages nurses to view themselves as partners in the implementation process.

7. *Maintain support after a "new" normal state is attained.*   Once the implementation phase is over, users still need support from expert resources. In addition to online resources, nurses should be able to access nursing and informatics specialists who are familiar with the technology. Unit-based super users can be particularly helpful during this time, as they provide an infrastructure for continued learning and for supporting staff through technology modifications and upgrades.

In the following sections, we provide some real-world case examples of how we have applied these recommendations in our technology implementation process. We believe the examples effectively demonstrate that practice provides a meaningful framework for developing technological competency in every type of learner, from technology-savvy nurses to patient care assistants with limited computer experience. Similarly, we have found that using practice as a context facilitates mastery of many different kinds of systems, from a multicomponent medication management system to a relatively easy-to-use patient education video program.

CASE STUDY #1: INTEGRATING A MEDICATION MANAGEMENT SYSTEM INTO NURSING PRACTICE

Mistakes in medication management and administration are among the most common medical errors, affecting an estimated 1.5 million people each year at a cost of billions of dollars (National Academies, 2006). Technology has often been cited as having the potential to dramatically reduce medication errors. However, to be effective, the technology must complement clinicians' workflow rather than require significant changes in practice (Ash, Berg, & Coiera, 2004), and must support each of the complex and interrelated steps involved in medication management.

At BWH, clinicians and information experts are engaged in a multiphase effort to implement a closed-loop, point-of-care medication management system that consists of multiple integrated applications and supports the process of medication management, from ordering through administration to surveillance. A multidisciplinary steering committee is overseeing the overall effort, with separate multidisciplinary work teams guiding the development, implementation, testing, and refinement of each component. A key part of the medication management system is the Electronic Medication Administration Record (eMAR) and bar-code scanning system. When this system was first introduced, nurse specialists helped evaluate it, but clinical nurses were not involved. As a result, the project ran into problems during the testing phase as nurses on the clinical units identified alarms and other design elements that were inconsistent with medication administration practice.

The eMAR implementation was already underway when the DON embarked on its vision-driven change process. The project quickly became a vehicle for change, as it allowed us to critique our approach to technology introduction and introduce a new approach grounded in practice. As a first step, the nurse specialist from the CNE who was helping to guide the eMAR implementation proposed adding clinical nurses to the eMAR work team. Working with nurse leaders on the pilot units, she invited several clinical nurses to join the eMAR work team and help it identify elements that should be changed to better support the medication administration process. The clinical nurses soon became project champions and played a critical role during the rollout on pilot units, helping to teach staff how to use the technology and serving as super users throughout the rollout period. The eMAR system was successfully implemented on the pilot units. Clinical nurses are now members of the project teams overseeing its implementation in new areas.

The eMAR project helped us establish the principles and practices that now guide our technology introduction efforts. Since changing our approach, we have consistently used practice as a framework to guide the project, as illustrated by the following examples.

1. Hardware and software design. The eMAR system automates the "five rights" (5Rs) of medication administration: right drug, right dose, right route, right time, and right patient. Validating the 5Rs is standard practice for nurses. The eMAR nurse champions played a critical role in identifying essential safety features, such as electronic advisories that alerted nurses to possible problems before a medication was administered. Nurses participating in this effort included individuals who frequently championed change, as well as nurses who were often resistant to and critical of new ideas. Including nurses with these different attitudes ensured that a broad range of issues would be identified and addressed during the design phase, and resulted in a system that satisfied even the toughest critics.

2. Testing and vetting in the clinical setting. Once the design phase was complete, eMAR was tested in the clinical setting. To prepare, the nurse champions helped develop detailed policies, procedures, and guidelines governing use of the technology, and assured that the procedures were consistent with existing nursing workflow and supported current nursing practice. Clinical nurses on the nursing units reviewed the guidelines and procedures, as did the Standards, Policies and Procedures Committee, which ensured that the policies were consistent with nursing practice throughout the organization.

The testing phase was a vital part of the overall development process, because the reality of complex medication management practices cannot be adequately captured in a simulated setting. Clinical nurses played an invaluable role during this phase, identifying numerous issues that required modification prior to broad implementation.

3. Education and training. Working with the clinical nurse specialist, the nurse champions ensured that the education and training provided to staff prior to implementation went beyond introducing eMAR's technical features. Teaching was provided in the context of patient care and included realistic examples of nursing workflow. Self-directed computer-based training (CBT) modules were useful in introducing the new technology, but were supplemented with hands-on classroom instruction to give nurses "real-life" experience in using the system and help them develop the critical thinking techniques needed to resolve problems in the clinical setting. During the go-live phase, the nurse champions served as super users, providing coaching and acting as resources and change agents among their peers. After the technology was fully deployed, the nurse super users resumed their original staff nurse roles, providing a matrix of technology expertise throughout the institution.

4. Assuring sustainability.   Once eMAR was fully integrated throughout the institution, the nurse specialist and nurse champions continued to provide real-time support to staff on the units. Staff also had access to backup technical and clinical resources via telephone 24 hours a day and to an online instruction manual.

Along with these resources, ongoing "Safety Rounds" also helped ensure the system's sustainability. Through Safety Rounds, multidisciplinary leaders on the implementation team met with staff on the units to hear their feedback about how eMAR was working and what elements needed to be improved. This feedback helped uncover unintended outcomes that had not been discovered during pre-implementation testing. Feedback provided by nurses also led to changes that improved how the system supports nurses' workflow, thus avoiding workarounds and other negative outcomes. As the eMAR implementation continues on other units, clinical nurses play a critical role, evaluating eMAR's fit with nursing workflow in each area and serving as instructors and super users in the unit. Involving staff in this way ensures that eMAR remains an effective tool for nurses, one that supports them in delivering safe patient care.

CASE STUDY #2: INTERACTIVE VIDEO TECHNOLOGY FOR PATIENT EDUCATION

Patient education is a critical part of nursing practice. By teaching patients self-monitoring and self-care skills, nurses empower patients to become partners in promoting health and managing disease. For teaching to be effective, each member of the care team must be involved in helping patients understand key concepts and acquire critical skills. For this reason, documenting teaching sessions is essential. Documentation assures continuity and consistency across teaching sessions and allows nurses and other care providers to identify what has been taught and assess the effectiveness of teaching strategies.

Given the intensity and short-term nature of most hospitalizations, inpatient nurses are challenged to find ways to teach essential concepts. In 2008, the DON secured the purchase of a computerized, interactive patient education video system to help nurses provide timely, individualized patient education. With its advanced functionality, nurses are able to select educational material/videos and assign them to individual patients using laptop computers. Patients can then access the assigned videos through the televisions in their hospital rooms. After viewing an educational video, a patient can use the television controller to indicate whether he or she would like to talk with the nurse about the information the video provided. The nurse receives the patient's request on a laptop computer, and after following up with the patient can document the patient teaching interaction through the video application's online reporting option.

Although the patient education video system is user friendly, it represented a significant change in the patient education practice of BWH nurses. In line with our principle that technology must support nursing practice rather than define it, the nurse director for patient education and nurse director for informatics, who were leading the system implementation, convened an advisory group to help them evaluate the potential impact of this technology on practice and develop recommendations for its introduction. In addition to the project leaders, the advisory group included clinical nurses, nurse directors, nurse educators, and nurse executive directors. The advisory group's goals are displayed in Box 13.1.

As a first step, the advisory group assessed the current state of patient education practices at BWH and agreed to a set of guiding principles to be applied across the organization (Box 13.2). The principles reaffirmed the accountability of clinical nurses for patient education and emphasized the importance of knowing the patient and knowing and using appropriate education resources and tools. By describing patient education standards and expectations for BWH nurses, the principles provided a framework for determining how the video technology could best be utilized to facilitate and support nurses in meeting the educational needs of patients and families, thus setting the stage for change.

The advisory group also developed recommendations for how the application should be introduced, used, and leveraged to support the work of the clinical nurse. The recommendations included: have expert clinical nurses review all video content; require nurses to ask patients whether they have questions after viewing a video (rather than having patients complete a formal test); have nurses use the system to create a report documenting which videos were recommended to a patient, which were viewed, the date and time of viewing, the nature of any follow-up questions asked by the patient, and nursing interventions prompted by the viewing experience; insert all reports into the medical record.

With these recommendations in place, the advisory group identified three intermediate cardiology units as pilot areas. The nurse director for patient education, nurse director for informatics, and a nurse director from an inpatient unit agreed to

---

BOX 13.1 *Patient Education TV Implementation Advisory Group Goals*

1. Articulate the current state of patient education practice at BWH and in the nursing literature.
2. Evaluate the application and its impact on the patient education practice of the clinical nurse.
3. Identify the workflow implications that result from having the application go live.
4. Identify policies that may be needed to support use of the application in the clinical setting.
5. Identify a process to prepare the environment for this change.
6. Identify a process and the necessary resources to implement this application.
7. Design critical implementation tasks with the Patient Education Task Force.
8. Guide the work of the Patient Education Task Force, solicit feedback from pilot users, and make changes as required.

BOX 13.2 *Guiding Principles of Patient Education at BWH*

- Accountability for patient education rests in every clinical nurse's role and is an essential part of the professional practice model.
- Every clinical nurse's responsibility is to provide, evaluate, and document education along the continuum of care.
- Patient education activities are communicated to the entire health care team through verbal and written methods.
- Knowing the patient/family is essential for effective patient education to occur:
  - Patient education is driven by the needs of the patient/family.
  - Patient education is provided following an interactive assessment of learning readiness and preferences.
  - Patient education is contextual.
  - Prioritized teaching is employed so that all patients are prepared to be safely transitioned/discharged from the hospital.
- Patient education best practice is more likely to occur when knowing the patient is combined with specialized clinical knowledge.
- Knowing the educational resources/tools:
  - Patient education is primarily provided through interaction and dialogue with the patient.
  - Patient education resources and tools are used to support the nurse/patient interaction.
  - The most appropriate educational resources and tools are driven by the needs of the patient.

---

oversee the pilot. In keeping with our practice of engaging clinical nurses in technology initiatives, the project leaders recruited clinical nurses and nurse leaders from the pilot areas to serve on a patient education task force. The task force took the lead in developing guidelines and mapping out a process for integrating the video/TV system into patient teaching and documentation practices. It also assumed accountability for monitoring use of the system and evaluating its effectiveness and impact on nursing practice.

Before the system was implemented on the units, the nurse director for patient education and nurse director of informatics trained 16 staff nurses as super users through a 90-minute classroom training session. Training for the rest of the staff took place on the unit and was supported by the super users. Throughout the 2-week go-live period, the units' nursing directors released one super user from staffing each shift to provide real-time, one-on-one training and support. The nurse directors for the inpatient units and the nurse director for patient education also made daily rounds to offer nurses additional assistance in using the technology within their practice, answer questions, and collect nurses' feedback. Nurses also provided feedback through an online option.

Through an observation audit conducted during the early stages of the pilot, the patient education task force learned that the majority of staff were not adhering to the newly crafted patient education documentation guidelines. Based on these findings, the task force initiated additional training focused on documentation and using the video education technology within the context of patient education practice. As the pilot continued, nurses reported that although the technology was easy to use during training, it was cumbersome to use in their daily workflow. In response to these findings, the pilot leaders and patient education task force worked with the vendor to implement more than 20 system enhancements and changes that made it easier for nurses to incorporate the system into both patient education practice and workflow. The enhancements included a "patient alert" message informing patients that a selection of videos was available and recommended for their viewing, easier system access for nurses via laptops, and a streamlined process for documenting the patient teaching interaction. After implementing the enhancements, the task force collected feedback that indicated nurses were satisfied with the usability of the system and the system changes. The task force also conducted an audit of patient education documentation that revealed a substantial improvement over documentation rates before the system was implemented.

Through this project, we reaffirmed the importance of involving clinical nurses and nurse leaders in technology introduction efforts. By leading efforts to create practice guidelines, serving as super users, and assuming accountability for monitoring compliance, nurse leaders and staff on the patient education task force demonstrated ownership of the technology implementation process, earned the buy-in of staff, and ensured that the patient education system supported rather than defined nursing practice. Acting on user feedback was also critical. In doing so, the project leaders and patient education task force sent the message that nurses' input was valued, and identified enhancements that improved how the technology fit into nursing workflow, facilitating its widespread adoption.

CASE STUDY #3: COMPUTER COMPETENCY AMONG PATIENT CARE ASSISTANTS

Patient care assistants (PCAs) are members of the staff in many clinical areas at BWH, working alongside nurses and helping them provide physical care and meet patient and family needs. Historically, PCAs have not had to interact with computer technology on the job. However, once the hospital computerized routine communication practices and administrative functions (e.g., benefit enrollment, electronic paychecks), and introduced an acute care documentation (ACD) project requiring electronic documentation of vital signs, ensuring computer literacy among PCAs became a priority.

In 2010, a nurse educator and nurse informatics specialist in the CNE created a work team composed of PCAs, clinical nurses, and nurse leaders, and worked with the team to design a PCA computer literacy program and pilot it in two clinical areas. As a first step, the work team established goals for the program, which included helping PCAs become competent in existing computer applications and preparing them for using the new clinical applications associated with ACD. Using PCA practice as a context, the work team then collaborated with the nurse educator and informatics specialist to define program content. Knowing that the computer skills of PCAs varied widely, the work team and project leaders created two separate classes: one for PCAs with minimal or no computer skills and another for PCAs with intermediate computer skills. We have found that grouping individuals according to their skills enhances participant satisfaction and enables educators to teach relevant information at a pace most learners can follow.

Both the beginner and the intermediate PCA computer literacy programs include a blend of classroom sessions and unit-based practice activities. The nurse educator, as the lead instructor, presents content incrementally, so that each teaching session builds on what precedes it. The nurse educator also incorporates real-life situations identified by the work team into the teaching sessions, and after each session assigns activities for participants to complete in their units.

The beginner class, 4 hours in length, introduces computer basics, including terminology (e.g., desktop, laptop, mouse), Internet basics, e-mail basics, and professional e-mail etiquette. PCAs at this level also learn how to use a mouse and navigate the keyboard. In the intermediate class, also 4 hours in length, PCAs learn how to use selected hospital systems, including e-mail, the human resources system used for benefits enrollment, and an online learning management program that BWH uses to provide required training. Those who participate in the beginner class proceed to the intermediate class once their skills are validated.

Seventeen PCAs from two clinical units, identified as ACD pilot units, participated in the pilot program. Before classes began, we asked the nursing leadership and the participants to describe their ability and comfort level using computers. We were specifically interested in their typing skills, familiarity with e-mail, and word-processing software, as well as their preferred language for learning. The project leaders and work team used this information to assign each PCA to the beginner or intermediate class. The nurse educator also used the information to address language barriers and to tailor the program's content and approach to build on the existing knowledge and skill level of our PCA learners.

To facilitate learning, participants each had a workstation to practice what they learned during the classroom session. The assignments on the clinical units further reinforced learning. The nurse leader and clinical nurses on the units provided coaching and supported the PCAs in completing their assignments, fostering team building as well as computer competency. The PCAs maintained a record of their practice sessions, recording whether they successfully completed the assigned activities and whether they needed assistance. The nurse educator met with the PCAs to discuss their experiences and any challenges they encountered in completing their assignments. The PCAs also completed online learning evaluation tools that reinforced the skills they learned and allowed the educator to identify areas where they needed more support.

Forty-one percent of the PCAs who completed the program participated in a beginner class. All participants reported feeling more confident using hardware such as a mouse and a keyboard. They also described performing more online activities such as "viewing their paycheck" and checking for new e-mail. PCAs stated they were grateful for the opportunity to learn these skills on the job and reported that they felt more "connected" to their "children and society" with improved computer skills. The instructors experienced the satisfaction of "making a difference." Our lessons learned included an enhanced understanding of the learning needs of adults who speak English as a second language. For these learners, we now present information using both audio and visual methods simultaneously and use more cuing during exercises. We have also created more opportunities to check in with them and assess their knowledge and skills through demonstration and feedback.

We believe that a key factor contributing to the success of this program was convening PCAs, nurse leaders, and clinical staff who work with PCAs together to help us define program content. Their input was critical in ensuring that the program met the learning needs of PCAs and was relevant to PCA practice. Having nurse leaders and clinical nurses provide coaching on the units was also critical.

This assured PCAs of real-time feedback and deepened nurses' understanding of PCA computer literacy needs and capabilities.

SUMMARY

Introducing new technologies into the clinical setting is a complex change process, one that requires a team involving nurse educators, technology and informatics experts, nurse leaders, and clinical staff. As noted at the beginning of this chapter, our efforts were guided by an essential principle: Technologies used in the clinical care setting must *support* nursing practice and patient care rather than *define* it, and must not compromise nurses' efforts to know their patients and ensure that their patients feel known by them. We believe our case examples demonstrate that practice provides a useful and important context for teaching nurses how to use a new technology. By helping them anticipate how the technology will affect patients and their workflow, using practice as a context helps nurses develop critical thinking and problem-solving skills required to safely integrate the technology into patient care. The case examples also illustrate the importance of seeking feedback about the technology from clinical nurses. As frontline care providers and the end users of many technologies, clinical nurses can offer invaluable insights and suggestions for improving the technology and ensuring that it supports nursing practice and safe and efficient care.

REFERENCES

Ash, J. S., Berg, M., & Coiera, E. C. (2004). Some unintended consequences of information technology in health care: The nature of patient care information system related errors. *Journal of the American Medical Informatics Association, 11*(2), 104–112.

Baker, C. (2001). Problem-based learning and technology: A caring pedagogy in nursing. In R. C. Locsin (Ed.), *Advancing technology, caring, and nursing.* Westport, CT: Greenwood.

Benner, P., Sutphen, M., Leonard, V., & Day, L. (2010). *Educating nurses.* San Francisco, CA: Jossey-Bass.

National Academies. (2006, July 20). *News from the National Academies.* Retrieved from http:// www8.nationalacademies.org/onpinews/newsitem.aspx?RecordID=11623

13.2 *Creating a Culture of Commitment Through Collaborative Multidisciplinary, Multiprofessional Simulation Training*

De'Ann McNamara and Michael G. Kyller

In the spring of 2010, the Centers for Diagnostic Interventional Cardiology and Interventional Radiology (CDIC/IR) at the Brigham and Women's Hospital (BWH) celebrated the completion of a year-long program to evaluate staff competency, foster teamwork, and enhance communication skills among staff in our divisions. This chapter describes what we were celebrating and why, told from the perspective of the two educators who made it happen.

FACING THE CHALLENGE

Two years ago, our individual departments were experiencing resource strain in maintaining documentation of yearly mandatory staff competency. Maintaining two separate staff competency formats was inefficient and frustrating to educators and staff. We had been working independently, each with a "cookie cutter" approach to skills evaluation that did not always apply to highly specific procedural/skill areas, and we were nearing creative bankruptcy. Efforts to track down staff to do competencies in a catch-as-catch-can fashion often failed outright. We were both properly exasperated, so we decided to commiserate. We asked ourselves, "Can we do this better?" We identified problems and began to brainstorm possibilities (although it looked like complaining and whining at first). The fatigue associated with repetitive lectures and demonstrating skills every year drove the creation of a new, innovative approach to teaching and practicing competency items. We developed a strategic plan, found executive resources for leadership support, and designed a competency program for our departments that was more interactive, conducive to learning, involved the technologists, and fostered team building.

IMAGINING A NEW APPROACH

We defined a new portfolio to encompass what providers in CDIC/IR need to know to be able to care for patients. Although many of the functions and skills of staff in procedural areas are similar to those in the inpatient hospital areas, much of the work and many of the skill sets are different. As a result, not only do we need to cover some content related to emergency equipment, infection control, and patient safety goals, but we also have to account for the fact that our patients receive contrast, need vascular access, and have specific sedation and medication needs unique to these areas. Our competency program would have to provide for this diverse array of needs among our participants.

We then sought out critical stakeholders. We shared our ideas with them, and asked them for resource investment, guidance, and approval of our objectives. The stakeholders included our departmental nursing directors and the directors of the Center for Nursing Excellence (CNE). The directors' support was crucial for coordinated efforts and reinforcement of both core hospital mandatory content and unit-specific content.

Our departmental nursing directors coordinated staff schedules for the program. Scheduling is critical to ensure a mix of staff from each area and discipline, which in turn ensures collaborative learning through sharing and exchanging viewpoints. For example, a nurse doing a similar case in IR, in contrast to the catheterization lab, may contribute a different approach, or a technologist may focus on a different point than a nurse. By sharing, both can broaden their perspective in caring for a patient in a similar case or situation.

Directors of the CNE acknowledged the validity of our creation and delegated authority for content presentation design, forecasting, planning, and scheduling. In a large institution like BWH, equipment acquisition and reservation is also a consideration, in addition to securing rooms, finding simulation labs, and scheduling personnel. They also agreed to support our efforts through the allotment of necessary program space, simulation resources, and administrative support to synchronize the whole effort. These leaders took a broad view of what this program could mean for the growth of the departments: efficiency, cost containment, commitment, and interprofessional team building. They realized, as we did, that this all meant additional benefits for our patients.

We embedded discussions about hospital policy in our content (e.g., infection control, risk management, quality, and safety). Stakeholders appreciated the potential hospital financial benefits that could result from having these policy discussions in the program. Aligning the program objectives with the vision of the CNE to develop a new culture in training and testing for competency was a central commitment in our approach to program creation and structure. A multiprofessional format emerged and began to simultaneously encompass multidepartmental, multidivision, multilevel, multipurpose appreciation. One of the caveats the CNE offered us was to have careful forethought for post-growth implications, such as the fact that others would want to be involved. At the time we had no idea what they meant ... but now we do!

DEVELOPING THE PROGRAM

Space allocations are on a first-come, first-served basis at BWH, and we did not want to find ourselves without a place to run the program. In early summer we made an assessment, identifying the number of staff members who needed to attend the competency program and the resources available to us. The latter included room and simulation lab availability, equipment, and staff who knew how to write simulation computer programs according to scripts we had not yet drafted. Thankfully, the CNE administrative and simulation lab staff were patient with us as we manufactured the first generation of this program. Meetings with the executive director of the CNE revealed mandatory requirements for general RN competency content, which drove the calculations of how much time and what areas we would devote to unit-specific content and simulation exercises. We felt strongly that simulation would enhance the learning of skills covered in "competency day" by providing an opportunity to practice skills with scenarios that we wrote for our areas.

Writing simulation scripts was a challenge because we had to consider the staff from various divisions when building the scenarios. We decided that basic patient care, monitoring, interventions, communication, and teamwork were the items that transcended all divisions, and so this is where we invested our efforts. Division practices vary. Loss of symmetry would not handicap our vision for a broader perspective and thoughtfulness outside individual units.

The CNE establishes mandatory content each year, but does not mandate how it is taught. They gave us guidelines for the content and we created how the content would be presented, along with the sequence of the modules. Each year it is mandatory for all hospital RNs to have skill check-off for Mannequin Practice involving Airway Management and CPR. In our divisions, however, nurses are also required to be Advanced Cardiac Life Support (ACLS) certified, and we felt it prudent to have a review of these skills to accompany these basic competency items. We began with Automated External Defibrillation (AED) and Mannequin Practice and then moved on to content regarding defibrillators, both manual and using defibrillation pads, with hands-on return demonstrations for each device. We then had a unit-specific transvenous pacing module. Some of this content was more applicable to certain areas than others; however, a pacemaker can show up on any patient in any division, and knowing the basics of pacemaker physics and troubleshooting is good for any nurse. We ended this module with an arrhythmia review and a test to evaluate the learners' understanding of arrhythmias and defibrillation, as well as ACLS therapy and meds.

We incorporated other hospital-required competencies as well as unit-specific content by designing a game to mimic the TV game show "Jeopardy." In this game we covered the Joint Commission's National Patient Safety Goals (NPSG), infection control policies (NPSG #7), and skin assessment and documentation using the Braden Scale. Other content included in this session were restraints, medications including anticoagulants (NPSG #3), and procedural access site care and issues. We devoted a specific category to radiation and laser safety. Although some of this content may not be applicable to the general nursing units, it is important for procedural areas that use x-ray and laser systems.

We also created a game for the cardiovascular systems review content. We divided the participants into two groups, then displayed PowerPoint slides showing basic cardiovascular anatomy to be identified. Each group was given a bell to ring when they identified as many blanks as possible from the PowerPoint slides. At this point in the day—about an hour after lunch—we found that chocolate was a great stimulant for participation.

IMPLEMENTING THE PROGRAM: INTRODUCING SIMULATION

Having completed the development process, we were ready to implement it, and were invested in a positive learning experience for our participants. To help break the ice and add a little humor, we donned wigs, hats, name-bands, and johnnies/hospital robes and were introduced as the patients. The "team" of participants was given the handoff of the patients, and the team now responsible for the patients was redirected to the mannequin as the patient. The mannequin was in the procedure area where the scenario began.

The simulation scenarios we wrote were complex and the patient, of course, never read the book. We used both common and uncommon situations that could occur in our areas as simulation scenarios; for example, a patient with sudden acute coronary syndrome, a carotid stent procedure with complications, and a patient with access site bleeding complications. The staff had to think critically, both on their own and as a group, to assess, treat, and summon appropriate resources to assist. Because seasoned groups were able to perceive problems quickly, they were speeding through the scenarios faster than the programmed scenario could unfold. As a result, the simulation control team had to be able to react on a millisecond's notice with these more experienced staff. We could not make the patient scene complex enough!

SO YOU LEARNED SOMETHING?

When a participant would say magical words such as, "Hey, I didn't know that!" or "Oh yeah, I had forgotten that was how . . .," we would invariably say, "Oh? So you learned something?" And one of us would scribble the comment on a notepad. The amount of scribbling was impressive by the end of the year!

Through the eyes of the participants, we created a needed tool to maintain competency requirements, communicate best practices through simulation, and apply skills directly where it matters most: at the patient's bedside. We have seen a marked change in the interactions between our staff and with us since installation of simulation into the program. This was not a computerized competency, but a human approach. Debriefing offered the opportunity to hear about the creative backgrounds of the participants through open-forum discussion. Participants were encouraged to query their colleagues about their practice and learn from each other. Changes in perception and perspective were made possible with the mix of technologists and nurses and the joining of CDIC and IR. Learning was evident through the sharing of stories from years of individuals' experiences.

We ended our day with evaluation of the program. We asked for honesty and suggestions. Some asymmetry regarding content for certain procedure areas was noted, which speaks to the diversity of our divisions. Overall, however, we received exceptional results, primarily ratings of 5 on a 5-point scale. Comments were equally affirming, as these examples demonstrate: "I wasn't sure at first . . . BUT I have to say the simulation was great!" "Honestly, one of the best competency days I have attended in the past 10 years! Good job!" "Interesting, fun, and helpful." "Simulation was excellent!"

WHAT WE LEARNED

Some people believe that competency day is simply about skills check-off and check boxes with no new material. However, we found that even as the checks are marked in the boxes, participants of our program have learned new things, made sharper and more accurate realizations about current practice, and received updated, evidence-based information to support current practice. We learned to adjust the painful parts and replace unremarkable styles of presentation by engaging the participants in creative ways, such as whimsical games that were found to be grounds for great learning! We also conducted the program off site, where staff were free from the pressure to interact with the workflow of the day.

From our lessons learned, we have generated a list of recommendations that others might find useful, and include them here as a roadmap for replication:

- Allow yourself to think differently.
- Seek collaborative nursing leaders to support creative endeavors for learning.
- Be prepared for forces of torsion, coefficient of friction, and inertia. We met expected resistance at times, but once the staff were submerged in the program, it resolved.
- Discuss objectives, content, and support with nurse leaders early in the process. They may see issues that from their perspective have to be addressed and/or reinforced.
- Try to have the program held off campus or away from the direct care area so staff are not distracted by patient flow during sessions.
- Consider early conference room, simulation lab, and equipment booking (including required audiovisual aids), especially if space is difficult to access. Crowded spaces and poor accommodations detract from the experience.
- If possible, use simulation to work on intangibles such as communication (briefing/debriefing) and team building. These interactions provide many teaching/learning moments.
- Incorporate skills into simulated scenarios appropriate to the participants' care/procedure area. This is great reinforcement of clinical use of the skills. It takes it to the next level closest to actual patient care.
- Chocolate and coffee breaks are a must!
- Include friendly team competition (well, sometimes it doesn't "look" friendly) in a game-style setting for dry (less appealing) content. Joint Commission safety goals became so exciting!
- Structure debriefing sessions to be led primarily by the staff with only "gentle facilitation" by the instructors. This is another rich medium for learning.
- Allow and document thoughtful evaluation with brutal honesty to be used for ongoing improvements. We changed a few things as we went, in addition to using comments to plan the next year's program.
- Invite other team members (e.g., procedure physicians, anesthesia physicians, nurse practitioners, physician's assistants, and house staff) to contribute, discuss, and bring about a more realistic situation. It's amazing how the different disciplines see things from a different perspective. Again, we frequently heard team members say, "I didn't know that" or "I never thought of it that way."

MOVING FORWARD

Our ongoing strategy is to develop a competency day that is capable of engaging physicians, physician's assistants, nurse practitioners, nurses, respiratory therapists, and patients as assistant team members in this captured, command performance.

Our goal is to enhance communication via complete team participation in the next generation of the existing program. The vision for our Department of Nursing is *excellent care to patients and families, with the best staff, in the safest environment.* We keep trying different methods and techniques to meet this vision through evidence-based practice. Once we find current best practice, we start looking at even newer data and technology to improve our program. This is how we will drive the next generation of innovative simulation productions to display, provide, and evaluate excellent care practice opportunities.

Change Through Synergy: Crafting Partnerships

14.1 *Academic Partnerships at Brigham and Women's Hospital: Our Commitment to and Capacity for Clinical Education*

*Linda A. Evans, Hallie Greenberg, Yolanda Harmuth,
Laura Mylott, and Patrice K. Nicholas*

*A*cademic partnerships at Brigham and Women's Hospital (BWH), crafted and sustained through the engagement and leadership of the Center for Nursing Excellence (CNE), are shaped by a philosophy, grounded in collaborative relationships, and open to possibility. We view them as critical to the future of the discipline of nursing and believe that healthy work environments must include comprehensive and creative educational opportunities for the next generation of nurses. We promote a philosophy that is responsive to the traits and values of the emerging generation.

Progressive technologies in education, including online learning, advanced approaches to electronic medication administration, recording and reconciliation practices, computer-based physician order entry systems, and online acute care documentation, must be embraced when structuring an educational curriculum for nursing students. We believe in the use of current, peer-reviewed, empirical evidence on the topics inherent to nursing education. We value the best educational practices in the United States and internationally. Additionally, in our setting we have integrated the key requisites of a healthy work environment identified by the American Association of Critical Care Nurses (AACN): skilled communication, true collaboration, effective decision making, appropriate staffing, meaningful recognition, and authentic leadership (see Chapter 3). These same requisites are implicit in our Department of Nursing (DON) vision statement: *excellent care to patients and families, by the very best staff, in the safest environment.*

More specifically, *we believe that*:

■ Respectful partnerships among patients, families, and caregivers are the foundation of care. Those learning in our setting must embrace this philosophy as well.
■ Individual and collective accountability are essential to achieve our mission.

■ All who seek or provide care in our diverse community, and all students engaged in a learning experience, deserve sensitivity, compassion, and respect.
■ Excellent practice is evidence based and is characterized by the development, application, and evaluation of knowledge.
■ Consistency, fairness, and integrity are essential in developing and mentoring staff.
■ The specific values stated here are indicative of our commitment to educate the future generations of nurses.

The leadership team of our BWH DON has a long history of commitment to the clinical education of nurses. This commitment evolved from an early model of diploma education at the Peter Bent Brigham School of Nursing into our current philosophy of baccalaureate preparation as a basis for professional nursing practice. The Peter Bent Brigham School of Nursing, one of the earliest schools of nursing in the northeastern United States, closed in 1985. However, the DON has continued to advance the teaching mission of our academic health care center with our commitment to academic partnerships.

Our BWH nursing workforce includes nurses who hold baccalaureate degrees in nursing (BSN) and others with earned master's and doctoral degrees. A substantial number of BWH clinical nurses, however, have not yet achieved a BSN. In support of a BSN-prepared nursing staff, we have instituted a key initiative. This initiative includes partnerships with academic institutions: an onsite BSN program with Emmanuel College, and an online RN-to-BSN program through the University of Massachusetts, Boston. We also participate in an RN-to-MSN program with Regis College.

Nursing education's evolution from hospital-based to university-based education supports learning experiences at a variety of clinical sites. Academic institutions and the agencies providing the clinical experiences must have shared goals and a common commitment. Ours include:

■ Development of nursing graduates with sound scientific, aesthetic, and ethical knowledge about the discipline of nursing
■ In-depth clinical expertise developed through real-life experience and in high-fidelity simulated laboratory settings
■ The ability to translate evidence-based findings into practice
■ An appreciation of policy issues as they apply to clinical systems, patient care, and health outcomes
■ Integration of sophisticated technologies in education, patient care, and outcome evaluation

The recent work by Benner, Sutphen, Leonard, and Day (2010), supported by the Carnegie Foundation for the Advancement of Teaching, calls for a radical transformation in how we educate nurses in the 21st century. Our response to this call to action began with crafting a DON position statement on academic partnerships to guide us in our future efforts. The outcome of our work follows.

GUIDING PRINCIPLES FOR CLINICAL/ACADEMIC PARTNERSHIPS AT BWH

■ The DON is committed to the education of the next generation of nurses and fulfills that mission through maintaining strong academic relationships and partnerships.

■ The creation of a robust clinical learning environment is essential for successful outcomes for student nurses.

■ Expectations of faculty and the clinical nursing staff should be articulated, implemented, and evaluated.

■ Creative learning technologies enhance learning for nursing students and complement direct interactions with patients, families, and staff on clinical units.

■ Our DON will continue to focus on developing academic partnerships that support our future professional workforce.

■ The student clinical learning experience must be guided by objectives that are shared by the nursing staff on the individual units.

■ Our future clinical/academic partnerships will promote relationships with programs that prepare nurses at the baccalaureate level. Educational opportunities will also be accessible to students pursuing a master's degree in nursing, or a research or practice doctoral degree.

■ Clinical/academic relationships will foster our mission to develop a multicultural nursing workforce which supports our diverse patient population.

THE ACADEMIC PARTNERSHIPS ADVISORY GROUP

The Academic Partnerships Advisory Group was formed under the guidance of the CNE in 2008. The focus was to promote creative initiatives through building on past strengths. This presented us with an opportunity to reevaluate and expand our outreach efforts to students. The overarching goals for the Advisory Group were to develop and implement innovative models to teach nursing students, while promoting BWH as a great place to practice nursing. Additionally, we hoped to ensure a pipeline of professional nurses to meet the needs of BWH patients and their families. The Advisory Group's early membership consisted of 15 nurses representative of multiple role groups from throughout the organization. The group was cochaired by Patrice Nicholas, Director of Academic Partnerships, and Linda Evans, at that time the nurse educator in the Operating Room. The Advisory Group began its work by formally describing our commitment to nursing students' education and defining the roles and responsibilities of BWH clinical staff within clinical and academic partnerships.

Although we knew BWH had a strong commitment to nursing student education, it was clear that we were using a variety of pedagogies to educate these students. To explore this issue, some members of the Advisory Group conducted a qualitative, descriptive research study utilizing a focus group methodology to examine the role and responsibilities of our clinical staff nurses in providing education to nursing students. Three learning models were explored: a clinical-faculty model where a faculty member oversees the learning experience of six to eight students; a preceptor-based model where an experienced nurse is paired with one student for an extended time period; or, as in a select area of our setting, a model known as the Dedicated Education Unit model (Moscato, Miller, Logsdon, Weinberg, & Chorpenning, 2007).

The findings validated the commitment of our staff to teaching nursing students. Findings noted critical factors that determined outcomes: the extensive time commitment teaching required, the great variability of the experience, the role of the school of nursing instructor, and the hospital's relationship with the academic institution. All the models of educating students appeared to assist nursing students to flourish. Most importantly, those who participated in the study, and who had served as clinical preceptors of nursing students, believed that teaching students positively influenced patient outcomes. This intensified the group's commitment to partner with academic institutions, to support the education process for students, and to support our colleagues in pursuit of attaining baccalaureate degrees.

ACADEMIC PARTNERSHIPS WITH THE CENTER FOR NURSING EXCELLENCE

Faculty Credentialing and Orientation

BWH annually welcomes approximately 100 nursing faculty, who complete a rigorous credentialing and privileging process granting them authorization to practice at BWH. We verify nursing credentials and mandate standards of nursing practice that align with the licensure requirements of the Commonwealth of Massachusetts Board of Registration in Nursing (BORN) and fall within the scope of the Nurse Practice Act. The CNE staff orient clinical nursing instructors using didactic, experiential, and clinical learning situations and formats.

Clinical Placements

Nursing students are welcomed to BWH in a variety of clinical settings. As an academic teaching hospital, the role of clinical education for nursing students is fully integrated into patient care. In early clinical immersion, students are taught in groups of approximately eight students per instructor. Student groups are assigned to most clinical units at the BWH except the intensive care units. One unique pedagogy utilized is the dedicated education unit, which will be described later in this chapter.

Senior practicum students enter BWH for a culminating clinical experience prior to graduation. This experience entails engaging in a one-on-one preceptorship with a BWH registered nurse for approximately 180 total hours. Each school has its own policy regarding length of the experience and student placements in areas of specialization such as Labor, Birth, and Recovery and the Operating Room. Schools of nursing also establish clinical hours based on curricular requirements for students to sit for licensure examination, or for certification board requirements for advanced practice nursing students. Nursing students in graduate programs also are assigned to clinical practica to develop advanced practice skills, and work under the direction of nurse-practitioner preceptors.

Partners HealthCare System/University of Massachusetts Boston Clinical Leadership Collaborative for Diversity in Nursing

One of our most innovative academic partnerships is the Clinical Leadership Collaborative for Diversity in Nursing (CLC). The leadership of the College of Nursing and Health Sciences (CNHS) at the University of Massachusetts, Boston, and Partners HealthCare System (PHS), including senior nursing leadership at BWH, were instrumental in the development of this initiative. Between 2007 and 2009, PHS and CNHS entered into a memorandum of agreement (MOA) to fund the effort. The first agreement supported 18 racially and ethnically diverse under-graduate nursing students, the second 19 students, and the third another 18 students. The grant also provided the CLC with administrative support funds during the second year of the program. Students are selected based on a competitive process assessing applicants' academic and clinical excellence, and includes an interview with members of the Steering Committee. The committee is composed of nurse educators from CNHS as well as nursing and human resource administrators and nursing directors from the PHS agencies, including BWH. The goal is for the students to obtain employment at a PHS institution upon graduation, and potentially, a future nursing leadership position. This will make a definitive, positive impact by increasing the number of culturally diverse professional nurses at PHS agencies.

Specific goals of the CLC are to:

1. Financially support diverse nursing students with tuition reimbursement and a stipend so that outside employment responsibilities are limited, allowing for full concentration on their studies.
2. Facilitate the smooth transition of CLC students to employment as a registered nurse at a PHS facility by:
   a. Ensuring a maximum number of clinical placements for CLC students at PHS agencies.
   b. Assigning CLC students to PHS agencies for their capstone preceptorship clinical experience.
   c. Assigning a PHS registered nurse mentor to each CLC student in order to support strategies for effectively managing the various racial, ethnic, and cultural issues the students may encounter in their professional career.
   d. Encouraging summer PCA employment opportunities at PHS agencies.

Mentors are racially and ethnically diverse volunteer registered nurses. Mentor/mentee pairings are determined by members of the CLC Steering Committee, with the goal of maximizing the experience for both participants. The mentors are orientated to the CLC program goals to ensure a mutually respectful relationship with their mentee, allowing for open communication and reflection. Mentors focus on development of leadership skills and provide guidance regarding becoming a successful multicultural nurse within the PHS. The pair continues to work together through the first year of employment of the newly licensed registered nurse. This provides continued support and guidance with transition challenges.

Dedicated Education Unit

The Dedicated Education Unit (DEU) offers an innovative way of partnering nurses situated in academe and clinical practice to create integrated clinical and scholarly learning experiences for students and clinical staff. Modeled after the "Portland, Oregon Program" described by Moscato et al. (2007), the BWH/UMASS's principal program objective is to transform a patient care unit into an optimal learning/teaching environment through the collaborative efforts of clinical staff, nursing leadership, students, and academic faculty. The clinical partnerships foster opportunities in which resources, knowledge, and experiences are both shared and reciprocal. The model enables nursing practice to inform student learning and nursing education to inform nursing practice and knowledge development.

The clinical teaching-learning experiences are immersive and designed to provide students with substantial continuity caring for patients/families, as well as with mentorship/team relationships. These relationships foster trust, enable the application of theoretical knowledge, promote the development of clinical knowledge and skills, and allow the student to experience membership within a health care team. The collaborating entities participate in the development of all phases of curriculum development, implementation (teaching didactic and clinical experiences, supervising, mentoring, and evaluating students), and program evaluation.

Clinical staff nurses are selected by the nurse director and prepared to be clinical instructors (CIs) through collaborative staff development activities. The CIs are the primary clinical teachers for the students. CIs develop clinical assignments in accordance with the academic learning objectives and real-time opportunities, provide feedback, and collaborate with the student and academic faculty in the design of all learning experiences that support clinical learning and goal attainment. The nurse director and nurse educator (with faculty support) assume the leadership of informing and preparing the nursing staff about the role of the CI, the goals of the program, and their roles in supporting of the CI/student dyad and in providing the day-to-day leadership for implementation of the model.

Students are assigned to the DEU by the academic faculty. The traditional academic faculty role is expanded to include a focus on the development and support of the CIs as teachers/coaches. The academic faculty member assigned to the unit is titled the Clinical Faculty Coordinator (CFC). The CFC partners with the CIs to encourage the use of evidence-based teaching/learning strategies, provide support, assure the student's attainment of expected clinical outcomes, and collaborate in the evaluation of student achievement.

SUMMARY

Our accomplishments at BWH are aimed at advancing academic partnerships that address the need for radical transformation on how we educate nurses for the complex patient environment. Through our creative partnerships and goal of educating nurses for today's practice, as well as advancing a process of lifelong learning, we embrace the mission of teaching in our academic health center. In this way we accomplish the very best care in the safest environment by our professional nursing staff.

REFERENCES

Benner, P., Sutphen, M., Leonard, V., & Day, L. (2010). *Educating nurses: A call for radical transformation.* San Francisco, CA: Jossey-Bass.

Moscato, S. R., Miller, J., Logsdon, K., Weinberg, S., & Chorpenning, L. (2007). Dedicated education unit: An innovative clinical partner education model. *Nursing Outlook, 55*(1), 31–37.

14.2 *The Nursing Department's Vision of a Baccalaureate-Prepared Nursing Staff: Development and Implementation of an Onsite Bachelor of Science in Nursing Program*

Linda A. Evans and Patrice K. Nicholas

*B*righam and Women's Hospital (BWH) has a long tradition of respecting and valuing exceptional professional nursing education. The legacy of the highly successful Peter Bent Brigham School of Nursing offered an historical framework for education in our Harvard-affiliated academic medical center. The Peter Bent Brigham School of Nursing welcomed its first class in 1912 and during its 75-year history educated many of the leading nurses in the Boston area. Carrie Hall, who served in World War I and received a British Red Cross medal for her service, was one of the early nurse leaders of the school. The Goldmark Report of 1923 challenged nursing education to move from an apprenticeship model to a university-based model, a change that evolved slowly. In 1985, the school closed, due to the increasing pressures to move toward baccalaureate education in nursing.

The focus on educational preparation of our nursing professionals was supported by BWH's executive nursing leadership (Mairead Hickey, the chief nursing officer, and Trish Gibbons, the associate chief nursing officer), and seen as a vitally important element of the department's mission statement—to ensure that patients and families are cared for by the *very best staff.* Our personal value for continuing education, and our professional roles within the organization, provided the groundwork for us to be champions of this work. This chapter describes our involvement in advancing the mission of a baccalaureate-prepared nursing workforce at BWH.

As co-chairpersons of the BWH Academic Partnerships Advisory Group, our interest focused not only on the traditional educational partnerships, which utilize our facility for the clinical teaching of nursing students, but also on mechanisms to enrich the professional lives of our currently practicing registered nurse colleagues. We value the experience and commitment of our staff nurse colleagues and have deep respect for those who find value in continuing their formal education, including those who are associate degree and diploma prepared and wish to pursue a BSN degree. To that end, we strategized with the other members of the Academic Partnerships Advisory Group—12 nurses who represent a variety of units and clinical roles. Our focus was on convenient, high-quality, and feasible options to support the efforts of these non-baccalaureate-prepared nurses who wanted to continue their formal education.

Recent research addresses the important outcomes related to baccalaureate-prepared nurses (Kanai-Pak, Aiken, Sloane, & Poghosyan, 2008; Kutney-Lee et al., 2009; Van den Heede, Clarke, Sermeus, Vleugels, & Aiken, 2007; Van den Heede, Lasaffre, et al., 2009; Van den Heede, Sermeus, et al., 2009). Aiken and colleagues have studied the relationship between educational levels and patient outcomes for more than two decades. Their research clearly indicates that hospitals with higher percentages of well-educated staff have lower mortality and failure-to-rescue rates. Aiken and colleagues found that after adjusting for patient characteristics and hospital structural characteristics (size, teaching status, level of technology), as well as for nurse staffing, nurse experience, and whether the patient's surgeon was board certified, a 10% increase in the proportion of nurses holding a bachelor's degree was associated with a 5% decrease in both the likelihood of patients dying within 30 days of admission and the odds of failure to rescue (Aiken, Clarke, Cheung, Sloane, & Silber, 2003).

The senior leadership members of the Department of Nursing (DON) hold the value, as we do, that the entry level into nursing practice at BWH be at the baccalaureate level. We were confident that the leadership support for this endeavor would also support creative efforts for the currently employed nursing staff without bachelor's degrees in nursing at our hospital. In order to encourage current staff members with educational preparation at the associate degree level or diploma level in nursing to begin to consider the added value of a baccalaureate education, we spearheaded discussions and endorsed programming and partnerships to provide convenient, high-quality, cost-effective educational opportunities for working professionals. Many staff had not participated in formal educational programs for several years. In addition, many also had the added responsibility of full-time employment and families. As co-chairpersons of the Academic Partnerships Advisory Group, we believed it was imperative that we approach the topic of returning to school with our staff nurse colleagues thoughtfully and that our discussions include our desire to provide programming that was convenient, cost-effective, and supportive. An academic partnership with Emmanuel College was launched at BWH in January 2009.

INITIAL STEPS

BWH has had many successful ongoing relationships with academic partners throughout the years. One highly successful partnership had existed with a neighboring college, Emmanuel College, where students at the former Peter Bent Brigham School of Nursing had enrolled in science courses. The academic dean of Graduate and Professional Programs at the College, along with the nursing faculty and department staff, expressed interest in recruiting BWH nurses for their existing RN-to-BSN degree program. Their interest in reinvigorating our partnership came just as we were all making the philosophical transition to an investment in BSN preparation for our nursing staff. Thus, it was a perfect opportunity to develop a program with appeal to both the DON and the College. In an effort to appeal to our nursing staff, several discussions took place between us and the leadership at Emmanuel College about how the program should take shape.

IMPORTANCE OF A GREAT PARTNER INSTITUTION

The advantages of education through a "cohort model" have been supported in the literature (Freiberg-Svoboda, 2003; Warren & Mills, 2009). Warren and Mills (2009) described the importance of a cohort model in the support of nurses' returning for further education. The cohort model involves tracking a group of students who share the same courses each semester and facilitate each other's success through sharing the educational experience. We believed the success of our staff returning to school would likely be associated with personal and professional development, as well as application of new knowledge in their clinical practice. However, many of our staff voiced concerns about their ability to be successful, their limited computer skills, and their anxiety about necessary writing and presentation skills. To address these concerns, we formulated a cohort model to offer student support and progression through an onsite program. In our view, if we could concentrate our early efforts on a single department with a number of non-BSN-prepared staff, we were confident that our initiative would be highly successful.

Because of the leadership support of the executive director of the Perioperative Nursing Division, Peggy Doyle, the Perioperative Division was chosen for a pilot site and recruitment efforts began. The first effort between the Academic Partnerships Advisory Group and Emmanuel College resulted in the creation of an online survey query of the nurses working in the Perioperative Division. This division had many associate degree and diploma graduate nurses, and we believed that they represented a group of nurses in the hospital who were cohesive and to whom a cohort model would be appealing. The results of the survey were very positive. The nurses were able to specify the type of program they would value. This input led to the nursing faculty at the College designing a program responsive to preferences for weekday and time for classes, class location, and the length of the plan of study. We quickly learned, with our partners at Emmanuel College, that the course of study plans could be developed to fit the needs of most of the prospective students. Individual review of transcripts by nursing faculty offered support for transfer of credits and was welcomed by the BWH nursing staff.

There was growing interest in an onsite program and the enthusiasm of a division-specific cohort began to build. Emmanuel College developed a plan of study. The faculty, administration, and staff of the College were eager to meet the needs of those nurses who expressed interest.

Recruitment activities within the division were robust, with the dedication of Helen Muterperl, enrollment counselor at Emmanuel, coordinating the efforts. We held several informational presentations for interested staff. Individual meetings with Emmanuel College faculty were scheduled for each staff nurse who was considering the program. The support and flexibility shown by the College were critical attributes of our productive partnership. A team of faculty members, led by Diane Arathuzik, met with the individual students to discuss transfer of credits from their prior educational experiences. A specific course of study was developed to meet individual needs and, most importantly, to offer encouragement and support to the prospective students.

Additionally, there was overwhelming support from the nursing leadership team in the Perioperative Division, thus accommodating the nursing staff meeting with college representatives, and offering support for potential students considering a return to school. As this planning progressed, we began the coordination efforts for reservation of classroom space, audiovisual equipment, and other supplies that would make it possible for nurses to conveniently transition from their workday to their school day.

CURRENT STATE OF ACADEMIC PARTNERSHIP

A full cohort—a potential 20 students—submitted applications for admission to the program. In an effort to make the partnership even more seamless and attractive to the nurses, Leo Buckley, director of Business Services for the BWH DON, and Judith Marley, dean of Emmanuel College's Graduate and Professional Programs, initiated negotiations to assess the feasibility of a direct-payment option between the hospital and the College. David McMahon, project manager in the DON, Rosaleen Riley, the administrative assistant from BWH, and Kathryn Mackintosh, director of Employer Partnerships at Emmanuel, were also instrumental in the implementation of the financial arrangement that emerged from these negotiations. Rather than the staff being billed directly by the College and then submitting for reimbursement from the hospital, the College agreed to invoice the DON directly.

The direct-payment arrangement was appealing to students. Hospital leadership thus sent a vital message of their support for the goal of a baccalaureate-prepared staff. Concurrently, interest in the program began to emerge from nurses and departments outside of the Perioperative Division, and the College agreed to expand its efforts to include a second cohort with a projected graduation date of May 2012. There were 51 nurses in these two initial cohorts of students—an overwhelming success for our neighbor, Emmanuel College, and the BWH's DON. In January 2010, we began our third onsite cohort with 17 students.

Although the nurses in their cohorts attend class onsite at BWH, they enjoy all of the benefits of the nearby campus and college community. These include library privileges, research support, access to the Yawkey Center's recreation and dining facilities, writing support, career counseling services, and access to on-campus cultural, athletic, and enrichment events. Our nursing staff report that they value the benefits of attending an onsite program balanced with a vibrant college community, and they embrace the role of student and learn new theoretical and clinical knowledge to apply in their practice.

The DON vision statement commits BWH nurses to *"excellent care to patients and families, with the best staff, in the safest environment."* We believe our onsite program story demonstrates the commitment we have all made to ensure not only that we have "the best staff," but also that we create the opportunities for that staff to become even better. The enthusiasm and commitment of our cohorts has assured us this initiative was a wise choice.

REFERENCES

Aiken, L. H., Clarke, S. P., Cheung, R. B., Sloane, D. M., & Silber, J. H. (2003). Educational levels of hospital nurses and surgical patient mortality. *Journal of the American Medical Association, 290*(12), 1617–1623.

Freiberg-Svoboda, G. (2003). *A study of informal learning in an adult degree-completion cohort program.* (Unpublished doctoral dissertation) Northern Illinois University, DeKalb, Il.

Kanai-Pak, M., Aiken, L. H., Sloane, D. M., & Poghosyan, L. (2008). Poor work environments and nurse inexperience are associated with burnout, job dissatisfaction and quality deficits in Japanese. *Journal of Clinical Nursing, 17*(24), 3324–3329.

Kutney-Lee, A., McHugh, M. D., Sloane, D. M., Cimiotti, J. P., Flynn, L., Neff, D. F., & Aiken, L. H. (2009). Nursing: A key to patient satisfaction. *Health Affairs, 28*(4), w669–w677.

Van den Heede, K., Clarke, S. P., Sermeus, W., Vleugels, A., & Aiken, L. H. (2007). International experts' perspectives on the state of the nurse staffing and patient outcomes literature. *Journal of Nursing Scholarship, 39*, 290–297.

Van den Heede, K., Lasaffre, E., Diya, L., Vleugels, A., Clarke, S. P., Aiken, L. H., & Sermeus, W. (2009). The relationship between inpatient cardiac surgery mortality and nurse numbers and educational level: Analysis of administrative data. *International Journal of Nursing Studies, 46*(6), 796–803.

Van den Heede, K., Sermeus, W., Diya, L., Clarke, S. P., Lesaffre, E., Vleugels, A., & Aiken, L. H. (2009). Nurse staffing and patient outcomes in Belgian acute hospitals: Cross-sectional analysis of administrative data. *International Journal of Nursing Studies, 46*(7), 928–939.

Warren, J. I., & Mills, M. E. (2009). Motivating registered nurses to return for an advanced degree. *Journal of Continuing Education in Nursing, 40*(5), 200–207.

14.3 *Preventing Patients From Falling: Achieving the Vision*

Patricia C. Dykes, Ann C. Hurley, Ronna Zaremski, and Diane L. Carroll

---

Our story of preventing falls in patients hospitalized in the acute short-term-stay hospital began with the Partners HealthCare System (PHS) Chief Nurse Council and the formation of a PHS-wide Fall Prevention Task Force (FPTF). The story closes, but does not end, with the good news that our team's intervention to reduce falls was the first randomized controlled clinical trial found to significantly reduce falls in this patient population. The story will end when national fall rates and falls with injuries of patients hospitalized in the acute short-term-stay hospital are markedly reduced.

BACKGROUND

Accidental falls are a public health problem worldwide (Chen, Warner, Fingerhut, & Makuc, 2009), and hospitalization increases the risk of falling (Evans, Hodgkinson, Lambert, & Wood, 2001) due to the unfamiliar environment, illness, and treatments. Falls with injury drive up hospital costs and lengths of stay (Fischer et al., 2005; Tinetti, Richman, & Powell, 1990). Despite more than 3 decades of published research on falls prevention, the need for hospitals to "do no harm" and a public policy denying reimbursement for treatment of injuries related to falls (Inouye, Brown, & Tinetti, 2009) remain a serious problem in U.S. hospitals, including PHS hospitals.

Partners HealthCare System Confronts the Issue of Patient Falls

I (first author, PD) was the PHS FPTF co-leader since 2004 and in that role worked with fall prevention teams at each of the eight PHS hospitals. The FPTF is an interdisciplinary team of fall prevention experts representing each PHS hospital. This team brings a wealth of expertise to the table. We knew that preventing patients from falling requires a combination of three factors: (1) system-level mechanisms to support patients and caregivers, (2) bedside caregivers with the necessary knowledge and resources, and (3) inclusion of patients/family/visitors in the fall prevention plan. Because an adequate fall risk assessment is needed to establish fall prevention interventions, our first action was to identify and implement standardized fall assessment methods across all PHS hospitals.

We examined and evaluated all published fall risk assessment scales, located through a review of falls prevention literature in English-language publications found in the MEDLINE (1966 to 2005) and CINAHL (1982 to 2005) databases using the search terms: fall prevention in hospitals, fall prevention qualitative, fall risk assessment, and nurse and paraprofessional perceptions of fall prevention. Our goal was to identify a "gold standard" scale, that is, a scale that had been prospectively validated to determine that it is accurate.

Of the five scales identified that had been prospectively validated, the Morse Fall Scale (MFS) (Morse, 1997, 2008) was selected because of its clinical credibility (being widely available, having a simple scoring method with variable weights based on a standard, and able to be completed in less than 1 minute), accuracy (sensitivity = 78% and specificity = 83%), and generality (tested in multiple settings and variables that were clearly defined). The MFS was implemented across all hospital sites during 2004–2005. FPTF members oversaw the development and implementation of competency programs and confirmed accurate use of the MFS, thus ensuring interrater reliability. FPTF representatives worked with site-specific documentation and safety committees and information systems staff to integrate the MFS into each hospital's documentation system.

THE OPPORTUNITY

In 2006, three conditions aligned to provide the impetus and resources for us to move forward to translate patients' fall risk status into interventions to prevent patient falls. First, the MFS was successfully implemented in all PHS hospitals, so patients' risks for falling were assessed accurately and their fall risk status was documented. Second, the communication between and integration among the PHS Chief Nurse Council and FPTF and PHS hospitals fall prevention committees provided ideal structural, organizational, and environmental factors to support going to the next level: development and implementation of an action plan to prevent patients from falling. Third, the Robert Woods Johnson Foundation (RWJF) issued a second call for proposals under the program, Interdisciplinary Nursing Quality Research Initiative (INQRI). The PHS FPTF next step of moving from standardized assessment of fall risk to using those data to prevent falls was an ideal fit with the goal of the INQRI program: to generate, disseminate, and translate research to improve the quality of patient care.

Developing the Fall Prevention Study

From our literature review, we learned that (1) poor communication is a leading root cause of patient falls in hospitals; (2) a gap exists between risk assessment and the application of interventions to alter ameliorable risk factors and/or the implementation of individualized fall prevention strategies; and (3) no link between evidence-based tailored interventions and a reduction in patient falls has been established in acute care, short-stay hospitals. We matched the specific goals of the INQRI with the three deficits identified here to develop our research study.

Our goal was to prevent patient falls by translating an individual patient's fall risk assessment into a decision support intervention using health information technology (HIT) and building on existing work flows. The intended outcome was an evidence-based toolkit to overcome barriers, strengthen facilitators, and improve communication of fall risk status to interdisciplinary team members, paraprofessionals, patients, and family members, as well as to translate an evidence-based fall prevention plan of care into practice. The 2-year study was reviewed favorably, funded, and begun in fall 2008.

Implementing the Study

We leveraged system-wide and individual hospital infrastructures to develop the organizational structure to conduct our study. As principal investigator, I (PD, then the PHS Corporate Manager, Nursing Informatics and Research) led the interdisciplinary research team with senior investigators representing nursing (authors DC and AH), medicine (Blackford Middleton), and biostatistics (Stuart Lipsitz). In addition to support from the PHS Chief Nurse Council, the PHS Clinical Informatics Research and Development Laboratory (directed by BM) provided heuristic evaluation and usability testing.

Each PHS chief nursing officer appointed a member from the PHS fall prevention task force to be a hospital-based facilitator to report to me (PD) to support conducting the study at each hospital. At each hospital, nurses were involved from the very beginning and provided essential support to lead to the study's successful implementation. At BWH, Escel Stanghellini, Quality Program Director for Hematology/Oncology/Bone Marrow Transplant, recruited nurses and assistants to participate in focus groups to learn what staff were currently doing to prevent falls. After randomization, unit champions on intervention units, such as BWH's Ronna Zaremski (nurse educator on tower 14cd), worked with the research team to introduce and sustain the intervention following the Institute for Health Care Improvement's Framework for Spread (FFS) (Massoud, Nielsen, Nolan, Schall, & Sevin, 2006).

LEARNING FROM KEY STAKEHOLDERS

We used both qualitative and quantitative research methods to identify and describe barriers and facilitators of existing fall risk communication patterns.

Patient and Family Interviews

Because patients who have fallen can offer unique views and directions for fall prevention, we interviewed nine patients who had recently fallen while hospitalized. In explaining why they fell, two fundamental reasons emerged: the need to toilet coupled with loss of balance and unexpected weakness (Carroll, Dykes, & Hurley, 2010).

Focus Groups

We wanted to hear directly from nurses and assistants about why patients fall: what barriers had to be overcome and what was currently working well to prevent patients from falling. With the assistance of hospital-based facilitators, we held four groups with 23 nurses and four with 19 assistants. They told us that a fall prevention intervention would have to carefully consider patient report, information access, signage, environment, teamwork, and involvement of patient/family (Dykes, Carroll, Hurley, Benoit, & Middleton, 2009). Our stakeholders told us loud and clear that more information was needed at the bedside to communicate to all team members (including patients and family members) why a patient is at risk and what specifically should be done to prevent a fall.

DEVELOPING AND TESTING THE INTERVENTION:
THE FALL PREVENTION TOOLKIT

We used HIT capability to link individual patients' determinants of fall risk, as assessed by nurses using the MFS, to an evidence-based and tailored plan of care to prevent falls. We developed a software package, Fall TIPS (Tailoring Interventions for Patient Safety), to integrate the Fall Prevention Toolkit (FPTK) into existing workflows without adding any extra steps by allowing nurses to enter the MFS electronically. The FPTK generates three outputs to communicate the fall prevention plan: an over-the-bed poster visible so that all who enter the room know of the risk and intervention, a patient handout, and the care plan for health team members. For example, if a patient is at risk for falls due to an impaired gait and the assistance of two people is required to get the patient up safely, the bed poster and plan of care would include the icon for "out of bed with assistance of two people." The patient handout would include the same icon and simple text reminding patients that they are at risk because they are "unsteady on their feet" and should "call for help to get out of bed."

FPTK Requirements

The wealth of information learned about overcoming barriers and strengthening facilitators during interviews and focus group meetings from key stakeholders was indispensable as we developed the initial prototype. For example, we were told about the limitations of the ubiquitous and generic "high risk for falls" sign that does not tell why the patient is at fall risk nor what to do to prevent a fall; we were assured that "a picture is worth a thousand words." These kinds of useful insights guided development.

We (PD, AH, DC) analyzed all transcripts to identify content and requirements for Fall TIPS and determined that icons supplemented with short, plain text would simplify and standardize communication across stakeholders. An illustrator developed a series of icons to represent each of the MFS areas of risk and the associated fall prevention interventions. With the assistance of the hospital facilitators, professional and paraprofessional caregivers were recruited to assist with validation and refinement of the icons/plain text during another eight focus groups, which yielded the final 11 icons to populate the FPTK (Hurley, Dykes, Carroll, Dykes, & Middleton, 2009). The simple text that accompanies the "out of bed with assistance of two people" icon described earlier is "Out of Bed with Assist of 2."

The final step before testing the FPTK on patient units was to learn recommendations from end users for making the Fall TIPS software user friendly. After usability testing was accomplished in the PHS Clinical Informatics Research and Development Laboratory (Dykes et al., 2009) and final modifications made (Zuyov, Benoit, Chang, & Dykes, 2010), the FPTK was ready to be tested in selected units in four PHS short-stay hospitals.

Unit champions (for BWH, unit 14cd facilitator, RZ, was joined by Nikki Shanley, Rachel Pozzar, and Sarah Imparato) were key to successful FPTK implementation, especially fidelity of the intervention. Not only did the champions encourage staff to use the FPTK, they so "bought into" the intervention that they shared the FPTK at several conferences, a poster session at the 2009 Annual NICHE (Nurses Improving Care for Health System Elders) Conference in Orlando, Florida

(Zaremski, Shanley, Pozzar, & Imparato, 2009) and podium presentations at the 2009 PHS Nursing Quality Leaders Conference and the New England Nursing Informatics Consortium.

A Little Serendipity

When we were reading the stories nurses and assistants told us about why patients fell and how to prevent patients from falling, we learned that staff put forth a great deal of effort to prevent falls; when they had the necessary resources and information, they were confident in their ability to prevent falls. Such confidence is the central component of the self-efficacy (S-E) concept, the belief in one's capability to carry out actions necessary to meet given situational demands (Bandura, 2001). We applied for and received funding through the BWH Lily Kravitz Nursing Research Award to develop and test the Self-Efficacy for Preventing Falls Nurse (SEPFN) and Assistant (SEPFA) scales.

Drawing on the qualitative data set obtained during the RN and CNA focus groups (four of each), we (PD, AH, DC) generated individual items for scale consideration and developed prototypes. We were joined by several nursing students in the Northeastern University Master of Science Program in Nursing and the Massachusetts General Hospital Institute of the Professions Doctorate in Nursing Practice Program, who were able to work with us obtaining hands-on research experience as a component of their research practicum. We carried out all the necessary steps to refine and confirm the SEPFN and SEPFA scales and have suggested that those scales be used at any site where fall prevention is a goal (Dykes et al., 2010). Kerry McColgan, the third author on the self-efficacy paper, contributed to and learned from developing the scales and is now a full-time graduate student. Lisa Colombo, the MGH IHP doctoral student, co-authored the paper that was recently published in the *Journal of Advanced Nursing* (Dykes et al., 2010).

RANDOMIZED CLINICAL TRIAL PROVES THE EFFICACY OF THE FPTK

We conducted a 6-month randomized clinical trial (RCT) to evaluate the effectiveness of the FPTK on reducing patient falls in four different PHS hospitals: BWH, Faulkner, Massachusetts General, and North Shore. Within each hospital, we had an intervention unit (5160 patients) and a control unit (5104 patients). The FPTK integrated existing communication and workflow patterns into the HIT application. A valid fall risk assessment scale (the MFS) completed by the nurse was the foundation from which the FPTK software tailored fall prevention interventions to address patients' specific determinants of fall risk. Three FPTK outputs were bed posters (composed of short text with the accompanying icon), patient education forms, and plans of care, all providing patient-specific alerts to key stakeholders.

The primary outcome was patient fall rate (patient falls/1000 patient days) adjusted for site and patient care unit. There was a statistically significant difference in the number of falls between control ($N = 87$) and intervention ($N = 68$) units. Site-adjusted fall rates were significantly higher on control (4.54 [confidence interval = 3.85, 5.37]) than on intervention (3.37 [confidence interval = 2.79, 4.08]) units ($p = .021$). The FPTK was found to be particularly effective with patients aged 65 years and older (rate difference = 2.29 [confidence interval = .63-3.95], p = .005). (The research aims, interventions, and outcomes may be viewed at http:// clinicaltrials.gov/ct2/show/NCT00675935.)

THE FUTURE

At BWH and PHS

We have an enormous amount of qualitative/quantitative data that we plan to "mine" to refine FTTK logic and will continue to write and submit publications as we further evaluate and extend our findings. For instance, some patients for whom the FPTK was used did fall. We do not know if any falls were associated with inaccurate assessment using the MFS, or if the FTTK was used incorrectly, or if the falls that occurred would be considered nonpreventable.

Beyond BWH and PHS

We applied and were selected to be included in the next edition of *Quality Profiles*™: *The Leadership Series*, published by the National Committee for Quality Assurance (NCQA) and Pfizer, Inc. Before publication of our results in *JAMA*, we were invited to participate in a media briefing at the National Press Club in Washington, DC, where *JAMA* released new research on aging (http://press.org/events/aging-jama-theme-issue-media-briefing). We hope that our generalizable model to improve communication of patient determinants of risk and to apply evidence-based, tailored plans of care to prevent falls will be used by others.

We recognize that when we prevent a patient from falling, we potentially prevent that patient from sustaining an injury. Therefore, we believe that by preventing falls using the FPTK, we likely prevented injuries as well. However, our study was not designed or powered to test the effectiveness of the FPTK on preventing injury-producing falls; additional research is needed to establish a linkage between the FPTK and prevention of fall-related injury. To test the FPTK for the capacity to prevent injurious falls requires time and resources beyond BWH operational funds. We are in the process of applying for federal funding to first mine the FPTK database and incident reports to refine the FPTK logic and then test the refined toolkit for effectiveness with falls and falls with injury on adult patients of all ages. We then hope to implement the toolkit across all PHS adult inpatient units.

CONCLUDING COMMENTS

The *JAMA* paper and the series of studies preceding the RCT also illustrate the many ways in which nursing scholarship was operational in the BWH clinical setting. Nurses (1) collaborated with other disciplines and across service/academic settings, (2) conducted research as principal investigators and mentored the next generation of researchers, and (3) willingly gave of their time to be research subjects and graciously facilitated the conduct of clinical research on busy patient care units. Collectively, these actions operationalize the BWH Nursing Department vision of *excellent care to patients and families, by the very best staff, in the safest environment.*

The authors acknowledge John Dykes for illustrating the icons, and the other members of our research team: Stuart Lipsitz, ScD; Angela Benoit, Bcomm; Frank Chang, MSE; Seth Meltzer; Ruslana Tsurkova, MSc, MA; Lyubov Zuyov, MA; and Blackford Middleton, MD, MPH, MSc.

REFERENCES

Bandura, A. (2001). Social cognitive theory: An agentic perspective. *Annual Review of Psychology, 52,* 1–26.

Carroll, D. L., Dykes, P. C., & Hurley, A. C. (2010). Patients' perspectives of falling while in an acute care hospital and suggestions for prevention. *Applied Nursing Research, 23,* 238–241.

Chen, L., Warner, M., Fingerhut, L., & Makuc, D. (2009). Injury episodes and circumstances: National Health Interview Survey, 1997–2007. *Vital Health Statistics, 10,* 241.

Dykes, P. C., Carroll, D. L., Hurley, A. C., Benoit, A., & Middleton, B. (2009). Why do patients in acute care hospitals fall? Can falls be prevented? *Journal of Nursing Administration, 39,* 299–304.

Dykes, P. C., Carroll, D. L., Hurley, A. C., Gersh-Zaremski, R., Kennedy, A., Kurowski, J., et al. (2009). Fall TIPS: Strategies to promote adoption and use of a fall prevention toolkit. *AMIA Annual Symposium Proceedings* (pp. 153–157). Bethesda, MD: American Medical Informatics Association.

Dykes, P. C., Carroll, D. L., McColgan, K., Hurley, A. C., Lipsitz, S. R., Colombo, L., et al. (2010). Scales for assessing self-efficacy of nurses and assistants for preventing falls. *Journal of Advanced Nursing, 67,* 438–449.

Evans, D., Hodgkinson, B., Lambert, L., & Wood, J. (2001). Falls risk factors in the hospital setting: A systematic review. *International Journal of Nursing Practice, 7,* 38–45.

Fischer, I. D., Krauss, M. J., Dunagan, W. C., Birge, S., Hitcho, E., Johnson, S., et al. (2005). Patterns and predictors of inpatient falls and fall-related injuries in a large academic hospital. *Infection Control & Hospital Epidemiology, 26,* 822–827.

Hurley, A. C., Dykes, P. C., Carroll, D. L., Dykes, J. S., & Middleton, B. (2009). Fall TIPS: Validation of icons to communicate fall risk status and tailored interventions to prevent patient falls. *Studies in Health Technology & Informatics, 146,* 455–459.

Inouye, S. K., Brown, C. J., & Tinetti, M. E. (2009). Medicare nonpayment, hospital falls, and unintended consequences. *New England Journal of Medicine, 360,* 2390–2393.

Massoud, M., Nielsen, G., Nolan, K., Schall, M., & Sevin, C. (2006). *A framework for spread: From local improvements to system-wide change.* Retrieved April 11, 2010, from http://www.ihi.org/IHI/Results/WhitePapers/AFrameworkforSpreadWhitePaper.htm

Morse, J. M. (1997). *Preventing patient falls.* Thousand Oaks, CA: Sage.

Morse, J. M. (2008). *Preventing patient falls: Establishing a fall intervention program.* New York, NY: Springer Publishing.

Tinetti, M. E., Richman, D., & Powell, L. (1990). Falls efficacy as a measure of fear of falling. *Journal of Gerontology: Psychological Sciences, 45,* P239–P243.

Zaremski, R., Shanley, N., Pozzar, R., & Imparato, S. (2009, February). *Fall TIPS (Tailoring Interventions for Patient Safety).* 12th Annual NICHE Conference, Orlando, FL.

Zuyov, L., Benoit, A., Chang, F. Y., & Dykes, P. (2011). Tailored prevention of inpatient falls: Development and usability testing of the Fall TIPS toolkit. *Computers Informatics Nursing, 29*(Suppl. 2), TC21–TC28.

14.4 *Interdisciplinary Leadership in the Oncology Service Line*

Patricia Reid Ponte

---

*B*righam and Women's Hospital (BWH) and Dana-Farber Cancer Institute (DFCI) have long collaborated to meet the needs of adult oncology patients and their families. In 1997, the collaboration moved to a new level when the two organizations agreed to combine their oncology services and locate all inpatient oncology care at BWH and hematology and oncology outpatient services at DFCI. This change prompted the organizations to integrate other support and clinical services as well, including oncology nursing, pharmacy, infusion, social work, pain and palliative care, and radiation therapy. The longstanding partnership between the two hospitals was ultimately formalized in 2004, when the organizations formed a joint venture creating the Dana-Farber/Brigham and Women's Cancer Center (DF/BWCC). Today, DF/BWCC provides the full continuum of adult oncology services and accounts for more than 280,000 ambulatory visits and 5,051 inpatient admissions annually. Fundamental to DF/BWCC's success is the two organizations' commitment to interdisciplinary collaboration. This commitment is evident in the interdisciplinary care teams that care for patients and families in the inpatient and ambulatory settings, and in the interdisciplinary leadership structures that guide clinical operations. Through these structures, responsibility for clinical operations is shared by teams consisting of a nurse, physician, and, in some cases, an administrator. Interdisciplinary leadership teams permeate DF/BWCC, overseeing operations at the organizational level and on the inpatient units and ambulatory clinics or "disease centers."

Sharing leadership responsibilities with members of other disciplines requires work and a high level of trust, communication, and collaboration. However, we have found that the effort that goes into establishing an interdisciplinary leadership model and making it work is well worth the effort. Interdisciplinary leadership facilitates collaboration and the sharing of ideas throughout the organization. Additionally, by ensuring that the perspectives and needs of all constituents are equally valued and represented at the table, the model strengthens decision making about priorities, resource allocation, improvement efforts, and the care environment (Reid Ponte, 2008).

In this chapter, I describe the interdisciplinary leadership model that guides operations at DF/BWCC, paying particular attention to the critical role played by nurses and nursing, and to the principles, processes, and structures that underlie the model and ensure its effectiveness. I also share examples that illustrate how interdisciplinary leadership helps advance oncology care and the vision of the Department of Nursing, by promoting collaboration among nurses, staff, and providers at every level and facilitating efforts to improve care and assure a safe and supportive environment for patients, families, and staff.

INTERDISCIPLINARY LEADERSHIP STRUCTURE AT DF/BWCC

Interdisciplinary leadership structures oversee DF/BWCC operations at every level.

Executive Level

At both BWH and DFCI, organizational operations are overseen by an executive leadership team consisting of the chief nursing officer (CNO), chief medical officer (CMO), and chief operating officer (COO). Each member reports to the president/chief executive officer (CEO) and works with the president and other senior leaders to guide organizational strategy, program development and approval, resource allocation, and policy decisions. With oncology as DFCI's primary focus, the executive leadership triad at DFCI is integrally involved in guiding DF/BWCC operations and facilitating coordination across the inpatient and ambulatory services. One way in which coordination is achieved is through cross-institutional committees and improvement teams, several of which are led by members of DFCI's executive leadership triad. The CNO, for example, chairs the DF/BWCC Quality Committee, the CMO chairs the DF/BWCC Service Line Committee, and the COO chairs the DF/BW Executive Leadership Group.

Coordination across settings is also supported by a unique nurse executive leadership and reporting structure. As the vice president of patient care services at DFCI, the CNO of DFCI oversees all adult and pediatric ambulatory nursing. (DFCI cares for children with cancer and their families through a partnership with Children's Hospital Boston.) In an unusual arrangement, the DFCI CNO is also the director of oncology nursing and clinical services at BWH, reporting to the CNO of BWH in this capacity. This unique arrangement acknowledges the responsibilities that the BWH CNO holds for all inpatient programs and services, including oncology, while also taking advantage of the special capabilities the DFCI CNO brings to the area of cancer care. It also positions the DFCI CNO to ensure standardization and integration of oncology nursing practice across the inpatient and ambulatory settings.

Interdisciplinary Leadership at the Service Level

The interdisciplinary leadership teams for the inpatient and ambulatory oncology services ensure a shared vision of excellence in patient care and a collaborative and interdisciplinary approach to quality and care improvement (Ponte, 2004). The leadership team for the inpatient service consists of a doctorally prepared executive nurse director and a medical oncologist, who share responsibility for program development, quality monitoring and improvement, and fiscal oversight and management. The team works closely with nurse directors and physicians on the inpatient units, collaborating with them to streamline work processes, evaluate and adopt new approaches to cancer care, and assure a safe environment for patients and staff. The executive nurse director of the leadership team is a member of the Nurse Executive Board at BWH and DFCI. This allows her to collaborate with nurse leaders at both institutions to support and guide the professional development of the DF/BWCC nursing staff.

The ambulatory program based at DFCI is also overseen by an interdisciplinary team. This team consists of a nursing vice president, a physician director who is a medical oncologist as well as the director of the breast oncology disease center, and an administrative vice president. The members of this leadership triad are jointly responsible for overseeing operations in DFCI's 12 disease centers, each of which specializes in a different type of cancer. The team also oversees the infusion areas, radiation therapy, and other cancer treatment areas at DFCI. The triad members jointly chair the Multidisciplinary Clinical Services Committee (MCSC), created to facilitate coordination across the clinical areas. The MCSC consists of nurse program leaders, physician clinical directors, and program managers of each disease center. The directors of centralized departments, such as Social Work and Pharmacy, also participate in the MCSC, using it as a vehicle for planning and introducing changes affecting multiple areas.

Interdisciplinary Leadership at the Unit and Disease Center Levels

Interdisciplinary leadership is also a hallmark of leadership at the unit and practice levels. We have found that an interdisciplinary model yields some of its most tangible benefits here, because this is where the "rubber hits the road" in terms of care quality and an interdisciplinary approach to care improvement is essential (Ponte, 2004). Each of the 12 disease centers is overseen by a leadership dyad composed of a nurse program leader and a clinical physician director, and is supported by an operations manager. The team members share responsibility for all aspects of operational decision making and are jointly accountable for the disease center's budget; managing and improving operations and systems; and meeting clinical, operational, and financial targets. They are also responsible for guiding the performance of staff and addressing personnel and performance issues (Ponte, Gross, Winer, Connaughton, & Hassinger, 2007).

The interdisciplinary leadership model outlined here has fostered an environment that values interdisciplinary and cross-institutional collaboration and shared decision making. Such an environment does not develop automatically, however. We have found that collaboration is ensured only if all members of the leadership teams commit to a core set of principles and adopt strategies and ways of leading to make these principles evident.

PRINCIPLES THAT GUIDE INTERDISCIPLINARY COLLABORATION AND LEADERSHIP

The following core principles form a foundation for interdisciplinary leadership at DF/BWCC.

Inclusion: Because every discipline cannot be represented on an interdisciplinary leadership team, leaders must possess a philosophy of inclusion and commit to developing mechanisms for involving all disciplines in problem solving and decision making.

Staff involvement in priority setting, decision making, and planning: Leaders must also commit to involving staff in governance activities. Involving staff in decision making contributes to a more transparent environment, while welcoming their ideas and input fosters the collaboration that is essential for improving care delivery. Staff involvement can be facilitated through forums that promote dialogue between leaders and staff, and by governance structures that promote staff participation in planning, policy development, and decision making (Reid Ponte, 2008).

Respect for differences: Listening intently and respecting others' ideas and suggestions are fundamental requirements of leaders on interdisciplinary teams. Individuals who are used to a more unilateral or hierarchical approach can sometimes find it difficult to truly listen and to factor others' ideas and experiences into decision making. If respect for differences is part of the organizational culture, however, and leaders have a chance to see it modeled by others, they quickly begin to appreciate its value and incorporate respect for differences into their own leadership style.

Patient- and family-centered care: As a philosophy and care delivery model, patient- and family-centered care embraces many of the same values as interdisciplinary leadership, including inclusion and respect for differences. In organizations that are truly committed to patient- and family-centered care, patients and families are valued as partners in every domain: The provider-patient relationship is marked by social equity, transparency, and joint decision making; and patients and family members work side-by-side with administrators and clinician leaders, helping to establish the organization's priorities, collaborating on decisions about the care environment, and participating in initiatives to improve care and service delivery. Leaders on effective interdisciplinary leadership teams recognize that patients and families provide a unique perspective and value their input and participation in oversight and improvement efforts (Reid Ponte, 2008).

Defined roles and functions: For interdisciplinary leadership to be successful, leaders must differentiate among areas for which they are jointly responsible, and areas where accountability rests largely with one discipline or another. These lines of accountability must be clear to the leaders and the organization as a whole. Although some domains are unique to one discipline, this does not mean that decision making in these areas always takes place in isolation from leadership colleagues. Rather, leaders recognize that adding other perspectives can sometimes strengthen the decision-making process by helping a discipline understand how its actions affect patients and families, interdisciplinary colleagues, and care systems (Ponte, 2004).

STRUCTURES AND PROCESSES FACILITATING COLLABORATION

Operationalizing an interdisciplinary leadership model can be challenging even for leaders who embrace the principles outlined here. A number of things can be done to improve a model's chances of success. These include carefully defining the leadership structures that are implemented, clarifying the responsibilities and accountabilities of leadership teams and their members, and developing processes to help leaders acquire the skills needed to work collaboratively and to turn the concept of interdisciplinary leadership into a reality.

Leadership Structures

Although no single interdisciplinary leadership structure is right for every organization and every level, we have found nurse-physician partnerships to be especially effective. Aligning nurse and physician leaders creates opportunities for synergy and for pursuing mutual goals related to patient care and care improvement. Nurse-physician partnerships also ensure a shared vision for excellence in patient care and serve as role models for other disciplines and individual clinicians (Ponte, 2004). Including administrative leaders on interdisciplinary leadership teams can further enhance a team's effectiveness by empowering it to address a broader range of service delivery and operational issues. Whatever structure is put in place, it must be accompanied by mechanisms for obtaining input from every discipline and engaging staff in decision-making and improvement efforts. Without such mechanisms, an interdisciplinary leadership model cannot fulfill its promise of promoting a truly collaborative environment.

Collaborative Practice Agreements

As a first step for a new leadership team, developing a collaborative practice agreement can be invaluable. Through such an agreement, members of the team define areas of accountability that are shared and those where accountability is held by one member of the group. Members of the leadership team can also use the agreement to outline mechanisms and parameters for decision making; to define expectations and methods for communicating with one another; and to specify how they will assess the team's effectiveness, including which metrics they will use and who will be asked to provide feedback. Collaborative practice agreements can be modified as the team gains experience. In the beginning, however, they help team members understand what interdisciplinary leadership means and can help prevent misunderstandings that arise from poor communication or making decisions "on the fly" (Reid Ponte, 2008; Reid Ponte & Peterson, 2008).

Team Training

Team effectiveness training focused on helping leaders acquire and practice skills required for collaboration and negotiating differences can be useful at any stage. When interdisciplinary teams are first established, team training can be used to establish guidelines for behavior and to equip leaders with useful communication tools and techniques. As the members of interdisciplinary leadership teams gain experience, team training gives them an opportunity to reflect on their methods of working with one another and identify opportunities for bringing collaboration to a new level. Leadership retreats that focus on broader issues can also be useful. From time to time, we have held retreats for all leaders in the organization, using them to reflect on the principles of interdisciplinary leadership and how they can be better manifested in the organization.

IMPACT OF INTERDISCIPLINARY LEADERSHIP MODEL
ON PATIENT CARE OUTCOMES

The greatest benefit of interdisciplinary leadership is the impact it has on patient care and outcomes, where it can help to ensure highly coordinated care that anticipates patient and family needs. It also establishes an environment in which an interdisciplinary approach to quality and care improvement is automatic (Reid Ponte & Peterson, 2008).

The interdisciplinary leadership model at DF/BWCC has been instrumental to our efforts to streamline and improve care across the continuum. The following two examples illustrate this well in terms of patient outcomes.

First, there is the role of interdisciplinary leaders at the service level. For some patients, chemotherapy must be initiated in the inpatient setting. Several years ago, a review of the admission process indicated that many oncology patients experienced long wait times in the admitting area, waiting for inpatient beds to become available. For these patients, the start of chemotherapy was delayed, sometimes until the following day. With their length of stay extended, patients and staff were dissatisfied.

Working together, the inpatient nursing director, medical director, and service line administrator developed a program to facilitate admission. In collaboration with clinicians from the inpatient and ambulatory settings, the team developed the ambulatory-to-inpatient clinical pathway or AICP. Through AICP, patients requiring admission for chemotherapy go first to DFCI, where a physician sees the patient and writes his or her premedication and chemotherapy orders. Pharmacists at DFCI prepare the first 24 hours of chemotherapy and nurses in the infusion area initiate treatment. Once the patient's inpatient bed is available, the nurse transports the patient to the unit and transfers responsibility to the inpatient nurse. Because of AICP, the start of chemotherapy is no longer delayed due to lack of an inpatient bed, and hospital lengths of stay and patient and staff satisfaction have improved.

Second, there is the interdisciplinary and cross-institutional collaboration fostered by the leadership model in use. Hypersensitivity reactions are relatively common among patients receiving chemotherapy. In the past, such reactions meant that some patients could not receive recommended courses of treatment. To address this issue, an interdisciplinary team from DF/BWCC developed a unique desensitization protocol through which patients receive a highly diluted form of the offending agent over 12 to 24 hours, gradually becoming desensitized to it. Because of the risk of hypersensitivity reactions, a special process was needed to ensure that patients would be closely monitored and treated at the first sign of an allergic reaction.

A team consisting of a nursing director, physician clinical director, an allergist, and nurse leaders and staff from the inpatient and ambulatory areas designed and implemented the desensitization program. Working together, they arranged to have patients receive their first desensitization treatment in the BWH medical intensive care unit (MICU). Assuming the treatment goes well (and most do), subsequent doses are administered in a special treatment area at DFCI. Before implementing the desensitization program, a nurse practitioner from DFCI, the nurse manager of the MICU, and the allergist trained MICU nurses in the procedure and coordinated communication with oncology providers, informing them of the treatment option and the required scheduling logistics. Because of their efforts, numerous patients have successfully received first-line agents that would not have been available to them in the past.

In both examples, the interdisciplinary leadership model was key to the development and successful implementation of innovative solutions directly benefiting patients and families.

SUMMARY

The oncology service line's interdisciplinary leadership model promotes coordination and continuity of care across settings and institutions, and ensures that the voices and expertise of all disciplines involved in oncology patient care are represented in planning and decision making. Although elements of the oncology leadership model were introduced before the BWH Department of Nursing embarked on its process of change, the two initiatives complement one another and work synergistically to achieve common goals. Both place the patient and family at the center and emphasize inclusion and respect for differences, and both are committed to achieving the DON's vision of *excellent care to patients and families, with the very best staff, in the safest environment.*

REFERENCES

Ponte, P. R. (2004). Nurse-physician co-leadership: A model of interdisciplinary practice governance. *Journal of Nursing Administration, 34*(11), 481–484.

Ponte, P. R., Gross, A. H., Winer, E., Connaughton, M. J., & Hassinger, J. (2007). Implementing an interdisciplinary governance model in a comprehensive cancer center. *Oncology Nursing Forum, 34*(3), 611–616.

Reid Ponte, P. (2008). Personal. In L. Adams Thompson & E. H. O'Neil (Eds.), *Nurse executive: The four principles of management* (pp. 217–241). New York, NY: Springer Publishing.

Reid Ponte, P., & Peterson, K. (2008). A patient- and family-centered care model paves the way for a culture of quality and safety. *Critical Care Nursing Clinics of North America, 20*(4), 451–464.

Expanding Our Clinical Lens: Integrative Care

15.1 *Integrative Care*

Patricia M. Reilly and Teresa M. Buchanan

The relationships nurses form with patients and families are critical to the healing process and to developing a healing environment (Green, McArdle, & Robichaux, 2009; Quinn, 1992). By listening to patients, responding to their questions and needs, and providing hands-on care, nurses humanize the care experience while enhancing patients well-being and the process of recovery (Samueli Institute, 2007). Given the rapid pace of today's acute care environments, however, nurses can find it difficult to develop such healing relationships. At Brigham and Women's Hospital (BWH), the challenges nurses face in being present for patients was highlighted when we experienced a decline in patient satisfaction scores in the early 2000s, which indicated that patients were less satisfied with their interactions with nurses and felt less cared for than in the past. Nurses in the charge nurse role offered a possible explanation: Due to the demands and stresses confronting direct-care nurses, many had "nothing left to give," and their connection to patients and families suffered.

We realized we needed to introduce changes that would replenish nurses and support them in being present for patients and families. One of the key strategies we introduced was the Integrative Care Program (ICP). This unique program offers a range of complementary therapies that benefit patients, families, nurses, and other staff throughout the organization. In this chapter, we discuss the development of the ICP, Patricia Reilly as the founding director of ICP, and Teresa Buchanan as the project manager who joined her part time in 2008, as the ICP became increasingly successful. We also describe how the ICP contributes to a healing environment for patients and families, while helping nurses realign their energy and regain a sense of balance, joy, and connectedness in their work.

PROMOTING HEALING THROUGH INTEGRATIVE CARE

Integrative care is a holistic approach to care that combines the best of complementary therapies with conventional treatments. In addition to addressing physical needs, integrative care attends to an individual's mind, spirit, emotions, and relationships

(Benor, n.d.). Evidence-based practices used in integrative care facilitate the creation of a healing environment and support the development of a transpersonal connection between nurses and patients that further strengthens a patient's healing abilities and advances the environment's healing qualities. The holistic approach embodied by integrative care complements nursing's historical commitment to caring for the whole person and is consistent with the caring model advanced by nursing theorist Jean Watson, which advocates for health care environments that embody human values, caring practices, and healing processes (Watson, 2006).

Based on the knowledge they develop about their patients, nurses are able to recommend and incorporate integrative therapies into their patients' plans of care, using these to alleviate stress, promote a sense of well-being, and create conditions that support healing (Williams, Davies, & Griffiths, 2009; Taylor, 2008; Bossi, Ott, & DeCristofaro, 2008; Beckman, Boxley-Harges, Bruick-Sorge, & Salmon, 2007). Nurses can also benefit directly from integrative care practices and use them to realign their own energy fields, reduce their stress, and attain a renewed sense of wholeness.

Our first steps toward introducing integrative care in the Department of Nursing (DON) involved a 2002 research study. With the support of Judy Hayes, the executive director of nursing practice, and under the lead of Carolyn Hayes, a nurse researcher, we conducted a randomized controlled study that examined whether complementary therapies commonly used in integrative care might be helpful in reducing stress among nurses. The study sample included nurses in the charge nurse role, clinical nurses from cardiology and perioperative care, and nurses from Children's Hospital Boston. Nurses randomized to the intervention group attended a 4-hour class on mindfulness meditation and meditated daily using a 17-minute progressive relaxation tape. The nurses' meditation practices were reviewed periodically to help them find ways to fit meditation into their busy lives. Beginning in the third week, the nurses also received a therapeutic touch treatment and carried a beeper at work that vibrated at random times, reminding them to take a minute and focus on their breathing to "center themselves." Nurses in the control group used their normal coping mechanisms to manage stress encountered throughout the day. A survey tool that measured perception of stress was administered prior to the start, and again at the end of the 6-week study. Survey data collected at the conclusion of the study indicated that, compared to nurses in the control group, nurses in the intervention group were significantly less stressed ($p = 0.001$) (Hayes et al., 2002).

For the DON leadership, the study provided a compelling demonstration of the power of complementary or alternative approaches to stress management, and piqued their interest in exploring how these therapies might be applied more broadly to support nurses and patients in the care setting. Thus, they created a new permanent position, that of program manager for integrative care. The founding director was hired in 2002 and charged with exploring opportunities for making complementary therapies available to nurses, patients, and families and integrating those therapies into patient care. This director, who was well versed in complementary therapies, also brought to her new position a background in nursing management, critical care, and perioperative nursing and was sensitive to the stresses and challenges inherent in the clinical nurse and nursing management roles.

The study also had a profound effect on nurses in the intervention group. After the study was ended, the nurses expressed interest in continuing with the intervention and asked for additional information about alternative approaches to managing stress. The director of the newly formed ICP recognized their interest as an opportunity and began offering classes about complementary therapies to help individuals stay centered and acquire greater self-awareness, rather than getting caught up in the chaos around them. In addition to meditation, the classes explored Reiki therapy, reflexology, therapeutic touch, and aromatherapy.

Nurses responded to the classes with enthusiasm. ICP added lunchtime meditation sessions in the hospital chapel, as well as Reiki training so that nurses could provide Reiki treatments to one another and their patients. We also introduced "Reiki shares": setting up a Reiki treatment area in a lobby or other public location where patients, family members, nurses, physicians, and any other member of the hospital staff could stop by and receive a treatment. The "Reiki shares" were very well received, attracting scores of individuals. We realized we were shifting a culture.

The ICP director also began to work with nurses in the post-anesthesia care unit (PACU) to help them manage challenges within the perioperative area. With 50,000 surgeries performed annually, the BWH PACU cares for a constant flow of patients and combines the intensity of an ICU with the turnover and pace of a busy emergency department. At any one time, up to 50 patients and 50 staff members might be in the unit, which is an open area roughly the size of several basketball courts.

The ICP director began working with the PACU staff and introduced the work of Don Miguel Ruiz, whose book *The Four Agreements* (Ruiz, 1997) has served as a guide to self-awareness and enlightenment for people around the world. We also helped them explore how they might "soften" the care environment and reduce the stress felt by nurses as well as patients. With the support of the ICP, the PACU nurses began learning meditation and therapeutic touch, and exploring how these could be integrated into their workday and the care they provided patients. For example, after learning about meditation, the nurses scheduled a weekly meditation session for staff on Wednesday mornings, when the operating rooms start late. Some nurses, physicians, and ancillary staff began taking advantage of slow periods by finding a quiet space for a meditation break. After learning about the calming power of music, nurses began bringing in CD players and offering patients the option of listening to favored selections as they recovered from anesthesia.

Nurses also began to explore Reiki therapy, receiving treatments and giving them to one another during the "Reiki shares" that were held on Wednesday mornings for members of the PACU and operating room staff. As they experienced Reiki's calming properties for themselves, nurses began offering pre- and post-operative Reiki treatments to their patients. Other members of the staff also came to appreciate the power of Reiki treatments. For example, anesthesiologists willingly waited until Reiki treatments were over before prepping patients for surgery, observing that Reiki's calming effects made it easier for them to insert intravenous lines and epidural catheters. After receiving a Reiki treatment for the first time, one surgeon found himself overwhelmed. In tears, he explained, "I touch people every day and no one ever touches me."

BUILDING AN INTEGRATIVE CARE PROGRAM

Through the introductory classes on complementary therapies, "Reiki shares," and presentations by PACU nurses about their successes with integrative care activities, nurses throughout the organization began to appreciate the benefits of integrative care and became interested in finding new ways to incorporate complementary therapy practices into their lives and the care they provide patients. The ICP emerged over time as we established a set of ongoing services. Some of the services we now offer through the program are highlighted here.

1. *Volunteer Reiki Service.* Although several hundred nurses and members of other disciplines were trained to use Reiki therapy through the classes offered through the ICP, most were not comfortable incorporating it into their practice. Instead, they contacted the ICP whenever they felt a patient would benefit from a Reiki treatment. Julie Hahn, a hospital chaplain, was among those who were trained in Reiki and saw its calming effects on patients. She began using Reiki in her sessions with patients. Recognizing Julie's interest in Reiki therapy, in 2009 we recruited and hired her to help establish a Volunteer Reiki Service.

Working with the Volunteer Office, Julie and the ICP director recruited 50 volunteers from a wide range of backgrounds. Each volunteer was trained to administer Reiki and was assigned to a patient care unit. We then worked with unit leaders to introduce the volunteers to nurses on the unit and to implement a system. Nurses identified patients who were interested in receiving Reiki therapy, obtained their consent for treatment, and placed them on the list of patients who would be treated by the volunteer. Although some units were initially slow to adopt the volunteer Reiki program, many welcomed it, and support for the service spread rapidly. Within 5 months, approximately 2,500 Reiki treatments had been administered to patients. Additionally, as nurses trained in Reiki observed the volunteers, they became more comfortable administering treatments on their own. Nurses and other staff also began requesting Reiki treatments for themselves. In response, we continued offering the "Reiki shares," making Reiki available to a broad range of patients, family members, visitors, and staff throughout the organization.

2. *Music Therapy.* Another program that the ICP director introduced in 2008 was the Music Therapy program. This program came about when Nancy Kleinman, a harpist who viewed her instrument as a vehicle for healing the wounded spirit, contacted the ICP and expressed interest in playing for patients and families. Aware of the harp's effect in ameliorating pain and anxiety, we supported the harpist's interest by introducing her to leaders and staff on the hospital units and using this as an opportunity to describe the benefits of music therapy. The harpist began playing in public spaces and patient care areas, including inpatient units, individual patient rooms, and even the operating room (OR) suite. Nurses immediately noticed how the gentle strains of the harp fostered a sense of tranquility and had a soothing effect on patients as well as staff. In the PACU, for example, nurses reported that the entire area, with its large number of patients and staff, immediately grew quiet once the harpist started playing. Even the phones seemed to stop ringing, they observed, as though respectful of the music's force. In the neonatal ICU, nurses reported a similarly calming effect on newborns and unit staff.

Nancy formed an especially close relationship with patients on the oncology units, who often experience long lengths of stay. Over time, she bonded with many individual patients and families, playing at wedding and birthday celebrations held on the unit, and at the funerals of patients who died.

3. *Pet Therapy.* The Pet Therapy service was initiated by a group of nurses who recognized the comfort and reassurance that pets can provide. Before long,

"Diva" the standard poodle and a cadre of other specially trained dogs were making rounds in the hospital units and waiting areas. Today, the dogs can often be found sitting contentedly next to patients, paw in hand, and dog biscuits are now part of the standard supply stock on many units.

   4. Wisdom Circles for Nurse Directors.   Maintaining a presence and developing self-awareness is as important for nurse leaders as it is for staff. Through their words, thoughts, and actions, nurse directors and executive directors set the tone for their units, communicate values, and influence nurses' attitudes toward one another and patients and families, as well as patient care. The power to create dissipates when leaders are not anchored in the present moment, when they are either too much ahead of their staff or mired in the past. Similarly, their power to shape the environment and turn it into something that is healthy for patients and staff is lessened when leaders are not centered, but instead spin and react to the multiple and various people and stimuli that pass through.

While working on the clinical units, we noted that some nurse directors and executive directors struggled to provide a vision and leadership and sometimes felt out of touch with staff needs. We knew that leadership development was a top priority for Mairead Hickey and Trish Gibbons, and we became interested in supporting ongoing efforts. After considering various options, we proposed forming "wisdom circles" for nurse leaders. The wisdom circles involved bringing together small groups of nurse leaders with the goal of creating a safe space for open and authentic communication, and for sharing and learning from one another.

   After proposing the idea of wisdom circles in late 2008, we invited interested nurse directors to contact us. Over the course of 1 year, first one and then a second wisdom circle was formed. Led by the two of us, the groups met weekly for 8 weeks. The groups began by examining core values that serve as a foundation for authentic leadership, such as courage, truth, and trust. Group participants then began sharing and examining challenges they faced as nurse directors. At the end of each session, the nurse directors were assigned homework, which often involved tackling a challenge that they might have avoided in the past. For example, in one instance the homework involved speaking with staff about the state's Nurse Practice Act. In another, it required the directors to confront a staff member whose behavior, practice, or attitude was creating problems on the unit.

   By participating in the wisdom circles, the nurse directors quickly realized they each had different strengths, and that coming together as a group created a synergy that fostered greater learning. As trust developed, the nurse directors grew more comfortable expressing what they truly felt and offering their thoughts and accepting each other's counsel. They also realized they could learn as much by examining their mistakes as their successes and found the "homework" especially helpful, even though the assignments produced anxiety for some and on occasion one would choose not to follow through. Once the circle reconvened and members shared their experiences, however, those who were most anxious often found the strength to act. The support, guidance, and power of the group not only gave them the courage to follow through on individual assignments, but also empowered the nurse directors to create units anchored in core values.

   After completion of the 8-week program, the wisdom circles continue to meet periodically. Participants value the support, counsel, and advice they access through the wisdom circles, and the opportunities they offer for sharing ideas and strategies for creating and sustaining a healthy and healing care environment for staff, patients, and families.

In addition to the programs described in this chapter, the ICP has introduced a variety of other programs and resources for nurses and patients. These include labyrinth walks for staff, which are a form of "walking" meditation. In our offerings for staff, we have included classes on aromatherapy, reflexology, forgiveness, craniosacral therapy, and the "Prepare for Surgery" program (Huddleston, 1996). Additionally, in 2009 we began co-sponsoring a nursing conference with Massachusetts General Hospital, "The Art of Healing Presence: The Essence of Nursing Practice," to facilitate discussion about spirituality in nursing and how it benefits patients, families, and staff.

SUMMARY

A wide range of nurses and other staff has embraced programs and therapies introduced by the ICP at BWH. For example, our Reiki Volunteer Program (which has moved from a pilot to an established program) has enjoyed widespread success, attracting 70 volunteers and providing 6,500 Reiki treatments to patients within only 14 months. Clinical nurses and nurse leaders frequently comment on how the ICP's initiatives and services have helped create a healthier environment for patients and staff by "softening" the environment and by easing the stress experienced by nurses as well as patients.

Perhaps the best indicator of the program's impact are the results of recent patient satisfaction surveys conducted at BWH. For example, in the last quarter of fiscal year (FY) 2010 and the first quarter of FY 2011, patient ratings of nursing care put BWH nurses in the 99th percentile of similarly sized teaching hospitals tracked by the national survey company (Press Ganey Associates, 2011). Although multiple factors contributed to these scores, there is widespread agreement that the ICP played a significant role. By helping clinical nurses and nursing leaders gain greater self-awareness and feel centered and in control, the program helps nurses be more present for patients and families and facilitates their efforts to establish healing connections.

A variety of factors have contributed to the success of the ICP. We believe that one of the most important was the background in integrative care, clinical practice, and nursing management the ICP director brought to our work. Additionally, our prior work experiences enable us to understand the stresses nurses encounter and the culture of clinical practice. We are thus able to tailor the support and services we provide to match the needs, interests, and readiness of various groups.

The support of Mairead Hickey and Trish Gibbons, the chief and associate chief of nursing, was also critical to the success of the ICP. In addition to providing required financial resources, they consistently verbalized support and respect for the program. This helped the ICP gain the attention and buy-in of nurse leaders and clinical nurses and paved the way for program services to reach patients, families, and staff throughout the hospital.

Finally, the approach used to introduce complementary therapies was crucial to the acceptance and the success of the ICP. By design, we carefully "tilled the soil," cultivating nurses' interest by responding to groups and individuals who reached out for help, selecting and introducing complementary therapies that could be applied in the work and patient care setting, and building on successes, finding ways to efficiently extend and expand program offerings. Today, services provided by the ICP are part of the fabric of the care environment. They exemplify the change process described in this book, its intent, and its impact. From Reiki treatments in the recovery room, to noontime meditation sessions, to music therapy, the ICP exerts a quieting influence that helps patients, families, and staff find moments of stillness and peace amid the bustle of clinical care delivery.

REFERENCES

Beckman, S., Boxley-Harges, S., Bruick-Sorge, C., & Salmon, B. (2007). Five strategies that heighten nurses' awareness of spirituality to impact client care. *Holistic Nursing Practice, 21*, 135–139.

Benor, D. J. (Ed.). (n.d.). *Wholistic healing research: Integrative care.* Wholistic Healing Publications. Retrieved July 29, 2010, from http://www.wholistichealingresearch .com/integrativecare.html

Bossi, L. M., Ott, M. J., & DeCristofaro, S. (2008). Reiki as a clinical intervention in oncology nursing practice. *Clinical Journal of Oncology Nursing, 12*, 489–494.

Green, M., McArdle, D., & Robichaux, C. (2009). Creating a culture of caring to foster a healthy workplace. *Critical Care Nursing Quarterly, 32*, 296–304.

Hayes, C., Chase, C. W., Reilly, P. M., Rich, C., Hayes, J., Moore, M. L., Ott, M. J., & Kruger, N. (2002). *The effect of a structured complementary healing intervention program on nurses' perception of stress* [Unpublished study]. Boston, MA: Brigham & Women's Hospital/ Children's Hospital.

Huddleston, P. (1996). *Prepare for surgery, heal faster.* Cambridge, MA: Angel River Press.

Press Ganey Associates, Inc. (2011). *BWH inpatient satisfaction survey report.* South Bend, IN: Author.

Quinn, J. F. (1992). Holding sacred space: The nurse as healing environment. *Holistic Nursing Practice, 6*(4), 26–36.

Ruiz, D. M. (1997). *The four agreements.* San Rafael, CA: Amber-Allen.

Samueli Institute. (2007). *Survey of healing environments in hospitals: Nature and prevalence.* Retrieved May 28, 2010, from http://www.siib.org/research/421-SIIB/version/ default/part/AttachmentData/data/Reportwithinstrument9-18.pdf

Taylor, E. T. (2008). What is spiritual care in nursing? Findings from an exercise in content validity. *Holistic Nursing Practice, 22*(3), 154–159.

Watson, J. (2006). Caring theory as an ethical guide to administrative and clinical practices. *Nursing Administration Quarterly, 30*(1), 48–55.

Williams, A. M., Davies, A., & Griffiths, G. (2009). Facilitating comfort for hospitalized patients using non-pharmacological measures: Preliminary development of clinical practice guidelines. *International Journal of Nursing Practice, 15*, 145–155.

15.2 *Implementing Alternative/Complementary Therapies for the Purpose of Stress Reduction in Nurses*

Alice O'Brien, Heather Hogan, Santina Wilson,
Mary Absi, and James Roche

Shortly after we experienced the joy of moving into the new Shapiro Building, a state-of-the-art cardiovascular center here at Brigham and Women's Hospital (BWH), our nurse director, Alice O'Brien, had an imaginative vision, an intuitive concept that she believed would promote ways to implement the changes that would further our Shapiro 8 unit nursing philosophy: "A professional practice unit demonstrated by our integrity, compassion, humor, optimism and respect for all." This mission emerged from our collective thinking and supported the Department of Nursing (DON) vision of *"excellent care to patients and families, with the very best staff, in the safest environment."* We believed that our nurse director's idea would assist all in furthering both our mission and the DON vision.

In focusing on the desires of both our patients and our nurse colleagues, we asked ourselves: "What gives Life?" "What is the world calling for?" "What do we want more of?" In promoting our theme of service to others, we began to organize our ideas around the appreciative inquiry model of "Discovery, Dream, Design, and Destiny" (Watkins & Cooperrider, 2000). Because health is not a steady state and we too, as caregivers, sometimes become the recipients of health care, we realized that our thoughts and ideas often mirror the needs and personal vision of the patients we serve.

In our professional nursing educational programs, we were taught that the human entity is a bio-psycho-social-spiritual-sexual being. While we realized that this was true, we had become acutely aware that in our complex work environment, we focus more time on the physical component of health and healing, and were not consistently integrating the composite needs of mind, body, and spirit. We realized that if there is a gap in any one area, then an imbalance is created. Some of our patients had begun to realize that their physical healing was far greater when their emotional and spiritual well-being were also addressed. Integrative therapies were on the horizon, and many of our patients had prior experience with selected healing modalities for a variety of health ailments.

Whether through guided imagery, therapeutic touch, healing phrases, or soft tones from a comforting music CD, there is one certainty: Most of us seek to be affirmed and comforted, to be valued by our health care providers, and to feel a sense of well-being from an experience that frees us from fear and infuses us with a profound spiritual energy. We believe that nurses should not be an exception to human reality. We too have the need and desire to experience caring, replete with an awareness of the emotional impact that another's kindness can have on us. We realized that this enables us, through awareness, to better give of ourselves in promoting quality care to others.

Through the direction of our very supportive nurse director, we started the process of applying for funding to help support our ideas. We created a research study and submitted it to the Lily Kravitz Foundation. Our title explained our goal: "Implementing Alternative/Complementary Therapies for the Purpose of Stress Reduction in Nurses While Improving the Quality and Care of Our Patients." We have provided our study abstract (see Box 15.2.1) to provide the reader with a summary of our proposed study. To our amazement, we were funded. Change was now imminent! This chapter describes the group work and decisions that led to this exciting opportunity to meet our mission and further the vision of the DON.

BOX 15.2.1 *Study Abstract: Implementing Alternative/Complementary Therapies for the Purpose of Stress Reduction in Nurses While Improving the Quality and Care of Our Patients*

Stress and stress-related illnesses are among the most significant health problems of the 21st century. The hospital care and work environment, rather than mitigating stress, often contributes to the stress of both the patient and the nurse. The Patient- and Family-Centered Care Model has begun to address the concerns of the patient, but little has been done to assist the caregiver in managing stress. The proposed research would attempt to answer the question: Does introducing complementary and integrative care techniques into the work environment of the nurse have a positive impact on decreasing the nurse's level of stress, improving the nurse's job satisfaction, and improving patient satisfaction with care? The research would be conducted using a quantitative, descriptive design. A series of integrative and complementary therapies would be integrated into the work environment and offered to nurses working on an intermediate cardiac care/vascular surgical unit at BWH as an intervention. The State Trait Anxiety Inventory for Adults and the Press-Ganey Patient Satisfaction Survey would be evaluated pre- and post-intervention to measure the impact of the intervention. Red Cap would be used to assess the satisfaction of the nurse working on the unit where the research is being conducted. Providing the nurse with the tools to mitigate stress has significant importance for the nurse as a person. This research also contributes to the knowledge of the nursing profession around the importance of self-regulation and self-care in the life of the professional caregiver.

BACKGROUND AND SIGNIFICANCE

Our first task was to create a context and rationale for our proposed study. In our proposal, we posited that a supportive practice environment that meets the social, spiritual, and physical needs of the nurse is essential to the nurse's role as provider of care. We noted that nurses care for patients during times of extreme disability, suffering, and sadness. Providing a compassionate response to patients requires a great degree of emotional engagement on the part of the nurse.

We believed that it was important to note that nurses actively experience the patient's emotional distress, and we found nurse experts who validated this conviction. Repar and Patton (2007) noted that over time, this intense sharing of the patient's emotional trauma can lead to chronic grief and compassion fatigue for the nurse. Inability to self-manage their own emotional distress often leads nurses to disengage from their patients. Disengagement can affect nurse-patient relations, patient outcomes, and patient satisfaction, as well as the nurse's perception of self as an effective provider of care.

In Cathryn Domrose's *Nurse Week* article, "Looking Out for No. 1," JoAnne Herman, an associate professor of nursing at the University of South Carolina, was quoted: "[S]tress or stress related illnesses probably will be the number one public health problem of the 21st century" (Domrose, 2001). Nurses will not be immune to these illnesses. Without the tools to manage the stress inherent in their own work environment, nurses will be at great risk for stress-related illness. For us, the question was clear: How do we care for our own caregivers? Creative solutions are needed to address these significant concerns. These resources and ideas helped us articulate the purpose of the research we wanted to initiate and are now currently conducting.

There is both historical and theoretical support in nursing for intervening in the environment to improve physical and emotional well-being. McElligott and colleagues (McElligott et al., 2003) remind us that Florence Nightingale saw nursing as inherently holistic and focused on caring for the body, mind, and spirit (Nightingale, 1969). Our exploration of available literature about integrative therapies validated that they are used for many reasons, including promoting relaxation and comfort, reducing anxiety, and maintaining wellness. This range of uses showed a fit with our conviction, supported by numerous experts, that it is essential to clinical practice in nursing to develop self-awareness and engage in self-care (McElligott et al., 2003).

Sister Callista Roy, a nurse theorist, was known for her "adaptation model" wherein she states that by manipulating the stimuli and not the patient, the nurse enhances the interaction of the person with the environment, thereby promoting health (Roy, 1991). This model builds on nursing theory's four domains: person, health, environment, and nursing. For Roy, *persons* are biopsychosocial beings whom she views as being continually in interaction with their environments. The person is an open, adaptive system that uses coping skills to deal with stressors. Roy also sees the environment as encompassing everything that surrounds and influences a person. What affects the patient affects the nurse. Roy's theory was helpful to us in presenting the significance of our proposed project: Her theory applies not only to the patient care experience but also to the experience of the provider of care.

We also were able to document the impact of neglecting to care for the providers of care. There are many factors in the nursing work environment that cause the nurse to internalize stress: poor work flow, unfamiliar technology, staff shortages, and unpredictable workloads (Zangaro & Soeken, 2007). Without positive intervention, burnout is the end result of chronic stress in the workplace (Schure, Christopher, & Christopher, 2008). We realized that we needed to identify and implement interventions that would help nurses experience stress in ways that are not harmful to their health. Although nurses cannot always control stress at work, they can increase their awareness of it and improve their ways of responding to stress by making healthy lifestyle changes and reaching beyond traditional Western medical practices through stress reduction and integrative therapies. With all this information as background, we were able to state what we wanted to study and what we wanted to discover.

OUR REVIEW OF THE LITERATURE

To prepare our research proposal, we collectively began a comprehensive search of literature that would guide our study. We quickly learned that there has been significant study regarding the role of integrative therapies in helping to reduce stress in the workplace (Hurley, 2007). "The National Institute for Occupational Safety & Health finds that stress-related ailments cost companies about $200 billion a year in increased absenteeism, tardiness, and the loss of talented workers. . . . [J]ob tension is directly tied to a lack of productivity and loss of competitive edge" (Der Hovanesian, 2003, p. 4). Noyce (2003) reports that employees experiencing stress are 25 percent more likely to miss work, use poor judgment, or make mistakes that can lead to injuries in the workplace. He points out that stress can decrease a person's ability to think clearly, thus having an impact on their emotional and intellectual skills. Intense pressure can leave employees feeling that they are powerless over their situations. Noyce also notes Bureau of Labor reports that worker's compensation claims have increased.

We learned that in response to this mounting evidence, some businesses have integrated concepts of stress management into their organizational culture and are now offering programs to their employees to help cope with busy minds and stressful lives. Texas Instruments, Raytheon, and Nortel Networks instituted programs that teach their executives meditation skills through one-on-one training (Der Hovanesian, 2003). Apple Computer, Yahoo!, and Google have expressed an interest in adding meditation to their wellness programs, which currently include onsite organic chefs and masseuses.

This new focus on employee wellness, we learned, is starting to filter into the hospital setting as well. White (2009) provides a useful analysis of this trend. He notes that meditation and wellness programs for employees have been shown to keep health care costs down, while increasing productivity, reducing absenteeism, and increasing employee satisfaction. He observes that the most attractive part of alternative therapies and wellness programs is that they are relatively low cost during tough economic times: By giving employees the opportunity to learn about healthier lifestyles, 50% to 70% of illnesses can be prevented. He proposes that management can demonstrate a commitment to staff that goes beyond a paycheck, by caring for their entire well-being. In reviewing these emerging services, we recognized—and found our recognition supported—that nurses are not socialized to care for themselves and are not prepared to sustain their own health as they attempt to promote patient health in busy inpatient settings (Raingruber & Robinson, 2007). We also agree with Hurley, who said: "The term 'self-care' can refer to nurses' participation in the healing of others and an awareness of ways of caring for oneself. By learning to self-care, nurses can care better for others, so that self-care and the development of caring relationships become intertwined" (Hurley, 2007, p. 16).

We found a pilot study (McElligott et al., 2003) that reported on the effect of touch therapy on nurses using AMMA Therapy® (a specialized massage therapy). This massage resulted in a positive experience for the experimental group. Nurses reported feelings of relaxation and less stress, and these feelings continued with them into stressful work situations and increased their ability to cope. "As nurses perform self-assessments, discover the mind-body connection, and recognize their own need for self-care, these concepts are transposed into the nurse-client experience" (McElligott et al., 2003, p. 57).

We also were able to find experts speaking specifically to the spiritual dimensions of self-care for health care providers. Having spiritual awareness at our center gives us the ability and hope that we can care for ourselves and provide healing to others (Andrews, 2009). Dr. Matthew Goodman, who teaches mindfulness at the University Virginia Mindfulness Center, states, "Patients need health care professionals to be well enough themselves to be in a healing space. If we're rushed, stressed and overworked, it's hard to connect with patients with compassion and empathy. We can retain our technical skills, but the compassion goes" (Bromley, 2005, p. 8).

BENCHMARKING

Our review of existing literature also provided further insights into the impact of self-care programs for health care providers as a dimension of hospital benchmarking practices. We learned that when staff are exposed to integrative therapies, they may begin to realize how beneficial they are and feel less stressed. With support from nursing, nurse leaders can advocate for staff by offering these therapies, addressing common workplace stressors, providing educational opportunities, and taking on renovation projects with a therapeutic milieu in mind. Two examples of hospitals that have incorporated this into their practice are the University of New Mexico Hospital and The Cleveland Clinic.

The University of New Mexico Hospital started a program in 2002 to encourage deep relaxation while at the same time stimulating participants' creative energies to bring nurses to greater awareness of and freedom from the pain and stress in their lives. This was done by offering relaxation techniques, including traditional massage, sound and guided imagery, walking meditation, and *acutonics* (the application of tuning forks to traditional Chinese acupuncture points on the body). Creative encounters were facilitated through guided-imagery classes, journaling, storytelling sessions, and clay workshops. Responses to the program were overwhelmingly positive (Repar & Patton, 2007).

Participants commenting on the program stated that they had "learned to relax" and "to be more aware" of physical and emotional issues. The nurses expressed a greater willingness to "take time for myself" and to "cut myself some slack." The program proved to be effective not only in learning to care for self but also in learning to support colleagues and improve a sense of community on the unit. One nurse wrote, "I feel I am more attentive and compassionate about my co-workers' stressors. I have started looking more at why people may react to certain situations and how I can help" (Repar & Patton, 2007, p. 185).

They also found that nurses were more attentive to how their own emotional and physical states could affect patient care. Another nurse commented, "As I was getting massaged and my body began to relax I envisioned entering a patient's room with that sense of calm and peace which in turn can be transferred to my patients. I have a much deeper understanding of the importance of self-care today than I think I ever had" (Repar & Patton, 2007, p. 185). Comments such as these have convinced the University of New Mexico Hospital that these relaxation programs can have a real and profound impact on the quality of nurses' work lives and the way in which they deliver health care in the hospital.

The Cleveland Clinic, as a part of its integrative care treatment modality, has created a healing services team of practitioners who provide relationship-centered care. The team uses a variety of techniques, including touch therapies, such as Reiki, Healing Touch, and massage; spiritual support and counseling; and healthy food and beverages. *Code Lavender*, which is a rapid response provided by the Healing Services team, offers a 10-minute Reiki session and Healing Touch to the nursing staff on the units to help decrease their stress. They also have an "Energized" program specifically targeted to enhance nurses' well-being, which addresses the issues of nourishment, movement, and self-management of stress. They provide free Weight Watchers® meetings and other nutritional counseling, free memberships to Curves®, free yoga classes, and educational offerings dealing with stress management. They also have their own Cleveland Clinic fitness center (Cameron, 2009).

The Cleveland Clinic conducted a pilot program for patients undergoing heart surgery, given visibility through coverage in *USA Today*. Half of the patients in this study opted for spiritual care, counseling, art, music, touch therapy, or guided imagery; 93% of these participants reported that the alternative services were helpful (Gill, 2008). In a report on the use of integrative therapies, a patient summarized what many experience: "Having the human touch and knowing that someone is paying very personal attention to you helps. It keeps everything from being so medical" (AHA reports, 2009). Another patient, who opted for Reiki therapy after open-heart surgery, commented that the treatment was "very relaxing and a gift toward my healing" (Gill, 2008).

We found ourselves fascinated with the extensive program initiated at The Cleveland Clinic, and contacted Michelle Cameron, the nurse who is the assistant director of Healing Solutions at The Cleveland Clinic. We shared with her our interest in visiting their facility, observing their programs, and learning how they implemented those programs. They are excited about sharing their work with us and have agreed to host us and give us a tour of their facility. We have this as one of the future portions of our project as we continue to pursue our goal of caregiver self-care.

The study of related initiatives in other hospital settings was encouraging, and helped us think through our goals with our research project. We wanted not only to start a program of care, but also to evaluate its impact. We set out to design a study that would make that possible.

OUR STUDY METHODS

We decided that all nurses currently working on Shapiro 8 East/West—approximately 60 nurses—would be offered the opportunity to participate in this study. Participation would be anonymous and voluntary. Staff would be contacted by e-mail to enlist their participation in completing surveys regarding anxiety levels and satisfaction with their job. Consent to participate would be implied by the nurse's completion of the survey instruments pre- and post-intervention.

The Design of Our Study and Our Planned Data Analysis

We designed our research using a quantitative, experimental approach. The study would last 1 year, would be a pilot study, and would use a questionnaire to collect data regarding nurses' satisfaction in the workplace and their stress levels pre- and post-intervention. We decided to use the State-Trait Anxiety Inventory for Adults (STAI) by Charles D. Spielberger to measure self-reported anxiety. In order to test our data, our plan was to issue a pre-survey to the Shapiro 8 East/West nurses through the use of Red Cap, which is a tool BWH uses for building and managing online surveys. Our plan was to then compare these results to a post-survey that would be given 6 months to 1 year after the program had been implemented. We also planned to measure patient satisfaction using the Press-Ganey Patient Satisfaction Survey results for Shapiro 8 East/West that BWH already administered throughout the hospital. This would give us some information about patient satisfaction without adding an additional data-generation burden on our patients. In all cases we would utilize standard statistical tools to examine our data.

Having identified our measurement tools, we set out to define our planned intervention. Our proposed plan was to introduce an integrative care program that would encourage nurses to use strategies to manage and overcome chronic grief, compassion fatigue, and burnout. The integrative care modalities we would introduce include, but are not limited to, massage, therapeutic touch, spirituality, Reiki, yoga, nutrition, reflexology, and lectures regarding compassion fatigue, burnout, and chronic grief. Our plan is to offer therapeutic treatments and alternative therapy healing classes on a monthly basis. These therapeutic treatment modalities will be offered as stress-reduction therapies and will be provided on Shapiro 8 East/West in a room designated as the "renewal room," specifically planned for caregiver well-being. Every month one treatment will be selected and offered to nurses on the unit in a 10-minute interval, including:

■ Massage and music: A chair massage treatment incorporating relaxing music.
■ Reflexology: Massage of pressure points on feet and hands that can heal pain in other parts of the body; often used to treat arthritis, back pain, and migraines.
■ Healing Reiki sessions: Reiki is an ancient healing art involving the gentle laying-on of hands; it is well suited for nurses who provide hands-on care to patients.
■ Group meditation/guided-imagery interaction.

We will also offer a once-a-month training session to those nurses interested in learning these techniques to implement in their nursing practice. Nurses will need to attend these classes on their own time and may use holiday or vacation time to participate. We are convinced that programs must be consistent and monthly in order to make a positive change in the lives of the nurses. It is our belief that by improving the lifestyle of the nurse, we will improve the quality of care given to our patients. If nurses are able to achieve balance in their lives through self-care, they are more apt to be in a positive mind-state and provide better care to their patients. Examples of full-day training programs we are planning include:

■ Therapeutic Touch: Learning Therapeutic Touch techniques followed by a hands-on experience of providing and receiving this treatment. Therapeutic Touch is a laying-on of hands to correct or balance energy fields in the body (Krieger, 1979).
■ Nutrition: Improving the diet of our nurses by bringing in a nutritionist for a training session that provides guidance for healthy lifestyle changes.

This would be followed by a hands-on experience of tasting and preparing heart-healthy meals by a heart-healthy culinary specialist.

- Lectures on chronic grief, compassion fatigue, burnout, and stress reduction
- Reiki
- Reflexology

One of the concepts that we are excited to be bringing to our nurses is a book called *Keys to Personal Success* (Lowry, 1992). This book details the program "True Colors®," which is valued by BWH. It has been used here for several years, with recognizable success, for improving relationships and communication in the workplace. Through this interactive program, core fundamentals of human beings are presented to improve work-life balance, team building, and communication. We believe that from this program we can expect to learn better ways to build more meaningful relationships in life, at home, and in the work environment.

Meeting Research Criteria

As with all research studies, we have also evaluated those components of our study that establish its value, potential impact, and assurance of protection of subjects—in this case, our nurses. Our plan is to use the post-survey questionnaire data to determine our study outcomes. There are virtually no risks or discomforts associated with our proposed research and our study does not include any invasive interventions. We do acknowledge that there are possible limitations to this study involved in the challenge of reaching out to and providing these therapies to the overnight staff and part-time nurses.

SUMMARY AND CONCLUSIONS

We believe that this project has significant implications for nurses and the profession of nursing. Due to the significant stress reported by nurses and its harmful consequences, it seems important to seriously explore effective means of supporting the caregiver at the bedside. Job burnout and distress have been significantly associated with decreased patient satisfaction, so incorporating wellness interventions and stress-reduction strategies for nurses ultimately have the potential to enhance patient care.

The BWH continues to be a leader in education and innovative health care. We believe our proposed study provides a wonderful example of that. Through the implementation of our program, not only are we following our Shapiro 8 nursing philosophy of integrity, compassion, humor, optimism, and respect for all, we are also supporting the DON's vision of *"excellent care to patients and families, with the very best staff, in the safest environment."* Excellent practice nurses nurture the body and minister to the spirit of patients, families, and each other. Bringing complementary and alternative education and learning experiences to deepen nursing practice will be of great value to the growth of nursing staff at BWH. *By implementing this program, BWH can reach beyond its mission statement to include not only the desire to serve the mind, body, and spiritual needs of patients, but to include meeting the needs of employees as well.*

REFERENCES

AHA reports increasing number of hospitals offer alternative therapies. (2009, January/ February). *Nurse Educator, 34*(1), 22.

Andrews, M. (2009, February 1). Meditate your angst away. *U.S. News & World Report, 146*(1), 84–85.

Bromley, A. (2005, January/February). Mindfulness courses reduce stress among doctors, nurses—lead to more compassionate patient care. *Inside UVA Online, 35*(2). Retrieved January 8, 2009, from http://www.virginia.edu/insideuva/2005/02/mindfulness. html

Cameron, M. (2009). Healing services "Code Lavender": Creating a positive environment for nurses and innovating patient care. *Notable Nursing.* Retrieved May 5, 2009, from http://my.clevelandclinic.org/nursing/notable_nursing_newsletter.aspx

Der Hovanesian, M. (2003, July 28). Zen and the art of corporate productivity. *BusinessWeek.* Retrieved June 7, 2010, from http://www.businessweek.com/magazine/content/ 03_30/b3843076.htm

Domrose, C. (2001, January 8). Looking out for No.1: Nurses extol the virtues of self-care in personal and professional life. *NurseWeek.* Retrieved April 14, 2009, from http://www .nurseweek.com/news/features/01-01/care.asp

Gill, L. (2008). *More hospitals offer alternative therapies for mind, body, spirit.* Retrieved February 8, 2011, from http://www.usatoday.com/news/health/2008-09-14-alternative-therapies_N.htm

Hurley, M. (2007). Managing stress. *Nursing Management UK, 14*(3), 16.

Krieger, D. (1979). The therapeutic touch: How to use your hands to help or to heal. Los Angeles, CA: Fireside Press.

Lowry, D. (1992). *Keys to personal success.* N.p.: Publisher unknown.

McElligott, D., Holz, M., Carollo, L., Somerville, S., Baggett, M., Kuzniewski, S., & Shi, Q. (2003, March). A pilot feasibility study of the effect of touch therapy on nurses. *Journal of the New York State Nurses Association, 34*(1), 16–24.

Nightingale, F. (1969). *Notes on nursing: What it is and what it is not.* New York, NY: Dover.

Noyce, J. (2003, August 22). Help employees manage stress to prevent absenteeism, errors. *Minneapolis St. Paul Business Journal.* Retrieved March 18, 2009, from http://bizjournals .com/twincities/stories/2003/08/25/smallb2.html

Raingruber, B., & Robinson, C. (2007). The effectiveness of tai chi, yoga, meditation, and Reiki healing sessions in promoting health and enhancing problem solving abilities of registered nurses. *Issues in Mental Health Nursing, 28,* 1141–1155.

Repar, P., & Patton, D. (2007, July/August). Stress reduction for nurses through arts-in-medicine at the University of New Mexico Hospital. *Holistic Nursing Practice, 21*(4), 185.

Roy, C. (1991). The Roy adaptation model in nursing research. In C. Roy & H. Andrews (Eds.), *The Roy adaptation model: The definitive statement* (pp. 445–457). East Norwalk, CT: Appleton & Lange.

Schure, M., Christopher, J., & Christopher, S. (2008, Winter). Mind-body medicine and the art of self care: Teaching mindfulness to counseling students through yoga, meditation, and Qigong. *Journal of Counseling & Development, 86,* 47–56.

Watkins, J. M., & Cooperrider, D. L. (2000). Appreciative inquiry: A transformative paradigm. *Journal of Organizational Development Network, 32,* 6–12.

White, A. (2009, March). Keeping employees healthy to save money. *Associations Now Supplement, 5*(3), 7.

Zangaro, G., & Soeken, K. (2007). A meta-analysis of studies of nurses' job satisfaction. *Research in Nursing & Health, 30,* 445–458.

15.3 *Reiki Practice:*
A Comfort for Patients and Nurses

Suzanne Silvernail, Margaret Costello, and Sarah Thompson

---

*T*hree of us, traveling different paths, converged on one very positive nursing care intervention we could provide to ease patient stress on our unit: Reiki therapy. Reiki is a Japanese technique that supports healing, promotes relaxation and well-being, and helps reduce stress. The practice of first-degree Reiki can be easily learned by anyone of any age. As self-practice is a foundation for all levels of Reiki, the practitioner also experiences all of the benefits of the energy healing (Miles & True, 2003).

Our nursing practice occurs in a 30-bed surgical unit at Brigham and Women's Hospital (BWH). Suzanne is the nurse director, Margaret is a nurse-in-charge (NIC), and Sarah is the clinical educator. Together and separately we learned about and experienced Reiki and realized it could be a very positive addition to the nursing care provided on our unit. We took different paths to reach that awareness, which converged in a shared conviction. We share our distinct stories of each path.

THE NURSE DIRECTOR PERSPECTIVE: SUZANNE'S STORY

Before becoming a nurse director, I first learned about Reiki from a colleague who incorporated the "hands-on" therapy in her clinical practice with women in labor. It seemed like a perfect fit in the labor room setting. As we began to get requests for Reiki from our surgical patients, I wondered if Reiki could become a part of the care nurses provided for our patients. Nurses on our unit recognized that our patients were experiencing a discomfort that could not easily be remedied by medications for pain or anxiety. The use of Reiki can provide the nurse with a tool to ease patients' discomfort and provide healing support while they are hospitalized. When a Reiki course was offered to the nurses at BWH, many nurses on 15CD, our unit, enrolled.

As our staff began taking the Reiki workshops, I had the pleasure of having the director of the volunteer department approach me about initiating a weekly Reiki program on our unit. The volunteers proposed visiting the unit for 3 hours weekly to provide Reiki to nurses and patients. As director, I eagerly accepted their proposal, and have been pleasantly surprised with the response from patients and staff: The Reiki volunteers have been a welcome presence for both. On "Reiki day" when the volunteer comes to provide treatments to our patients, there is a calming effect over the entire unit. For a short period, patients can experience peace of mind as the Reiki effect takes over. As nurses who had never heard of Reiki before began to see the effects of treatments, more nurses expressed an interest in signing up to become Reiki certified. The nurses saw this as a way they could provide patients with a helpful service. I was happy to support the nurses in achieving their goal of Reiki certification and am currently in the process of becoming certified myself.

THE NURSE-IN-CHARGE PERSPECTIVE: MARGARET'S STORY

I took the Reiki courses and was eager to begin providing Reiki therapy for my patients. Despite my interest in Reiki, I remained timid about using my new-found skills on actual patients, except for those patients who knew about it and requested a Reiki treatment. I was thrilled when I was informed that Reiki practitioners would be visiting our unit on a weekly basis to provide care to our patients. As an NIC, my job includes both unit-wide organizational responsibilities and providing direct care to patients. I am expected to ask the patients if they would like to receive a treatment from the practitioner. Some patients have an idea of what to expect and others have not heard about Reiki and require an explanation.

The Reiki volunteers provided colorful pamphlets that offer a simple explanation of Reiki for patients. Patients who have a treatment by the volunteers describe the experience of having Reiki as very positive. At times, some patients report that Reiki provides them with relief of their pain or anxiety, and usually patients report that they feel much calmer and more relaxed after a treatment. Having the Reiki volunteers on our unit has influenced practice for each of us. It has also increased our comfort using our Reiki skills with patients. Seeing the benefits Reiki had in relaxing patients has made us more confident in our abilities to provide healing Reiki treatments to our patients. The following story provides a good example of how Reiki is practiced with our patients.

I recently cared for Marie, a 26-year-old woman who had been discharged from our hospital 2 weeks earlier following gastrointestinal surgery. She was readmitted to the hospital with intractable vomiting and abdominal pain. On the first day I met Marie, she was very distraught. When I walked into the room, she was sitting up in a chair with a pink basin close by. She had been up all night with severe nausea. I asked her if I could give her any medicine for pain or nausea. She said not to bother because none of the multiple medications she had been given for her symptoms worked. A tear came down her cheek and she put her head down. "I am just so tired," she said. "If I could only get rid of this nausea, I could sleep." Marie looked so forlorn sitting in her chair. I decided I would offer her a Reiki treatment, which she accepted.

I began the treatment by centering myself, focusing on my breath, as a method of becoming present in preparation for providing a Reiki treatment. I then placed my hands on Marie's shoulders and just breathed with her before embarking on the treatment; I began the process of allowing healing energy to flow through me and into her. As Marie's breathing became deeper and more even, I could feel the Reiki energy calming and relaxing her. Her eyes closed and by the sound of her rhythmic breathing I could tell she was asleep. I was just delighted. However, when Marie did not wake up I did get the slightest bit concerned, prompting a few extra visits to her room to make sure she was okay. Hours later, Marie walked past me on a stroll around the unit. She had a big smile and she gave me the thumbs-up sign. "This is the best I have felt in days, thank you so much!" she said happily.

Stories such as Marie's are getting more common on our unit. As the benefits of Reiki become more evident, more nurses are seeking out opportunities to learn about the practice. It is very helpful to have strong advocates of Reiki to support the practice on the unit. One of the greatest supporters on the unit is Sarah Thompson, our nurse educator, who joined our shared commitment through a very personal experience.

THE NURSE EDUCATOR'S PERSPECTIVE: SARAH'S STORY

Before I ever became involved in the Reiki treatments on our unit, I had a personal experience with integrative therapy modalities that influenced me. I had read the book *Prepare for Surgery, Heal Faster* (Huddleston, 2007) and utilized the author's relaxation tapes and the power of positive thinking as I prepared for my own surgery. The morning of surgery, one of BWH's social workers, Kristyn Morrissey, who was trained in Reiki therapy and therapeutic touch, gave me a treatment while I waited as a patient in the pre-operative area. I found the experience relaxing and I was able to calm my worried thoughts about my impending surgery. As a result of my experience I became Reiki certified.

As a nurse educator on 15CD, I have grown to appreciate the profound effects of Reiki therapy on patients. After taking Pat Reilly's Reiki I and II classes at the BWH Center for Nursing Excellence, I wanted to get comfortable with this integrative therapy before I tried my new Reiki skills on patients on 15CD. So, at Pat's and Margaret's suggestion, I practiced Reiki on several family members over the next couple of months—especially with my 8-year-old daughter, trying to help her relax enough to go to sleep.

My comfort level with Reiki grew and I eventually felt confident enough to try Reiki on BWH patients. In the beginning, when a patient on 15CD requested Reiki, I would call another trained practitioner. When she came to visit the patient, I would be present and observe her Reiki session. Several times, Margaret and I would also provide a Reiki treatment together on a patient. Before long, I was comfortable enough to offer Reiki on my own. As an educator, I plan to model the "buddy" technique to help train other 15CD staff members once they complete the two Reiki classes. Over the last 6 months, I have provided Reiki treatments for many patients. When I find patients in pain on the unit, I ask them if they know about Reiki and if they would like a Reiki treatment in addition to their pain medications. Recently, one patient's mother stopped me in the hall and asked me to please go visit her daughter again, that the Reiki treatment was so wonderful! She said her daughter has had so much pain after the surgical removal of most of her quadricep secondary to cancer. Her mother said it was the Reiki treatment that made her sleep for a few hours and gave her some peace. I visited this patient two more times during her admission. She felt her Reiki treatments were of such great benefit to her health that she was interested in pursuing treatments as an outpatient.

SUMMARY

We are happy to share our personal introduction to Reiki, as we believe all nurses should have an understanding of the value of Reiki as a healing modality. As the demand for integrative therapies such as Reiki continues to grow, we feel confident that our program will be able to meet the need. It is wonderful to be part of an institution and a unit where such patient-focused practice is supported.

REFERENCES

Huddleston, P. (2007). *Prepare for surgery, heal faster.* Cambridge, MA: Angel River Press.
Miles, P., & True, G. (2003). Reiki: Review of a biofield therapy history, theory, practice, and research. *Alternative Therapies, 9*(2), 62–72.

16

The Development of a Critical Care Leadership Team: Where We Have Been, Where We Are Now, and Where We Are Going

Matthew Quin, Teresa Moore Buchanan, Catherine Paccioretti,
Joyce Thomas-Browning, Kathleen M. Leone, Shaun Golden,
Karen Reilly, and Karyl J. Davenport

*I*n May of 2007, the seven intensive care units (ICUs) at Brigham and Women's Hospital (BWH) were collectively over budget by more than $1.9 million in nursing salaries. Each ICU was operating as an "island," with very little awareness of the other units' operations or impact on the overall organization. There was very little understanding of staffing needs and patient acuity across the ICUs. In an effort to ensure that our patients always had the right nurse caring for them when needed, while at the same time managing resources wisely, the associate chief nurse sponsored a work group to examine staffing to volume and acuity in the ICUs.

This work group included all the ICU nurse directors as well as the executive nurse directors from each area. We began to have daily meetings at noon to examine patterns of staffing across each of the ICUs and, in doing so, quickly realized that the current system had each director operating in isolation with little or no data or coordination of efforts. We quickly realized that to achieve the departmental vision of providing excellent and safe care to patients and families with the very best staff, we needed to improve our processes and communication.

The initial charge given to our group was to develop a method to staff based on patient volume and acuity while maintaining the ability to accept admissions without delay. This one goal has led our group down an unexpected path that includes strategic planning, data-driven decision making, advancing the goals of a healthy work environment, leadership development, fiscal responsibility, and an expanded emphasis on patient-focused care and patient outcomes. This chapter tells the story of our work group's experiences on our shared path.

FIRST STEPS

We began by using our daily meetings to project daily and weekly staffing needs in each ICU. This forum provided directors with the opportunity to share critical information required to plan across ICUs while ensuring the staffing needs were met in each ICU. In addition, we were able to support each other on a daily basis when an individual director was dealing with staffing challenges. Prior to the formation of the ICU Nurse Director work group, each director had been receiving weekly reports for retrospective analysis of budget, staffing, and acuity variances. Planning for staffing resources was largely day-to-day or short-term, and planning was carried out with limited knowledge of issues that could affect staffing requirements across all ICUs. The central resources that supported our ability to be flexible were shared; yet we functioned as if each director alone could plan only for the needs of his or her individual unit. As a result of these daily meetings, it became clear that long-range planning was critical if we were to move from a reactive to a proactive mode.

A project manager role was advanced by the executive directors to support our work as we began more complex data analysis and predictive modeling. The project manager assisted us in organizing, retrieving, and analyzing data, and in facilitating the group process. Data reports were created so that directors had timely staffing information, both on a daily and weekly basis. As our work progressed, many variables were identified that complicated our ability to plan and manage fluctuations in staffing requirements. Predictive modeling (looking at current and historical data for patterns and trends in order to predict staffing requirements) was used as a method to help the group improve the ability to forecast staffing needs. Those variables for which data were collected included shifts in ICU census, acuity, and workload; ICU length of stay; ICU admissions (analysis of time of day and day of week); floating of nursing staff; use of nonproductive time (sick or medical leave, vacation); and unfilled positions. Other variables were also identified that were not known or necessarily quantifiable. These included physician conferences, service line initiatives that affect volume and acuity, changes in physician staff, plans for new programs, blocks to throughput, reliability of acuity measures, tools for budget building, and changes in insurers that might impact census and patient populations.

STAFFING TO VOLUME AND ACUITY

Based on the initial analysis of our historical data and current staffing patterns, we recognized opportunities for greater efficiency and cost-effectiveness. In an effort to be ready for a possible admission, each ICU was staffing an extra nurse. This translated into seven extra nurses, 24 hours a day, waiting to care for potential patients. This had a large impact on the ICU nursing budget. At the same time, we acknowledged that any solution had to have the principle of the "right nurse for the right patient" as an underpinning.

We made the decision to staff the ICUs based on actual volume and acuity, and together crafted solutions for staffing unplanned admissions. We created a Designated ICU Nurse role (DIN) to meet the needs of any unexpected ICU admission, thereby removing the need to staff at the unit level for potential admissions. This new role did not require any additional staff, as we assigned an existing ICU float pool nurse to that role at the start of every shift. This nurse would carry a beeper and would be deployed to the first ICU receiving an admission that required assistance. The ICU requesting the DIN would page the staffing office nurse director, or nurse administrator on the off shifts, to request the DIN. The DIN status would be reevaluated every 4 hours beginning at 7:00 AM, and a new DIN would be assigned as needed. For example, if the DIN was assigned by 9:00 AM, we would appoint another float-pool nurse to this role at 11:00 AM.

There were a number of ways to refill the DIN role once the first floating nurse was deployed. To create more staffing flexibility, we altered our staffing pattern to allow for more float-pool nurses to come in at 11:00 AM. Also, as units reviewed their staffing every 4 hours, float-pool nurses were sometimes returned to the staffing office for use elsewhere in the hospital.

We knew from the start that this would be a huge shift in culture for our staff, and that much preparation would be necessary to get this new initiative off the ground. All nurse directors worked to update and educate their staffs about the changes. We focused on the plan to staff responsibly rather than concentrate on cost as a main driver. Many staff expressed doubt that they would get a nurse when they needed one for an unexpected admission. We reassured them that they would always have a nurse available for every admission. We realized that the true test of our plan would be in the rollout, and with that in mind, we chose a date to begin.

This new staffing initiative promoted regular exchanges between the nurse directors and charge nurses. The nurse directors reviewed staffing every shift and also helped to dispel rumors and correct inaccurate information in real time. We continued to meet daily as a group to discuss overall ICU staffing, as well as review DIN deployment and any staff concerns from the previous day. This kept all feedback to staff current and allowed for immediate follow-up of any issues.

Staff knew nurse directors were very committed to making this work and each time a unit asked for the DIN, one was available. The trust of the staff in this new initiative and in nursing management became increasingly strong each time we were able to fulfill their requests. Since inception of the DIN role, there has only been a very rare occasion when we could not immediately provide the nursing personnel resource, and as a result staffing to volume and acuity has become comfortable for the staff and is now built into the culture of the healthy work environment. On the infrequent occasion when a DIN has not been available, the hospital "stat" nurse (a float-pool nurse who provides support hospital-wide for a multitude of clinical situations) becomes a backup resource.

JUST WHEN EVERYTHING SEEMS TO BE GOING FINE, A NEW CHALLENGE

As we moved forward, we continued to explore additional options to meet our work group's goals. We realized that one of the challenges of staffing to patient volume and acuity arises from variations in census. In the midst of our work, the ICU census fell in some ICUs while it remained high in others. As a result, the need to float nurses from the inpatient specialty areas where they typically worked to another inpatient specialty area surfaced. It became clear, as floating frequency increased, that there were varying degrees of comfort and satisfaction with this process among frontline unit-based staff nurses. In our daily meetings, the nurse directors discussed the challenges nurses from our ICUs experienced when floating. We recognized that to ensure patients were receiving the best care, we needed to listen to our staff nurses and make certain that we were providing the right nurse for the right patient. In a hospital of highly specialized care, this meant that "a nurse is a nurse is a nurse" way of thinking would not support the type of care model that we were advancing in the ICUs.

We made a commitment within our work group to support our staff nurses by listening to their concerns and soliciting feedback about their floating experiences. We also recognized that this was a big area of dissatisfaction for our nurses, and wanted to make this process as smooth and pleasant for them as reasonably possible. We agreed that all directors would engage their staff in both formal and informal discussions to begin understanding what it was about floating that troubled staff nurses.

The feedback we received had two themes requiring the attention of our work group. First, the nurses acknowledged that there were many patients they could competently and safely care for in other units. In these cases, the care seemed more like the care they provided to patients in their own unit. However, there were patient populations for whom they did not feel they possessed the knowledge and skills needed to provide good care. The second theme that emerged from the feedback was less about the type of care they were providing and more about the environment of care they experienced while floating. They described how some ICUs were better to float to because of how they were treated by the staff in that unit.

Through our commitment to listening to our staff, we were able to begin understanding what was challenging for our nurses when floating amongst the various ICUs. We decided to brainstorm around how decisions were made on where nurses floated. We found that these decisions were primarily based on the thinking that ICU nurses had skill sets transferable to any ICU or step-down/intermediate care area, especially since these nurses routinely cared for the sickest patients in the hospital. As we spoke to our staff on the units, we began learning that nurses on particular units seemed to have higher comfort levels when floating to some units and lower comfort levels when floating to other units. Much of this comfort level was related to similarity of patient populations or units that typically cared for overflow patients from the other ICU. We began to map out these floating preferences among the various units, identifying where nurses from particular units felt most and least appropriate to float. This document became known as the *ICU RN Floating Guidelines*, and since its inception it has gone through continuous evaluation and revision based on the input of our nurses. It now acts as a compass for the floating process in our ICUs, as floating is now driven by where nurses feel most competent in providing good care. If staff members asked to float feel that they cannot safely care for the patient(s) they are assigned, they always have the option of contacting the nurse director or nurse administrator to help them work through their concerns.

We then needed to begin thinking about addressing the environment for floating, which was identified as the second major source of concern for staff nurses. In order to better understand what challenges staff nurses faced upon arrival at a unit, we pulled together a focus group that we called the ICU Welcoming Committee. This was a group of ICU staff nurses and two nurse director facilitators charged with better understanding the challenges of floating from one ICU to another as it related to patient populations and environment of care. Each nurse director was asked to choose a nurse from his or her area who would be able to speak to the floating process on behalf of the staff.

The group met and discussed the challenges faced when floating. The feedback was then presented to the ICU work group to be discussed and evaluated. The Welcoming Committee members detailed a wealth of valuable information about the floating experience. They noted that many times the problem is not the type of patients nurses are assigned to care for. Rather, it is how float nurses are planned for and supported by the staff in their assigned ICU that makes the float experience good or bad. With the recognition that there are nuances of care between the various types of ICU patients, this group of nurses felt strongly that with a more supportive environment a nurse floating from one ICU to another could take excellent care of the critically ill patient to whom he or she was assigned. The recommendations of the ICU Welcoming Committee are summarized in Box 16.1.

BOX 16.1 *Summary of Recommendations From "The Welcoming Committee"*

Assignment consideration required prior to arrival of float RN:

- Charge RN should know where the RN is floating from and make sure the assignment is appropriate for the RN. For example, if there is a patient in the cardiac surgery ICU who is experiencing some form of mental status changes and the unit is receiving a float RN from the neurosurgical ICU, it may be a good match to assign that patient to the floating RN, assuming that the patient does not have intensive cardiac surgical issues that require a specialized cardiac nurse.
- The complexity of the patient assignment for a RN floating to an ICU should be taken into consideration prior to the start of the shift. A floating RN should not be assigned a highly complicated patient with needs specific to that discipline of nursing. In addition, a float RN should not be assigned a patient that has a highly complex family/social dynamic that is known to the nurses on the unit. Nurses floating from another ICU should be assigned a less complex patient(s) and when possible would benefit from having a single patient assignment.
- Patients should not have consecutive shifts with a float RN assigned to their care, when possible. This will help to improve the continuity of patient care and decrease the potential for any missed care opportunities due to lack of patients being known by their nurse.

From the recommendations of this group, we were able to create a float support sheet that detailed the information identified as important to know for a nurse floating from one ICU to another. This sheet is given to the float nurse at the beginning of the shift. It includes the names and contact numbers of the attending physician, charge nurse, unit coordinator, patient care assistant, respiratory therapist, pharmacist, and other support staff, as well as any pertinent information the floating nurse might need to know. Listed on the back of this sheet are guiding principles of care that are specific to that patient population, along with nuances and details of care identified by the staff of the unit that would be important to know for a nurse floating to that area. There is a space on the bottom of the form for feedback on the float experience. The float nurse is encouraged to provide such feedback on this form, which goes to the nurse director of the area. On many occasions this has been done by e-mail or in person.

To prepare for the changes in float nurse experience we were planning, directors met again with their staffs to discuss the changes in the environment that had to be made to better support nurses floating to their unit. They discussed the plan of unit familiarization and ensured that the recommendations from the Welcoming Committee were in place on their unit.

Once all this work was in place, the directors provided real-time feedback to their staffs as to how others perceived their experience when floating to that specific ICU. We also spoke with our nurses after each float experience to gain any feedback that would be helpful. In addition, each director personally checked in with nurses floating to their area at the beginning of the shift to see how their experience was going and to make sure they had the support they needed to care for their patients. All the feedback was brought back to the daily ICU nurse director meeting to be shared. Thus, we were able to debrief each float experience that failed to meet our expectations and, when necessary, make changes and address issues until we reached a place where we felt comfortable that nurses were supported in all ICUs when floating. In addition to ensuring the quality of the float experience, we found that this process served to build confidence in one another's units and the ability to support nurses who floated.

The group did recognize that we might not always be in a position where we would be able to meet the nurse's preference as indicated in the floating guidelines. In every instance that we needed to float an RN outside of the guidelines, we committed to a brief communication with the nurse who floated. What we learned from these conversations was that, as we began to fix the environment of floating in each ICU, there was a higher comfort level from our nurses who floated to units outside the guidelines. This emphasized the important role a supportive environment of care played in a nurse's ability to provide excellent care to his or her patient. Although this is an added benefit, we continue to hold the floating guidelines as a guiding principle when determining where nurses will float.

We did meet some resistance to floating from a few small groups of nurses who felt that they should not float for a variety of reasons. In these instances the nurse directors of those areas met to develop a plan to address the resistance. In one instance there were a few nurses from one ICU who had previously had difficulties floating to a particular ICU; the directors of each area discussed the potential concerns to check the assignment and make sure it was appropriate for the nurse who was floating. The nurse directors would then be able to describe the assignment to the nurses prior to their floating. This helped to assure the nurses that they would get an appropriate float for their skill set. This proved to be a successful process. After several positive float experiences, the nurses developed a level of comfort floating to that area without the need for director intervention. Box 16.2 provides a sampling of recent feedback we have received from nurses who have floated since our work on the floating guidelines and our Welcoming Committee work.

BOX 16.2 *Float Nurse Feedback on Improved Float Guidelines and Practice*

"The patient I picked up was a stable post-op. He had an ICD placed and was doing very well. I received a thorough and complete report from the night RN. Then she brought me around the unit and showed me where things are. Everyone was pleasant and very helpful. The charge nurse continually checked in on me to ensure my comfort level and make sure I didn't need anything." —*MICU nurse describing float experience to CCU*

"I just wanted to drop you a quick note to let you know what an awesome floating experience I had. I had a great assignment and every nurse that was here made sure I was doing okay. Great crew and a great experience. Thank you." —*SICU nurse floating to MICU*

"Greeted by charge nurse. Paired with Shapiro nurse. Tour/overview of room and general population. Took care of a stable POD#2 patient. Having a card for the med room would have been very helpful. It was very helpful to have a nurse designated a 'resource person' for help and questions. As long as people can help you and show you around there shouldn't be an issue." —*Nurse floating to Cardiac Surgery ICU*

"I was warmly received and greeted by the day and night charge nurses. I received a great hand-off report and was given a tour of the unit and had all resources made available to me. Everyone from the Charge Nurse to the unit secretary made it a great experience— would not mind picking up some time over here." —*Burn/Trauma nurse floating to Cardiac Surgery ICU*

"Just a few positive remarks about my float on Friday night. I was given an appropriate assignment, a little busy, but the people I was working with acknowledged that and helped out when I needed it. . . . Kathy, George, Lon, Feliza, and a couple more whose names escape me all made it a point to make me welcome, offer help, and even jump in and do some vital signs or make out a flow sheet for one of my patients when I was busy in my other room." —*Nurse from Neurological/Neurosurgical ICU floating to Cardiac Surgery ICU*

"Just wanted to reinforce what I'm sure you know. You have a team of true professionals and this is reflected in the way they work and in the way they treat their floats. They did a great job of alleviating my anxiety about floating and made it a positive experience. Thanks." —*Note from nurse floating to the nurse director of unit where he/she was floated*

"Very impressed with all the support and help offered to me instantly as I walked through the door. RN reporting off took time and went in depth about unit specifics without asking. Very appropriate assignment." —*Cardiac Surgery nurse floating to CCU*

"I just wanted you to know how terrific your nurses were last Friday night. Four of your nurses floated to us, and they were saviors. Truly, we appreciated their professionalism during a very busy night. We had 6 admissions; their flexibility and selflessness did not go unnoticed." —*To nurse director of Neurological/Neurosurgical ICU from MICU charge nurse*

We have certainly experienced a change in culture about floating in our ICUs at BWH. This change came from the work group's willingness to listen to the voices of staff nurses and make system changes to address their concerns. We now have a culture where nurses feel supported in the floating process and patients are receiving the best care in the safest environment by the appropriate skilled nurses, thereby supporting the departmental vision. We are able to effectively utilize floating as a technique to address census fluctuations in our ICU. While we recognize that floating can be used to address census fluctuations, our goal of limiting the overall amount of floating required continues to be central to this process.

BROADENING THE SCOPE OF OUR WORK

As our noon meetings continued, so did the breadth and depth of our work. Meeting 5 days a week for an hour over lunch provided the opportunity for the group to grow and mature as a leadership team. This growth was fostered by both formal and informal mentoring provided by our executive sponsor, the associate chief nurse, Trish Gibbons, as well as our executive directors. It would have been very easy for senior leadership to just assign the next project, give a deadline, and expect results, but they consistently provided the support, resources, and direction that made our success possible. This made it easier to identify and prioritize issues that had to be addressed and then approach these issues in a systematic, confident manner.

Another major factor in the effectiveness of our group was the diversity of our members. Group participants had a wide range of nursing experiences and backgrounds, as well as cultural, gender, and generational differences. From our leadership development work, we understood how generations approach situations differently, and capitalizing on this knowledge has been enormously helpful to us as we examine projects and issues from varying perspectives.

Much of our work and many of our initiatives were situations generated by changes in the organization, or were a product of one of our "brainstorming" sessions conducted over lunch. As we worked on each challenge, we began to truly understand the power and influence we had as individuals and as a group on improving patient care in our respective units, as well as hospital-wide.

We realized that we could do more than successfully address the challenges we shared by creating effective floating practices. We could also anticipate new types of float nurse challenges that could emerge. To illustrate, one year into our project the hospital was preparing to open a new cardiovascular building that would house both the cardiac surgery and cardiac care intensive care units. As preparations were made for the move to this new building, the two directors involved would periodically present plans that were being developed to ensure a safe and efficient move. They would solicit feedback from our group and consider implications of the plans on the ICUs as a whole. One concern identified very early by our group was how to manage floating from the current building to the new building, as the patient care environments were quite different. We realized that floating would still be necessary, due to volume and acuity fluctuations, and so agreed that it was important to address this early rather than during the move into the new building.

We decided on a two-pronged approach, involving both short- and long-term strategies. For the short-term solution, the entire ICU float-pool staff was familiarized with the new building so that they could support the ICUs during the early stages of the move. Creating a long-term plan to provide support for nurses who floated from ICUs in the existing building to the new work environment was a bit more challenging. In the new building, the floor plan and location of supplies and equipment were drastically different, although the equipment nurses were using to deliver care was the same.

In the past, nurses were accustomed to being "oriented" every time a new initiative, product, or practice change was introduced. Therefore, the "easy" solution would have been to create a 4-hour orientation for all nurses before they cared for patients in the new building. This, however, did not feel like the right solution. After discussion of what was really needed, we decided on a different approach. Because the nurses already knew how to use the equipment and were familiar with the patient populations, they were not in need of an "orientation" to provide care; rather, they needed to become familiar with the new care environment before floating. Therefore, we decided that any nurse who floated to the new building for the first time would need to be familiarized. We invented and adopted the term *building/care environment familiarization* to describe the process. This process occurred immediately when a nurse was floated, before he or she actually cared for a patient. The familiarization included a structured tour and explanation of the floor layout, including where supplies were located, how the alarm and telephone systems worked, what information was needed for initiating a code, and instructions for accessing the medication area and staff locker room, as well a thorough review of the patient area and patient- and family-centered care environment. The nurse was also provided with a staff support sheet and asked for feedback on the familiarization in order to improve the process. The permanent staff of the unit to which the nurse was floated would act as the experts for the new environment, having received an in-depth orientation prior to the move.

BROADENING THE SCOPE OF OUR IMPACT

Our work as an ICU leadership team has encompassed a wide variety of situations and challenges, many directly connected to our initial charge from the associate chief nurse. Over time, influenced in part by past success and in part by our engagement in the DON vision, we began to identify other venues where we could have a positive impact. We have included here a few select examples to demonstrate the power, effectiveness, and efficiency of such a team in achieving results.

Addressing a "Staffing Mismatch"

Though we staff our units using both 8- and 12-hour shifts, most of our nurses work 12-hour shifts. Over time, we realized that this was creating a "staffing mismatch" between 3:00 PM and 7:00 PM, with the units consistently experiencing a staffing deficit between these hours and struggling to find coverage. Ironically, this was usually the busiest time of the day, which only magnified the problem. We had been dealing with this situation by requesting that nursing staff remain for additional 4-hour shifts, using overtime and relying on the float pool to address this problem.

As volume and acuity increased, it became more difficult to cover these staffing needs. We realized that we needed to address the problem at its root cause. Working with a consultant, we conducted multiple brainstorming sessions and a concentrated analysis of the situation, examining ways to correct the 3:00–7:00 PM staffing holes that plagued us. We came up with many strategies, including:

- Hiring more 3:00–7:00 PM shift nurses
- Increasing rotation to evenings
- Increasing the number of 12-hour shifts

■ Creating an 11:00 AM–7:00 PM shift
■ Moving 3:00–7:00 PM education to mornings
■ Converting 8-hour shifts to 12-hour shifts

Though there was nothing on this list that was surprising, going through the brain-storming and analysis process allowed us to focus on solutions and correct the problem through utilization of these identified strategies. As a result, we now rarely have issues with a 3:00–7:00 PM staffing mismatch.

Communication Between Charge Nurses and the Central Staffing Office

Our process for staffing each shift involved the charge nurse communicating staffing needs to central staffing office via phone, followed by a return call from the central staffing coordinator to communicate the plan for staffing office support (or lack thereof) for the next shift. As the majority of charge nurses have a patient assignment, this meant that the charge nurses would need to interrupt patient care to make or receive calls regarding staffing. After recognizing the inefficiency of this system and soliciting feedback from our charge nurse staff, we recognized that this method had to be refined. We established for ourselves the goal of developing a reliable staffing tool that would reduce the number of phone calls to and from the Staffing Office.

Utilizing staff input, we worked with a departmental expert who helped in the development of a staffing tool. We invested a great deal of time in determining functional requirements, and then consulted on the design, testing, and refinement of a computerized staffing program. This program allowed charge nurses to electronically document shift-by-shift staffing requirements without having to leave or be called out of a patient's room. The charge nurses were educated on necessary time frames for entering the data, but had a wide time span in which to do so, making it possible to perform this task on their schedule. This provided ample time for the staffing office to weigh the staffing needs of the ICUs against available resources, and still develop contingency plans.

This new computer system eliminated the inefficiencies and inconveniences of the phone-call method, and reinforced with our staff our joint commitment to keeping the focus on the patient. Of course, implementation was not without challenges, as it necessitated a change in practice and acceptance of the new system. We realized that without compliance and reliability, this new process might not only fail to work, but might also create a dual system of calls and electronic data entry. Therefore, our implementation plan included education of all permanent and intermittent charge nurses on use of the program and the time deadlines necessary for accurate staffing assessment.

Education occurred prior to implementation over a 3-week period on all three shifts and the weekend, utilizing both permanent and temporary trainers. Once implemented, we tracked compliance with the staffing tool and initially had directors paged if staffing numbers were not entered on time. This feedback loop made real-time staff intervention possible during the rollout process. With rapid cycle improvement methodology, we were able to perfect this tool in the ICUs, and now the staffing office is rolling this out to inpatient intermediate care units using a tested and proven process.

Communication With the Emergency Department

An important detail we identified during our initial explorations as a work group was that we could not fully address appropriate staffing if we did not know when our next patient was coming. To help with understanding ICU admission patterns, each director received an in-depth analysis of all admissions to their unit by source, day of week, and time of day. Using this information, we divided the admissions into two basic types, predictable and unpredictable.

Our evaluation of the data made it obvious that the unpredictability of admissions from the Emergency Department (ED) was a major factor affecting the medical, trauma, and neuroscience ICUs more than the other intensive care areas. We evaluated the emergency room length of stay for the patients admitted to these areas and identified an opportunity to improve this time through better communication between ED and ICU nurses about potential admissions. We initiated a collaborative effort among ICU and ED nursing leadership and ED care facilitation nurses in an effort to improve predictability and communication.

Our task force examined the key personnel and systems involved in the process, mapping the flow of these patients once they enter the ED. A key factor recognized in this assessment was that the structure between 4:00 PM and 8:00 AM provided for good communication between the ED and the receiving ICU, unlike the time period from 8:00 AM to 4:00 PM, when there was no central nurse administrator to coordinate and ensure that this communication occurred. It became clear that resolving this was the task of our group.

In the ED, physicians, charge nurses, and care facilitators all shared information regarding ICU admissions. The task force designed an 8:00 AM to 4:00 PM process to improve communications between the ED and ICU. This flow of information involved the ED charge nurse informing the ED care facilitator of any potential ICU admissions. The care facilitator was charged with discussing and clarifying the service/team assignment with the ED physician, and then notifying the ICU charge nurse of the impending admission. If the care facilitator experienced problems in communicating with the ICU charge nurse, a text page was sent to the ICU nurse director. Receiving this information earlier has resulted in ICUs being able to better arrange staffing for unplanned ED admissions, leading to more timely transfers and less discomfort for patients.

Bed Turnaround and ICU Throughput

Consistently we have been struck with the importance of patients moving without impediment through the system during their hospital stays (*throughput*), and the impact that good throughput can have on effective, timely, and seamless care. Therefore, we conducted an analysis of bed turnaround times by day of week and time of day to help us to understand the impact of inefficiencies on patient flow. This assessment allowed our group to partner with leadership from Environmental Services in identifying areas of opportunity and possible solutions. Additionally, work has been done at the unit level in identifying throughput issues related to each area. For example, the ICU nurse director group agreed on a set of ICU charge nurse responsibilities as they relate to throughput for all ICUs, but have individualized how these are implemented at the local unit level.

Staffing, Continuity of Care, and Unscheduled/Sick-Time Usage

As an ICU leadership group, we have worked on many projects that have crossed unit boundaries, affecting not only the ICUs but all inpatient areas. A good example of this is our grappling with the issue of sick-time usage and its impact on staffing. As a department of nursing, we have struggled with the realization that our nurses' sick-time usage was higher than national trends. Staffing challenges related to use of unscheduled time arose periodically as we worked on various projects around staffing and continuity of care. As a result, over time we developed a consistent voice on how to deal with and approach sick time within the ICU group. We also found that only a small percentage of the staff actually utilized excessive unscheduled time. Once identified, we were able to work with and support these staff members in exploring solutions that could potentially reduce their use of sick and Family and Medical Leave Act (FMLA) time. After this work, a hospital-wide task force was put together to revise the policies concerning unscheduled time off and sick calls. We now have a new hospital-wide attendance policy that gives directors direction, strategy, and support in ensuring that our patients and families have the staff to provide for their nursing care needs.

AN INFORMED JOURNEY

As we developed as a leadership group, we realized that having the right information at the right time was crucial, not only for ensuring that we were taking the correct path, but also for measuring progress and knowing when to adjust our course. Therefore, from the outset we decided to collect information that would help us manage, assess, and sustain our quality gains. To illustrate, we recognized the importance of quantifying and qualifying the outcomes of our work with ICU floating and the Designated ICU Nurse. To that end, our project manager created and managed databases, recording when and where ICU nurses floated, and generated a weekly report containing this information. This allowed us to touch base with staff, particularly when they floated outside the set guidelines.

Similarly, use of the DIN was tracked, detailing the time, length, location, and reason for each "deployment." These databases allowed us to compare activity over time, and assess where changes were indicated. For example, we found that heavy DIN utilization occurred Monday through Wednesday between 7:00 PM and 7:00 AM. Knowing this, we worked with the off-shift nurse administrators in planning for a second DIN during these periods, based on actual acuity and volume for a given day.

Putting structure and process around receiving and reviewing data were also a key strategy for our group. As mentioned earlier, we were provided with daily information on volume and acuity, as well as weekly productivity metrics. However, we realized that evaluating collective and individual ICU data over time would provide an opportunity to identify consistent or changing trends not always recognizable in the moment.

Over the course of the project, we discovered that monthly volume, as well as historical and current sick-, FMLA-, and vacation-time utilization are good predictors of potential staffing challenges. Therefore, together with our executive directors we conduct a quarterly data review identifying service line initiatives and changes that affect nursing workload, allowing us to proactively manage staffing in a dynamic environment. In addition, we engage in a yearly review that includes not only the quarterly metrics, but also ICU floating, DIN utilization, ICU length of stay (LOS), and admission patterns as compared to previous years.

Our group has become increasingly sophisticated in data utilization, with the idea of quality-versus-quantity as a key driver in new data requests. In other words, we challenge each other when making new data requests to see if this information will really shed light on the topic at hand and/or help us measure the success of our efforts. This leads us to what information is actually needed. A good example of this in action is evaluating the effect of admissions, transfers, and discharges (ADT) on nursing workload. We decided that understanding the "churn" on our units was essential, and discussed a number of measures to help capture this activity. After discussion, we were able to pare it down from many to a few metrics that allow us to track and assess ADT, and better inform decisions regarding staffing plans.

BENEFITS: POWER OF THE TEAM

Working daily side by side has not only improved ICU staffing, but has also allowed us to see a view of all the ICUs, rather than just our own specialty. We are able to understand the differences and similarities that we were facing as ICU directors. This understanding has enabled us to explain to our nurses why staffing variations exist on a particular ICU or follow up on rumors presented to us. Being able to investigate issues concerning our units and provide quick feedback to staff not only helped us to build credibility as a group, but also showed that we were committed to supporting our staff. As the project's success continued, we were able to be a resource to each other as needed.

Another benefit that developed from our work group was the opportunity to work directly with our associate chief nurse, the executive directors, and the nurse administrators who cover the evening, night, holiday, and weekend shifts (see Chapter 19). The nurse administrators were able to help us implement changes that came out of our work group. They were aware of what we were saying to our staff about changes being introduced at the unit level, and utilized consistent language in communicating with our staff when reinforcing these changes. They also provided us with real-time feedback so we could achieve timely follow-up with staff as needed.

As a group, we were all committed to the departmental vision of a healthy work environment for our nursing staff—one that respects the voice of the nurse and allows the best care possible to be provided to patients and their families. This vision has helped us to keep the patient and family at the center of our decision making. We have had situations where a patient needed care by another specialty in addition to our own staff specialty. Because of the relationship building within this group, we have had been able to support each other when we needed a nurse with a competency that staff on our unit may not have. For example, on the Thoracic ICU, a patient arrived from the OR with a balloon pump. The Cardiac Surgery ICU nurse director was notified, and responded by sending Cardiac ICU RNs who were trained to monitor the balloon pump to the Thoracic ICU to care for this patient. In the Neurological/Neurosurgical ICU, the nurses are not trained to perform continuous veno-venous hemofiltration (CVVH), as they rarely have patients who require this therapy. The agreement between the Neurological/Neurosurgical ICU and the Medical ICU (MICU) is that the MICU nurses will provide the CVVH for their patients. If the MICU staff is unable to go, then another ICU, such as the Surgical ICU (SICU) or Thoracic ICU, sends RNs who can provide CVVH for the patient. We have made the commitment to base our decisions on what is best for the patient and family. Do we move the patient to the caregivers or caregivers to the patient? What is best for the patient and family?

Collaboration with our physician leaders has also been a focus and positive outcome of our group. We like to know what is in the future so we can strategically plan and not be required to respond on an emergency basis. For example, if a specific medical service is hiring a new physician and our patient population is likely to increase as a result, knowing this in advance helps us to carefully examine our staffing patterns. Conversely, if one of the leading surgeons is preparing for sabbatical, then we know that our census and volume may decrease during this time.

Collaborating with other departments has also helped us, as a group, to manage our areas more efficiently. For example, positive collaborations have resulted from meeting with Human Resources to better understand the FMLA process, meeting with the Admitting Department to understand changes in admitting patterns, and meeting with Environmental Services to see how they can best deploy resources during our peak times and at change of shift.

Currently, we feel that we are a unified group of critical care nurse leaders who have become more effective in leading our areas, embraced the concepts of a healthy work environment, and more effective in our communication skills. We can attribute our success to the team building that came from this group, and the knowledge that we have gained from each member of the group. We have developed a trusting relationship among group members and know that we can rely on each other to focus on the vision of the nursing department and make it a reality.

We believe that this model of collaboration that we have developed can be used in other areas, such as the step-down and intermediate areas. As a leadership group, we continue to focus on providing safe, quality care for our patients and families and on making sure our staff has the knowledge and resources to provide excellent nursing care, and to feel supported by us while doing so.

MAPPING OUR FUTURE PATH

The future holds many questions for all of us in the health care industry. As nurse directors in this dynamic environment, it is crucial that we position ourselves to respond to changes from all directions—legislative, political, scientific, technological, demographic, and socioeconomic—while being clear about our core work, which is patient care. The ability to remain agile is dependent upon our ability to understand all the relevant factors and their impact on our patient volume and nursing workload.

One of the more challenging issues we have uncovered has been to recognize that the tools we have been using to understand our staffing needs have told us only part of the story. Specifically, our most immediate task is to understand what *acuity* means. We have had an acuity system in place for several years, but each unit audits and classifies very differently. Furthermore, each unit has its own unique culture that approaches staffing decisions on the unit level in specific ways. We realized that this made our determinations of acuity less valid. We used the opportunity of a recent classification system upgrade to improve the way in which we instruct nurses across the institution to interpret the indicators.

As we improve the quality of the data, we improve our ability to interpret and utilize the data. Once we have a better understanding of acuity as an institution, we can more accurately quantify patient needs and then place resources where they are needed, by setting a reliable and meaningful hours per workload index (HPWI). Our group put forward a recommendation to the nursing department to hire a program manager to oversee patient classification and support the nurse directors in accurately quantifying the nursing workload of any given unit. We proposed starting with the ICU group, given our already established working relationships as directors and the flexibility that has germinated within our staff. This was consistent with our initial goals as a group to find the right nurse for the right patient.

Nursing workload is a multifaceted product of patient acuity, volume, and turnover. To bring better understanding to the variables that influence workload, we have begun to add features to our weekly director reports, which include *Average Daily Census, 24-Hour Contact Census, ADT Index, Acuity,* and *Sick Calls.* The project manager for this initiative has been given the task of building consistency among our units when we evaluate nursing workload. This is no small undertaking. Our intent is to have a given patient receive the same acuity score no matter what unit the patient happens to be in. The ability of any given nurse to care for that patient is going to vary according to the nurse's individual experience, expertise, or ability, but the patient and the care this patient requires should not vary. The project manager is going to have to change the way we monitor and audit our units to build a more reliable data point. This requires an intensive and comprehensive re-education of staff about application of the indicators across the institution.

The ultimate goal is to understand and quantify the staffing requirements necessary to meet the nursing care needs of our patients, and accurately incorporate this into our budgeting process. The growth in our sophistication as we build our own reports allows us to understand the impact of changes in acuity and volume. This knowledge positions us to better support the work and vision of the department in a financially responsible and patient-centered way: the very best staff providing excellent care to patients and families in the safest environment.

Our expectation going forward is that we can use the process established within our group to tackle other issues common to the ICUs. New technology rollouts can be managed with greater efficiency, and new administrative policies related to sick-time management or FMLA time can be handled with greater consistency, thereby reducing misinterpretation and manipulation. Our ability to communicate with each other and hear the concerns of each nurse makes us a better support to our staff in caring for patients with highly specialized needs. It is a journey that is fluid, but the view improves as we get farther down the road. The pavement is smooth and our ability to avoid potholes in the road has improved. We are laying the course as a leadership group that gains strength which each new brick we tackle.

Amen!

17

Building Anew

Mary Lou Moore and Catherine Saniuk

" The new building will be called the Carl J. and Ruth Shapiro Cardiovascular Center." The long-awaited decision about the clinical focus of the new Brigham and Women's Hospital (BWH) building had been determined and the leaders chosen. That, we realized, would be us. The Cardiovascular Nursing Executive Director, Mary Lou Moore, new to the director role, had been a part of the design process from the outset and was now leading a newly formed Cardiovascular Nursing Leadership Team, composed of the nurse directors, assistant nurse managers, and clinical educators. We would be the people in the nursing leadership roles in the new Shapiro building.

Some members of our team had a long history of shared professional practice; others were new to the hospital or to their positions. We were initially concerned because we were asking them to participate in a time-consuming and demanding construction project as well as transition to new roles. However, the opportunity to shape the environment of care was compelling and there was a growing sense of confidence that our team had the capacity and the passion to meet the challenge. A natural work flow emerged while people flexed their strengths and creative abilities.

The building would be devoted to the care of cardiovascular patients, both inpatients and outpatients. It would include 136 inpatient beds, provide new outpatient clinics, and house many of the services that support the cardiovascular patient population. The existing cardiac operating rooms and cardiac diagnostic and intervention center (CDIC) areas would be moved to new, updated quarters. Even food delivery would be changed to an all-room-service menu. Our team would work with multiple services and vendors to design care delivery spaces in the building and ultimately prepare staff to move into these spaces. For those of us in leadership roles, the process was an awesome responsibility, both exciting and overwhelming. We knew that the opportunity to participate in this process would be a once-in-a-lifetime career event and we were committed to producing something extraordinary.

How does a team inexperienced in such a process gain the expertise, confidence, and courage to do this? The answer to that question is complex. We were strongly supported and guided by the vision statement of the BWH Department of Nursing: "A commitment to providing excellent care to patients and families delivered by the very best staff in the safest environment." This vision is not the exclusive prerogative of nursing, but is organizationally shared and embraced. Because of the mutuality of that commitment, the building of Shapiro would be the highest priority for those of us working closely on the project, and this accountability would be organizationally endorsed. We would return to the vision statement repeatedly throughout the journey we were then beginning—a commitment that would serve to ground us as we worked to realize outcomes to support stakeholders and, ultimately, those patients who were to receive their care in the new building.

THE PATIENT ROOM

The design of many of the elements of the building had been long thought about by those who came before us within the context of patient-/family-focused care. All inpatient rooms were to be private, spacious, and have a sleep space for a family member to stay overnight. From the outset, hospital leadership also demonstrated a clear recognition that nursing expertise was essential to the design of the room and, finally, to managing the occupancy of the building. To explore design aspects and enhance the learning process, a model patient room was constructed to the same scale as the planned inpatient rooms. When the space occupied by the mock room was needed for another building project, the hospital accommodated our efforts by reconstructing the room a second time in a space more readily available for training and meetings. This was a powerful message about the value of our work and the hospital's commitment to creating the safest possible environment for patients.

With repeated redesigns in response to feedback from all the disciplines involved, both model rooms involved numerous hours of work. Nurses, physicians, biomedical engineers, vendors, contractors, and respiratory, physical, and occupational therapists all weighed in. Planning sessions were held in the mock room on day and night shifts to maximize everyone's opportunity to participate and familiarize themselves with an environment in which they would soon deliver care. Although some preliminary blueprint decisions had already been made, the design details became our work. The room would be divided into three spaces: a family space, a patient space, and a clinical space. Refining each space was our job.

As the plan for the room emerged, clinical events were simulated to challenge the room design. How would the room support the care of the patient being resuscitated or requiring bedside continuous renal replacement therapy? Where should the bed be positioned during resuscitation? How would the mobile boom facilitate 360-degree access to the patient? To answer these questions, we held mock clinical events to determine functionality. The nursing staff came together, often working with nursing staff unfamiliar to them or with a discipline other than nursing. Not all these interactions were simple or smooth, given the diversity of disciplines, opinions, and styles. But once again the underlying commitment to serve patients and families in the safest environment would help defuse escalating emotions and refocus us on shared values.

Over time, a subtle but real change became apparent as the staff developed and deepened relationships with each other. Equally as subtle and as real, the nursing staff became more invested. This transformation was not surprising, given the amount of time we shared, the energy we invested, and our awareness of the commitment by hospital leadership. And it was pivotal. The nursing staff began to feel a sense of ownership and pride in the building and the work. It was their building! They were no longer being asked to consult on a process, but instead were the architects of their own environment. This truly was a turning point. Most importantly, the nurses felt valued, included, and respected. During this process the leadership team coalesced, coming together with a deepening commitment to the project and each other. All were essential to delivering a well-designed room and supporting the engagement of nursing staff with the project and the leadership team.

We learned also that an individual has a finite ability to assimilate multiple changes. The room had a new boom, new headwall, and a new custom-designed IV pole. The pole design was a culmination of many ideas and trials, but there remained functional limitations. Within this process, we came to appreciate how difficult it is to be sufficiently analytical while in the midst of a multiplicity of changes, including a finite ability to successfully introduce new information. This knowledge would serve us well, keeping us more balanced and realistic when our natural temptation was to do too much. With the multiplicity of the tasks waiting to be done in a compressed time period, we may have been overly ambitious. In the end, our enthusiasm was tempered by real safety concerns: Lesson learned.

We polled all providers and found that the main physical concern for physicians, mid-level providers, and nursing staff was visibility and audibility of cardiac monitor alarms. Our facility has never used monitor technicians. Alarm monitoring and response is a shared responsibility. Nurse directors worked with the vendor and Biomedical Engineering to fashion a solution. As a result, the decentralized workstations were equipped with fully functional central monitoring stations, along with "slave" monitors mounted in the hallways so that there were no blind spots for viewing the patients on cardiac monitoring.

PATIENT/FAMILY-CENTERED CARE

As determinations were made about the clinical focus of Shapiro, the leadership of BWH developed a philosophy statement regarding Patient/Family Centered Care (PFCC). The purpose was to frame and support the progress toward universality of this value at BWH.

> BWH commits to placing patients and their families at the center of care and considers patients and their families to be partners in the care team. Through this partnership, the priorities of patients and their families help guide each patient's care. This includes tailoring our approach to meet each patient's definition of family and supporting how his or her family will be involved in care and decision making. We empower patient and families to be active participants rather than passive recipients of care. We seek to understand and meet the needs of our patients and their families, striving to deliver information, which is open, timely, complete and understandable to them. We extend this contract with attention to the dignity of and respect for the patient's and family's preferences, culture, capacity and abilities in determining care. To maintain the vitality of commitments to patient's and families, BWH recognizes the need to incorporate patient and family advisement in operations,

policy development, and at all levels of care delivery. We wholeheartedly support all who work here in order to make this possible.

Throughout the hospital's clinical settings there were examples of individual efforts to provide PFCC as described by this philosophy. The practice, however, had not been universally embraced or integrated, and the physical design of much of the hospital made family presence difficult. The Shapiro building plans had a range of features supportive of family presence beyond the inpatient room design. Each inpatient floor had a large, comfortable waiting area. These shared spaces had televisions, computers, and an inviting space for children to play in. Private consult rooms were readily available. If a family member wished to stay around the clock, he or she could sleep in the patient room or in the family area on a convertible couch. All of this was in stark contrast to much of the rest of the hospital, designed before family presence had been a norm of care.

Although PFCC was not yet a consistent practice, there were clinical units that were front runners in adopting and integrating this approach to care. The inpatient oncology units were an exemplar. The Dana-Farber Cancer Institute PFCC Advisory Council was established in 1998 and had been actively involved in the oncology inpatient units at BWH. The Neonatal Intensive Care Unit also has had an active parental advisory group. However, the cardiovascular units had not previously been a part of any focused effort to move to a PFCC model. PFCC practice within the cardiovascular nursing staff was as it was elsewhere at BWH—largely determined by the individual delivering care. Because each patient would invariably receive care from multiple nurses during a hospitalization, the patient and family might be exposed to a number of individual philosophies regarding family involvement and presence. This inconsistency had been a longstanding concern and had led to misunderstanding between staff and family on numerous occasions.

The building of Shapiro and the organizational commitment to PFCC were timed to provide an unparalleled opportunity for implementation of PFCC in a building that could optimally support family presence. Still, it would take a dedicated institutional effort to ready the Shapiro staff for PFCC. Here we drew on the expertise of the BWH Center for Clinical Excellence (CCE) Performance Improvement Group to facilitate this change in practice. The CCE's work is devoted to improving quality and safety at BWH through a number of direct and consultative initiatives. The Performance Improvement Group specifically is skilled in the art and science of change. First they held numerous focus groups. All those who would be working in the inpatient units and in the CDIC were involved. The nurses raised specific concerns about the patient and family involvement in the change-of-shift report and physician rounds. They also explored the implications of family access to the patient's medical record. Family presence during procedures and resuscitation, and private clinical conversations and care while patients had a family member/support person with them 24 hours a day, were also identified as concerns.

Nurses expressed the need for a consistent message about what PFCC meant and expectations for family behavior. They emphasized the significance of appropriate staffing and intradisciplinary buy-in for PFCC. They raised the importance of nursing assessment and decision making about family presence and questioned how to go about asking a family to leave when appropriate. They agreed that patients and family needed updates and should be involved in the plan of care, but there was considerable variance in thoughts about how best to accomplish this. At the conclusion of the series of sessions, the leadership team and the staff received a summary of the discussion. The magnitude of staff concern sensitized us to the tenor of the staff. This information guided plans for the orientation classes which we called "Connecting with Care." This was our effort to respond to these identified issues and to support the staff's first step in the process of adaptation to PFCC. In the richness of life in the Shapiro building, this work has evolved and continues.

THE SHAPIRO NURSES PREPARE

Moving would be a big day and a big change. We remained focused on the singular long-term outcome—safely moving patients into the building—through a series of short-term, time-limited, predetermined agendas that were continually affected by the construction schedule. The education planning began with multiple brainstorming sessions about current care provision. What worked well? Were there common difficult concepts across services? How could we use this gift of education time to ensure a safe environment for the patients on move day and beyond, *and* build on skills to spawn a stellar Shapiro cardiovascular nurse? We imagined how care delivery in the building would be different. How would we preserve the best of the physical environment we were leaving, the intimacy of the smaller units, the inherent safety of patients and nurse being so proximal and always visible? Assignment structure and flexing the new nurse call system to its fullest capacity would be critical on day one.

Many of the transformative stages would overlap. We planned the sequencing of the classes on the notion that the staff needed time to plateau each learning curve before another was piggybacked on top. They needed time to process and unfreeze before moving toward practice changes. We set saturation goals for each part of the training.

The Cardiovascular Expert Nurse

We asked ourselves a new question based on this opportunity for change: "What if the nurses identified the patient's stay as being more than this diagnosis, this shift, and were able to anticipate, teach, and in some instances care for patients throughout their heart disease journey?" To answer this question, we first identified expert practices appropriate to our patient populations, including high-risk, low-volume technologies.

We then strove to create a curriculum that would foster a continuity of knowledgeable concern from all nurses providing care during the patient's stay. Heart-failure patients provided the blueprint: They were "frequent flyers" to all our services. The care these patients required already connected the nurses to one another's care practices. Ultimately the class included common concepts such as anticoagulation and cardiac pacing, and practice "pearls" regarding care of each cardiovascular patient type.

Technology Training

We knew that training staff in new technologies—a new nurse call system, new beds, new IV poles, updated cardiac monitors, and a variety of other accessory equipment in the patient rooms—was imperative. We learned that it would be challenging to accomplish this training within the context of the construction schedules. Everything was new. These embellishments presented demanding and overlapping technology learning curves, each subtly nudging how the work would be done. For instance, we elected not to use the inpatient room digital clock to its fullest capacity because it would change how we documented during codes.

Through past hospital-wide technology conversions, we had learned that it is not enough to simply present the buttons and menus of a new gadget as training. The inservice must recognize and highlight key differences from old technology. We also recognized how crucial it was to remain within our care values to prudently leverage any new technology. An equipment vendor generally will not be able to speak to practice, yet emphasizing practice changes is critical to safety. The Shapiro classes were always scripted and hosted by BWH experts as well as the vendor representatives to ensure that accurate technology information was coupled with comprehensive practice information.

The cardiac monitor training was the most time-consuming topic to plan and execute. A consulting group was brought in to assist in brainstorming. Interestingly, because our group was already leading and working intuitively, we grew impatient with their time-consuming discovery process, which only revealed the shared values and desires we already held and recognized. Nonetheless, for cardiac monitoring training, Biomedical Engineering set up a remote training site using the monitors and computerized network slated for the new building so that nurses could leave their floor for several hours to concentrate on the updated equipment. The time with the monitors was invaluable, but the monitors then went into the building and we did not have access to them again for months. Yet another challenge!

In the class, we wanted to cover the new monitor functions as well as address all current cardiac monitoring practice stumbling blocks. We used demonstration and return demonstration techniques combined with case-study analysis. The new system would stretch the monitor functionality because each intermediate care room in the Shapiro building would have a built-in bedside cardiac monitor. If a patient on telemetry became acutely unstable, the nurse could quickly access the cardiac rhythm from the room, and immediately have access to oxygen saturation probes and noninvasive blood pressure monitoring. We knew that this would be a powerful aid in treating an unstable patient. We recognized that the translation of the button training into practice, especially in an acute event, would require more than the class. Once settled in the building, we refined the procedure and held periodic practice sessions and produced many revisions of bedside cue cards.

Thirty nurses attended a "master" class on the monitoring system, so they could serve as "super users" in the new building after the move—with sufficient expertise to ensure safe cardiac monitoring and support practice changes on the unit. Unfortunately, with class size too large and content too dense for the time available, this was the one class that was less than successful. However, once in the building, the super users, immersed then in hands-on experience, were able to fulfill their roles.

We timed the technology classes as close as possible to the move. This was vital for learning retention and yet challenging because of construction rules and vendor/equipment availability, which created an ever-changing timetable. From a scheduling perspective, this was an immense challenge. Flexibility was key. We used the mock room to test and train on as many technologies as we could before the move. Our goal was to familiarize the nurses with the buttons, knobs, locks, poles, and alarms while stimulating feedback born out of imagining using the device. We used scripted, problem-oriented scenarios to foster critical thinking.

As soon as we could bring people into the building without hard hats, the clinical educators hosted familiarization tours. We were sensitive to the increase in expenditure of nursing time during care provision because of the size of the floor and the length of the hallways. There were redundant spaces for medication and supplies. On each floor there were two nursing units and three medication rooms, to reduce the number of steps. Each supply room had two doors, on different hallways. We spent a lot of time planning and stocking these spaces so that nurses could access care resources easily. Nurses were concerned that moving to a rectangular environment from the intimate BWH semicircular pod would make their work flow difficult. We created a building inservice that specifically took the nurse through a workday, from entering the building through tasks at the nursing station and into the patient room. They needed to be familiar with both the mundane (new lockers) and the high tech (new call system). We did our best to build on the excitement and even had some fun with a scavenger hunt competition, while every button and knob was revisited.

We staffed our RN super users 24/7 after the move to support practice, along with vendor coverage to work out any technology issues. Two technologies most central to care delivery were revisited in depth, requiring major revision and repeated inservice after the move: the nurse call system and the cardiac monitors. We had not anticipated how our patient care assistants would interface with the cardiac monitors in the room and had not included them in the monitoring classes. Once again, education came to our aid. In the end, we learned that the classes had only laid the groundwork. A great deal of learning occurred after we got settled into the new space.

MOVE DAY

Having the right team together meant having a big team. Redundancy was our friend. We explored team dynamics. BWH's Security Operations Manager, Robert Donaghue, was the conductor of our virtuoso staff. His 32-year Marine career and his experience in planning amphibious landings framed his thinking. His primary objective was to create a strategic, logistic, and communication plan that would leave the clinicians completely free to care for the patients. No detail was so minute that it wasn't considered. Our preparation included focus groups, tabletop drills, and mini-drills, culminating in three full mock drills in which we moved beds and equipment through long hallways under street level. We analyzed each drill to reveal the good and bad. We simulated moving an ICU patient with every piece of equipment that could possibly be involved in life support. It took 15 minutes and

2 elevators. We learned the human and equipment resources required to transfer each patient and ready the team to deploy for the next patient.

We all intuitively worked backward from the concrete outcome of a safe move. Across the institution, we had zero tolerance for a "normal accident" in this tightly coupled event. Perrow (1999), in describing a *normal accident*, states that "given a system's characteristics, multiple and unexpected interactions of failures are inevitable." We understood that we were dealing with an inherently chaotic environment and project. There were variables we could try to anticipate, but not really predict. We remained flexible and patient focused. Our shared values of safety and patient centricity emerged in all conversations, and created our intentionality. Stacey describes a view of intention:

> When one comes to regard intention as a theme that organizes the experience of being together, it becomes clear that intentions emerge in the conversational life of a group of people. A single individual does not simply "have" an intention. Rather, the intention an individual expresses has emerged in the conversational interaction with others. Intention and choice are not lonely acts but themes organized by and organizing relationships at the same time. (2007, p. 15)

Our intentionality allowed us to experience all themes, overlapping and paving the way for forward movement over the years of planning and learning despite chaotic circumstances.

Health care providers may be more accustomed to working in (if not planning for) chaos because of the dynamic nature of our work. We had multiple contingency plans. If a patient was too ill to be safely moved, the progression of the day would not be interrupted and the patient would be reevaluated at a later time. We agreed that on move day patients would be admitted directly to Shapiro. We had teams of nurses and physicians in each building, those receiving and admitting patients and those moving patients. ICU patients were moved in the freight elevators to the underground hallways under the street that separated the two buildings. The CDIC recovery room marked a halfway point, which was equipped for emergencies. A safety pause was held and then the patient moved on into Shapiro. Intermediate patients moved in pairs with their nurse through the above-ground enclosed bridge, which was closed off to other foot traffic. Elevator mechanics were available all day, which turned out to be a talisman that warded off elevator trouble. The patients moved in orchestrated waves. We finished the move at 16:42, safely, efficiently, and with a welcoming message for all.

Recalling the move day, one staff nurse said, "I brought my patients over in their new (Shapiro) bathrobes when it was my turn. Funny, I remember these shoes were new that day. I remember the whole day. We got here and just continued with our day." Another observed, "It was so calm, I didn't feel nervous, I knew what to do and I knew who to call if I didn't. I had been involved with the drills so I knew how many people were working on this." Describing the transfer of one of our most acutely ill patients, her nurse remarked, "We moved this patient who was so sick, but everyone recognized the risks, was ready to respond, crash carts in the hall on the way, the security guys with their walky-talkies—it felt like a long walk, but it was safe. Then when we got to the new room, the receiving team helped settle her in and it was seamless." Late in the afternoon, there was a code on a patient freshly admitted from the operating room in the cardiac surgery ICU. We had all the correct equipment available. The staff all knew where to find what they needed in a timely manner. The patient did not suffer any delays in treatment related to distractions of the new environment and the excitement of move day.

TRANSFORMATIONAL SPACE

Finally, the culmination of an immense body of work, the orientation, and the complex move itself, were behind us. We had relocated into the new building. From the outset, we had a commitment to optimizing the aesthetics in our new work environment: the design, the furnishings, the color choices, and the presence of art all supported an optimal experience in the building. The architects had incorporated large expanses of glass along the exterior walls, which filled the space with natural light and afforded superb views of the city. The inpatient units and the entire building provided openness and breathing space. This diminished the concentration of people and dramatically reduced the noise level. We saw patients sleeping better and using call lights less. The presence of family members in the patient room normalized the environment for the patient. Family members were able to be present throughout the night, offering familiar reassurance, and were present during the day as they would be at home. All of this was in profound contrast to the environment the staff, patients, and families had come from, and gradually we all began to adjust.

Once the initial first few weeks in the building were over, the staff began to comment on the spaciousness and quietness of the environment. They felt more relaxed and associated the new environment with a decrease in stress. A design environment that had once been concerning to them because of the size and their perceptions of isolation was instead affording them with both visual and auditory uncluttered space. The patient care environment was truly changed, and it was creating a new experience not only for patients and families but for the staff as well. The staff still delivered the same kind of nursing care, but they were able to have a more reflective and focused practice. Something about this change in environment was resulting in a less frenetic, more engaged, more thoughtful, and more deliberate nursing staff and care delivery process.

One nurse director and her staff created a staff renewal environment that would take advantage of the building attributes. Caring practices can extract a toll. A nurse who is attentive to self-care would have deeper care reserves for patients and families. Thus, there was an intentional effort to create a renewal space that would be used by staff, patients, and families for meditative practices, Reiki, or quiet rest. The spirit of this undertaking has clearly influenced the care on the involved unit and its influence has spread and permeated the climate of care. It has encouraged all of the cardiovascular leaders to examine the environment on their units and look for opportunities to create a similar experience.

The initial adjustment process is now behind us, though we remain in discovery mode. This new environment has created so much change, and continues to present opportunities that never could have been previously realized. There remains much work to do, but the staff have been energized and renewed by the opportunities that the building naturally creates.

Individuals and groups of nurses have achieved national certification and awards, participated in global humanitarian outreach, developed new skills, weathered losses, and reexamined their practices for the next developmental steps that are unique to each individual nurse and unit. We look forward to what it is we will discover as we further evolve in this new space that has proven to be transformational for both people and practices.

The authors extend thanks to the following persons who provided input into our chapter: Janet Razulis, MHA; Dorothy Goulart, MS, RN; Robert Donaghue; Alice O'Brien, MS, RN; Jacqueline Gagnon, MSN, RN; and all members, past and present, of the Cardiovascular Nursing Leadership Team.

REFERENCES

Perrow, C. (1999). *Normal accidents: Living with high-risk technologies*. Princeton, NJ: Princeton University Press.

Stacey, R. D. (2007). *Strategic management and organizational dynamics: The challenge of complexity* (5th Ed.). Upper Saddle River, NJ: Prentice-Hall.

Thompson, P., Parenti, C., & Peterson, L. R. (1990). Planning the move of patient activities at a large medical center. *Hospital & Health Services Administration, 35*(3), 443–460.

Woodward, H. (1994). *Navigating through change*. Boston, MA: McGraw-Hill.

18

Neuroscience as Exemplar

18.1 *The Intersection of the BWH Department of Nursing Vision Statement With Nursing Theories, Theorists, and Practice*

Vincent M. Vacca, Jr.

More than 30 years ago, while working as an aide assisting patients and nurses in a tuberculosis sanitarium, I decided to pursue a career in nursing. My decision to become a registered nurse was based on the realization that nursing represented and strengthened my personal values. The decision emerged from both consideration and personal reflection about what I wanted to do with my life and education.

The process of personal reflection was inspired by experiences and interactions I had with the tuberculosis patients and nurse role models. As I assisted nurses delivering care to these patients, I learned the importance of addressing and meeting patients' practical and physiological needs, or the *how* of nursing. I also learned the importance of making a personal connection, the *why* of nursing. It was the why of nursing that appealed to and fit my personal temperament. Learning and mastering the practical skills one must have to be an effective professional nurse is essential, as nursing is a fast-paced, results-oriented endeavor, but scheduled care can leave little time for reflection on the philosophical and theoretical dimensions, or the why of nursing.

The most inspirational nurses I have encountered over the years demonstrated a balance between meeting the demands of timed events, such as medications and treatments, and making a personal connection with their patients. They were adept at both communicating and demonstrating clearly through words and actions what it took to provide complete and responsive nursing care for another person, a patient. I admired these nurses who got to know patients as individual people, beyond just their diagnoses and medical plans. These nurses became my role models and mentors.

As a nurse, I have practiced in a variety of specialized care environments. All required meeting precise scheduled activities, such as assessments, vital signs, medications, procedures, treatments, and documentation. In addition to becoming proficient in those important skills, I had not forgotten the significance and value of making a personal connection with patients that I learned from the nurses in the tuberculosis sanitarium.

MY INTRODUCTION TO NURSING THEORIES

Years later, in graduate school, I became aware of and acquainted with the domain of nursing theory and nurse theorists. My research into this domain reminded me about the importance of making a personal connection with patients and families. Hildegard Peplau, a past president of the American Nurses Association, was the first nurse, in 1952, to blend concepts from other disciplines into a nursing theory that she named: Theory of Interpersonal Relations (Peplau, 1997). Peplau believed that nursing is both a healing art and an interpersonal process between two or more people sharing a common goal. She proposed that strategies including education, problem identification, problem solving, and therapeutic interactions between nurse and patient would lead to the shared common goal of healing. I believe Peplau's work advanced nursing from a job with a set of skills to a profession with its own structure, language, and theoretical basis. Many nurse theorists have built on her work, which was done more than 50 years ago.

A few years ago, I came to Brigham and Women's Hospital (BWH) as a travel nurse assigned to a new and unfamiliar specialty—the neuroscience intensive care unit (ICU). At that time and stage of my nursing career, I was eager to accept the challenge of learning a new and complex specialty from the ground up, and that was exactly the situation I had accepted. In the neuroscience ICU, I discovered a care environment that was as challenging as I expected, but I also experienced much that was unexpected. Despite the newness and complexity of neuroscience nursing to me at the time, I realized that this nursing environment also felt vaguely familiar. These feelings of familiarity soon became an unexpected revelation for me. My challenge as a staff nurse in this specialty of neuroscience ICU nursing both energized and inspired me with a force I had not felt for many years. Perhaps it could be described as déjà vu, as I recognized and understood that these feelings were similar to what I had experienced as a nurses' aide learning the how and being introduced to the why of nursing in the tuberculosis sanitarium.

As I built my practice in the neuroscience ICU, I found myself wanting to better understand the principles described by Peplau, and by Faye Abdellah, who, 50 years ago, stated that nursing as a profession is a "service to patients, families and therefore to societies" (Basavanthappa, 2007, p. 55). Abdellah described a nurse as possessing qualities including kindness, a caring nature, intelligence, competence, and technical preparation to provide nursing's unique service to all who need it (Basavanthappa, 2007, p. 55). Abdellah advocates that nurses, by knowing their patients, are better able to act on behalf of their patients and families as problem identifiers, decision makers, and problem solvers. For me, Peplau and Abdellah defined a framework that provided structure and support centered on the essence of nursing practice.

I realized that understanding the teachings of Peplau and Abdellah would benefit me as a nurse, and benefit my patients as I cared for them in the neuroscience ICU. This realization led me to revisit and discover the work of other nurse theorists. I had some limited awareness of nursing theories and nurse theorists from graduate school years ago, but my knowledge of this body of work up to this time was cursory at best.

FURTHER DEPTH IN MY EXPLORATION OF NURSING THEORIES

My intention to explore the theoretical basis of nursing marked the beginning of a quest for me. I revisited the writings and teachings of nurse thinkers and theorists.

Lennart Fredriksson, from her work on suffering, makes the distinction between nurses "being with," which she says is a "gift of self" from nurses, and "being there," which she describes as a "physical presence" (Iseminger, Levitt, & Kirk, 2009). Timely treatments can heal a patient's wounds, and medications can control their symptoms, and even cure a disease, but establishing a relationship, or providing the gift of self as Fredriksson suggests, can be as valuable and important to patients and families as healing a wound or curing a disease.

Fredriksson and Abdellah, like Peplau before them, incorporated and built upon what Florence Nightingale meant when she expressed, more than 100 years ago, that nursing as a caring profession goes beyond the sciences to be holistic in its approach to caring. She was the first to suggest that nursing knowledge is separate and distinct from medical knowledge, and described the goals of nursing care as restoration of health and health maintenance by providing fresh air, warmth, cleanliness, a quiet environment, and proper nutrition (Basavanthappa, 2007, p. 42).

Jean Watson, a past president of the National League for Nursing, states in her theory that "Caring is the essence of nursing." Watson defines *caring* as occurring during any "nurse–patient interaction" (Drenkard, 2008, p. 404). Karen Iseminger, in her work, captured the importance of knowing a patient as the basis of an empathic relationship between nurse and patient, one that "fosters collaboration, cooperation, and healing" (Iseminger et al., 2009, p. 448). Martha Rogers, in *The Science of Unitary Human Beings*, echoed Nightingale, stating that professional nurses seek to "promote symphonic interaction between man and environment, to strengthen the coherence and integrity of the human field, and to direct and redirect patterning of the human and environmental fields for realization of maximum health potential." She too advocated a holistic approach to delivery of nursing care to promote recovery or maximum health potential (Dossey & Keegan, 2009, p. 53).

FROM THEORIES TO PRACTICE: GUIDED BY A VISION

In my nursing practice as staff, and now as the service line nurse educator in the neuroscience ICU, I use knowledge gained from these nurse theorists to establish a framework as I provide care for patients and families and support to my nurse colleagues. Although there are similarities and overlap among many nursing theories, there are also significant differences. The challenge of how to capture and articulate a blend of many disparate nursing theories into one vision statement has been addressed and accomplished by our BWH chief nursing officer (CNO) Mairead Hickey. Working with all levels of the BWH Department of Nursing (DON), she crafted a nursing vision statement that is inclusive of both the how and the why of nursing practice, as well as the supporting structures necessary to create, expand,

and sustain it. This vision statement both challenges and supports every nurse practicing at BWH: *"excellent care to patients and families, with the best staff, in the safest environment."*

Hillman and colleagues state that the intent and benefit of an organizational vision statement is to define and support the structure and culture of an organization. The vision statement serves to influence motivation, behavior, cooperation, performance, teamwork, and relationships (Hillman, Chen, & May, 2009). Our DON vision statement, by defining the culture of nursing practice, affirms that every nurse at BWH will be fully supported with effective and responsive leadership, educational opportunities, and environmental and workplace safety as they provide care to patients and families. Covenants are explicit: Nurses will be supported and empowered to provide the gift of self, to be with patients and families, and to get to know patients and families, with care rendered through a nursing presence and nurtured with full support from the larger organization. The concept of nursing presence can lead to and create what Owens suggests is a therapeutic relationship that promotes healing: "Healing requires integration of psychological, emotional, spiritual, and social components, which are beneficial to patients and families even when a cure is impossible" (Iseminger et al., p. 449).

The DON vision statement challenges each nurse to understand that nursing care is most effective when the nurse knows his or her patient, beyond the diagnosis and plan of care, as a unique human being. Knowledge of the patient, in the manner that the DON vision statement envisions, encourages the nurse to integrate the biological, physical, emotional, psychological, spiritual, and social dimensions of each patient in a safe care environment. The vision statement is strengthened by Watson, who suggests that the nurse is essential to "preserve humanity and sustain caring in situations where it is threatened" (Watson, 2006, p. 50), and by Farley, who defines a *therapeutic relationship* between nurse and patient as a partnership requiring "caregiving skills, skilled communication, respect for autonomy and diversity, and shared decision making" (Iseminger et al., 2009, p. 449). Farley also suggests that success in developing a therapeutic relationship requires "energy, effort and moral courage" (Iseminger et al., 2009, p. 449). Rogers said that in the service of patients and families, *energy* is the "fundamental unit of the living system" and therefore "it is not that human beings have energy, but rather that human beings are energy" (Rogers, 1992, p. 30). For me, the DON vision statement captures what Peplau, Abdellah, Rogers, Watson, and others convey when it asserts that all nurses will be encouraged and supported to channel their energy and effort to develop and sustain the courage and ability to provide comprehensive nursing care to a diverse population of patients and families.

AN IDENTIFIED PRACTICE CHALLENGE EMERGES

In our 20-bed neuroscience ICU, with support from our nursing director Shaun Golden, and CNO Mairead Hickey, we created a partners-in-care (PIC) team, led by staff nurses, to strategize and develop interventions designed to improve and sustain the quality of nursing care delivered to all of our patients and families. The PIC team develops initiatives designed to strengthen nursing practice at the bedside (see Chapter 18.2). One of these is the nurse-to-nurse handoff.

The Joint Commission (TJC), the Institute for Healthcare Improvement, the Agency for Healthcare Research and Quality, and the American Association for Critical Care Nursing (AACN) have position statements specific to many aspects of nursing practice. One such shared focus is the nurse-to-nurse handoff process. These organizations and BWH nursing department leaders emphasize both the timing of and content discussed during nurse-to-nurse handoffs as essential to promoting seamless delivery of nursing care and creating a culture of patient safety. The AACN synergy model supports and identifies the importance of nurse-delivered patient care as follows: "Nurse competencies as defined by the synergy model include clinical judgment, advocacy and moral agency, caring practices, facilitation of learning, collaboration, systems thinking, response to diversity, and clinical inquiry" (Marzlin, 2011, p. 44).

It is essential that nurses discover, develop, and direct practice changes designed to create a sustainable culture of safety and caring. Often nurse-to-nurse handoff can be variable in content, length, organization, and structure. Variability of nurse-to-nurse handoff can result from a combination of factors, including patient acuity, readiness of the departing nurse to hand off the patient, prior knowledge of the patient by the receiving nurse, and the handoff process itself. In 2005, TJC reported that poor "communication is the most frequent cause of sentinel event that is evaluated by the Joint Commission" (Odom-Forren, 2007, p. 233). In 2001, the Institute of Medicine (IOM) reported that "it is in inadequate handoffs that safety often fails first" (IOM, 2001, p. 45). TJC recommends a handoff process that includes interactive communication, including opportunity for questions and clarification, up-to-date information specific to the patient's care, verification of information between sender and receiver, an opportunity for the receiver to review data, and minimal interruptions (Friesen, White, & Byers, 2008).

THEORIES, PRACTICE, VISION, AND CHANGE: AN EXAMPLE

Our PIC team accepted the challenge of development, rollout, and implementation of a structured, standardized, comprehensive nurse-to-nurse handoff tool called FASTHUGSBID. It is a comprehensive template that creates a bidirectional exchange of all essential patient information in a timely fashion between nurses at every handoff opportunity.

Authorities in organizational management theory warn that changing or modifying existing systems can be challenging. Kotter describes organizational change as a process designed to "create awareness and acceptance for the intended change." He recommends "creating a sense of urgency, designating a change leader, developing a clear vision for the intended change, communicat[ing] the change in clear language, empower[ing] organizational members to accept and facilitate change, generat[ing] short-term wins to promote acceptance of the change, and finally anchor[ing] the change into the culture"(Hillman et al., 2009, pp. 104–105).

FASTHUGSBID, found in Box 18.1, is an adaptation of a tool originally developed by a group from the Department of Intensive Care, Erasme Hospital, Free University of Brussels, Brussels, Belgium, who created this mnemonic device for managing a handoff. Each of the letters denotes a specific piece of information essential for a handoff (Vincent, 2005, p. 1226). Acknowledging Kotter's principles for organizational change, the neuroscience ICU set out to integrate FASTHUGSBID into our nursing culture. Nurse-to-nurse handoffs are common; they can and do occur several times a day, every day. Done poorly, they can result in a gap in care that could have negative effects for nurses and patients. In fact, nurses may be found legally liable for failing to report necessary information during handoffs. Therefore, a sense of urgency existed to create a standardized, comprehensive nurse-to-nurse handoff process that would meet TJC standard for handoffs: "An effective end-of-shift report is accurate, concise, complete, specific, relevant, and timely" (Welsh, Flanagan, & Ebright, 2010, p. 148).

BOX 18.1 *FASTHUGSBID* for Your Patients, by Our Nurses, With Every RN-RN Handoff

- ■ F: Feeding and Nutrition > Adequate to meet metabolic requirement?
- ■ A: Assessment > Targeted and comprehensive?
- ■ S: Skin and Safety > Interventions for prevention and treatment and for all safety risks?
- ■ T: Thromboembolism > Appropriate ambulation, compression, mechanical, chemical prophylaxis?
- ■ H: Head of Bed > Elevated ≥ 30° or appropriate to patient condition?
- ■ U: Ulcer (Gastric/Stress) > Prophylaxis provided?
- ■ G: Glucose > Glycemic control utilizing oral agents, subcutaneous or intravenous insulin?
- ■ S: Support > Provided as needed by interprofessional team to all patients and families?
- ■ B: Bowel Regimen > Appropriate to patient condition?
- ■ I: Infection Control > Surveillance, identification, practice, and education?
- ■ D: Documentation > Completed; all forms — Paper and electronic?

Utilizing the established structure of the PIC team as recognized, accepted, and empowered change leaders, we believed that the concept of FASTHUGSBID could be effectively communicated, providing short-term gains by improving the quality of communication between nurses for the benefit of nurses, patients, and families. We were convinced that FASTHUGSBID would positively influence the standard of practice, leading to integration of FASTHUGSBID into our nursing culture.

MAKING THEORY MANIFEST IN OUR PRACTICE

FASTHUGSBID facilitates a relationship between nurses and patients, recognizing that the patient and family are the focus and recipient of nursing care, as Peplau, Abdellah, Watson, and other nurse theorists have described. FASTHUGSBID is designed to be comprehensive, yet sensitive to the time demands nurses face at shift change and other handoff instances. It is structured to overcome existing barriers to an effective handoff, such as disorganization, inadequate or inaccurate information, and failure to communicate essential information. FASTHUGSBID is a tool that is simple to learn and use, and will result in improved satisfaction with both giving and receiving report during nurse-to-nurse handoffs. It represents a clear transfer of responsibility from one nurse to another by providing all essential and relevant information, facilitating improved nurse awareness of the patient and family, promoting seamless delivery of nursing care, enhancing patient satisfaction, and fostering a culture of safety.

FASTHUGSBID is a face-to-face encounter and exchange that can be delivered at the bedside or during walking rounds. It provides a bidirectional opportunity to seek clarification and ask questions. If interrupted during nurse-to-nurse hand-off, FASTHUGSBID enables picking up where handoff stopped, but also provides a clear and simple structure to avoid the possibility of omissions or incongruence of essential patient information. TJC, in 2008, added elements for performance specific to the handoff process. They suggest that the handoff be structured to have consistent information communicated in a consistent pattern and that it be standardized with opportunity to seek clarification and ask questions (Riesenberg, Leitsch, & Cunningham, 2010).

An understanding of the theoretical foundation of the nursing profession can strengthen the care that nurses develop, organize, and deliver to patients and families. FASTHUGSBID invokes the spirit of Nightingale, Peplau, Watson, Abdellah, Rogers, Fredriksson, and others by putting the patient at the center of nursing care, and creating a culture of safety. FASTHUGSBID complements and is supported by the DON's vision statement, which advises that nurses get to know their patients and provide a therapeutic use of self to be with and provide comprehensive care for patients and families using scientific knowledge, intellectual judgment, moral courage, and imagination: "Excellent care to patients and families, with the best staff, in the safest environment."

REFERENCES

Basavanthappa, B. T. (2007). *Nursing theories*. New Delhi, India: Jaypee Brothers Medical Publishers.

Dossey, B. M., & Keegan, L. (2009). *Holistic nursing: A handbook for practice* (5th ed.). Sudbury, MA: Jones & Bartlett.

Drenkard, K. N. (2008). Integrating human caring science into a professional practice model. *Critical Care Nursing Clinics of North America, 20*(4), 403–414.

Friesen, M. A., White, S. V., & Byers, J. F. (2008). Handoffs: Implications for nurses. In R. G. Hughes (Ed.), *Patient safety and quality: An evidence-based handbook for nurses.* Rockville, MD: Agency for Healthcare Research and Quality, 2-285–2-289.

Hillman, K., Chen, J., & May, E. (2009). Complex intensive care unit interventions. *Critical Care Medicine, 37*(1) S102–S106.

Institute of Medicine. (2001). *Crossing the quality chasm: A new health system for the 21st century.* Washington, DC: National Academy Press.

Iseminger, K., Levitt, F., & Kirk, L. (2009). Healing during existential moments: The "art" of nursing presence. *Nursing Clinics of North America, 44*(4), 447–459.

Marzlin, K. (2011). Structuring continuing education to change practice: A nurse-driven initiative. *Dimensions of Critical Care Nursing, 30*(1), 41–52.

Odom-Forren, J. (2007). Accurate patient handoffs: Imperative for patient safety. *Journal of PeriAnesthesia Nursing, 22*(4), 233–234.

Peplau, H. E. (1997). Peplau's theory of interpersonal relations. *Nursing Science Quarterly, 10,* 162–167.

Riesenberg, L. A., Leitsch, J., & Cunningham, J. M. (2010). Nursing handoffs: A systematic review of the literature. *American Journal of Nursing, 110*(4), 24–34.

Rogers, M. E. (1992). Nursing science and the space age. *Nursing Science Quarterly, 5,* 27–34.

Vincent, J. L. (2005). Give your patient a fast hug (at least) once a day. *Critical Care Medicine, 33*(6), 1225–1229.

Watson, J. (2006). Caring theory as ethical guide to administrative and clinical practices. *Nursing Administration Quarterly, 30*(1), 48–55.

Welsh, C. A., Flanagan, M. E., & Ebright, P. (2010). Barriers and facilitators to nursing handoffs: Recommendations for redesign. *Nursing Outlook, 58*(3), 148–154.

18.2 Partners in Care: Quality Improvement at Work in the Neuroscience Intensive Care Unit

Shaun Golden

T he Neurosciences Institute, one of the five centers for clinical excellence at the Brigham and Women's Hospital (BWH), offers the most innovative and advanced treatments and therapies for all diseases of the nervous system. As an integral part of the Institute, the neuroscience intensive care unit (ICU) is dedicated to delivering the highest quality of nursing care to all of our patients. In recent years, the emphasis on improving the quality of care provided by hospitals has increased significantly, and continues to gain momentum with pressure and influence from regulatory bodies, accreditation agencies, and quality improvement organizations such as The Joint Commission (TJC), Centers for Medicare and Medicaid Services (CMS), and Leapfrog. The 90 nurses on staff are committed to providing high-quality, evidence-based nursing care in our 20-bed ICU. With the formation of the Partners in Care (PIC) Committee, and its precursor, the Care Improvement Committee (CIC), our frontline nurses are playing a pivotal role in continuous quality improvement. In this chapter I describe the development, functions, and impact of the PIC Committee on our ICU.

Prior to 1997, the BWH did not have a neurosciences ICU, but with increasing demand, the necessity for a neuroscience-dedicated unit became clear. With the opening of a 10-bed neuroscience ICU, I was afforded my first leadership role at BWH as the permanent day nurse-in-charge (NIC). This opportunity allowed me to work closely with my nurse manager, Maureen McGrath, and learn the importance of strong nursing leadership, relationships, and the need to be a passionate advocate for my staff. For the next 7 years, as the NIC, I continued to advance my clinical competency and leadership skills, mentored by Maureen. In August of 2004, when Maureen retired, I was asked to take her position and so became the nurse manager (now the nurse director) of the neuroscience ICU.

Shortly after I became the nurse manager, patient volume dramatically increased and there was a pressing need to expand neuroscience critical care to 20 beds. With the doubling of the unit size, we initiated a massive recruitment and hiring initiative to support the new 10-bed unit that opened in January of 2005. Concurrently, I was asked to be the interim nurse manager of the troubled radiology department. Challenges abounded, change was rapid and intense, and all our quality improvement work was reactive and "in the moment," with very little proactive quality improvement. Even though the Institute of Medicine report *To Err Is Human* had been published in 1999, we were still looking at the incident and not the systems that allowed the event to happen (Institute of Medicine, 1999). However, the transition to the concept of "bad systems and not bad people lead to most errors" was beginning to take hold across the institution (Berwick & Leape, 2005).

We knew safe care was being delivered, but believed evidence-based nursing care was limited, with care based on historic practice. Personally overwhelmed and getting discouraged with the limited amount of time I could give to any quality initiatives, I lobbied for the help of an assistant nurse manager. Thankfully, my efforts paid off with the addition of Matthew Quin to the leadership team. This timing was perfect, because as a Department of Nursing (DON), engaged in a change process under Mairead Hickey's leadership, we had just finished defining our mission, vision, and values and were moving to the next step, "Finding the Good" (see Chapter 2). Matthew stepped right in and took on this project, enabling us to understand what was good in the care that we were delivering and what the nurses in the ICU needed to deliver excellent care. This was our first glimpse into where opportunities for improvement could be identified in the neuroscience ICU.

As a hospital, we were preparing for a 2006 TJC visit, so there was an increased emphasis on audits. Audit teams were being established at the unit level throughout the hospital to carry out medical record and blood administration audits. Up until this point, audits were thought of as a tedious task with very little benefit. We felt that the results did nothing other than point out what had not been done or had been done incompletely by a colleague. Audits and an audit team were not high on the priority list for the unit. In fact, it was not until someone noted that I did not have a team doing the audits, but rather my clinical educator, Vince Vacca, that I was asked about my plan for audits moving forward.

What happened next was my good luck at the expense of someone's bad luck. Paula Trabucco, a neuroscience ICU staff nurse, broke her leg. BWH's occupational health professionals indicated that she could not return to giving care at the bedside while wearing a cast, but noted that if I had any projects to work on, she could do these. In bright neon lights the word "AUDITS" was flashing right in front of me. It was a win-win: Paula could get back to work and we now had the beginnings of an audit team in the unit. Shortly after Paula returned to the bedside, Occupational Health issued new policies, ones that would have excluded Paula from project work in the unit. As you will soon see, if that had been the case, this chapter would probably never have been written.

By the fall of 2007, among Mairead Hickey's initiatives for change, the DON was embarking on establishing a hospital-wide committee structure to bring together professional nurses from different practice areas and roles to shape, influence, and recommend and/or approve decisions to improve the clinical practice environment. In an effort to mirror the work of the hospital, we established a committee to improve care in our ICU with Paula, Vince, and I as founding members. Sticking with the grassroots philosophic approach that was so successful in the "finding the good" work, we asked for volunteers from our nursing staff. We set fundamental expectations regarding meeting frequency and time commitment for the members. Skepticism was blatantly obvious from the small number of staff that initially stepped forward to join the team, but those who did set the stage for others to follow. The mission, values, goals, and expectations of the membership were established during the first few meetings, and these have been crucial to the success of the team. Critical to goal achievement by the new CIC were two important factors: leadership and committee composition. Each one of these contributed to the development and culture within the committee.

LEADERSHIP

Every committee needs leadership and organization to be efficient and productive, but the kind of leadership that is needed may vary significantly among committees. As the nurse director, I am ultimately responsible for all clinical and administrative functions that take place in the unit. It would have been very easy for me to manage the CIC and dictate what and when projects should be started and completed, but that was not the approach I took. That approach harkens back to an outdated style of management that Porter-O'Grady described perfectly: "Managers have learned the science of control and how to do it humanely so that people ultimately do not mind doing what they are told. Role parameters have been clearly defined, as has the subordinating character of each job" (Porter-O'Grady, 1999).

I believed that leadership and the human element of mentoring and coaching were essential to the success of this committee. I asked Paula to chair the CIC and Vince to serve as the content and practice expert; I was the advisor, mentor, and coach. As the inaugural chair of the committee, Paula brought what is often referred to as "street cred": She is personable, approachable, confident, and an expert practitioner who is always patient focused and above all respected by the staff (Benner, 1984). These attributes made Paula the perfect nurse to lead this committee through its beginning growth. She carefully planned and scheduled each meeting, always including an organized agenda with timely follow-up on action items from the previous meeting (National Academies, 2000). Because this was our first effort at a unit-based care improvement initiative, there was excitement and enthusiasm at the early meetings, but it was Paula's unique ability to harness this energy and convert it to productivity that ensured success.

Vince's contributions to the early committee work were immeasurable. As the content expert, he would research and provide the most up-to-date evidence-based literature for any initiative embarked on by the committee. To make it easy for the committee to understand and incorporate the literature into the plan, Vince would condense all of his research into a "Cliff Notes" format, with all of the highlights and outcomes that were relevant to the work of the team, and send it to the members in advance of any meeting. In addition, he would also provide information regarding practice and policy changes that were being generated at the DON level.

As the advisor to this committee and as the leader of the ICU, it was my job to help the committee focus on a common vision and improve safety and the care of our patients. Leadership that focuses on the merging of goals and ideas of the staff and manager into a common cause is the hallmark of transformational leadership (Sullivan & Decker, 2009). Indeed, Sullivan and Decker posit that nurse managers may experience transformational leadership as a natural model. No leadership theory can explain every situation, but we were committed to using a transformational leadership approach and we believe it produced results. Staff nurses working at the bedside 24 hours a day, 7 days a week, 365 days a year, know their patients and have the insight and knowledge to elicit needed changes in practice to improve outcomes. We knew this and we trusted it.

CIC COMPOSITION

By far the most amazing aspect of the CIC is its composition and the diversity of its members. As noted earlier, members were volunteers; no management pressures determined the membership. We were fortunate, from the beginning, to have representation from all shifts: Getting every shift's input and feedback are critical because there are noteworthy differences in nursing practice demands from shift to shift. More impressive to us, the CIC membership is a reflection of today's multigenerational workforce. Although I do not think I have any staff that are members of the World War II or the veterans generation, I do know that I have baby boomer, generation X, and millennial generation nurses working side-by-side on this committee (Sherman, 2006).

As part of our leadership seminar series in the DON (see Chapter 5), Phyllis Kritek provided workshops in part focused on generational diversity in the workforce. Working with Phyllis, I realized that each generation's life experiences were formed by the events of their time and are reflected in their attitudes, beliefs, drive, work ethic, and aspirations. Each generation has unique workplace characteristics; thus, each contributes in its own unique way. The challenge is to lead this diverse, multigenerational group of nurses so that the richness of each generation can be captured for all to benefit from them (Sherman, 2006; AARP, 2007).

I believe the CIC has truly captured the benefits and strengths of this multigenerational workforce through the natural evolution of the team. A swing in culture that in the past would not have happened was adopted and fully capitalized on by the team. Moving from a cultural mindset of "your input is not important until you've put your time in at the bedside" to a culture of "everyone has important contributions to make and patients and families may lose out if everyone's ideas are not heard" was a monumental change in culture. Some of the benefits, recognized early from this change in culture were increased flexibility, innovation and creativity; thinking outside the box; and decisions made that reflect the multigenerational patient population that we serve (Sherman, 2006; AARP, 2007). A resource published by the American Association of Retired Persons (AARP), entitled "Leading a Multigenerational Workforce," lists characteristics common to each generation (AARP, 2007). It includes the following categories: assets, liabilities, the type of manager they prefer to work for, motivation, messages that motivate, rewards, preferred method of communication, how to recruit and retain, and, for managers the most important characteristic: what we as managers do that drive them crazy. This resource was useful to us in maximizing our opportunities in the work of the generationally diverse CIC.

FROM CIC TO STAFF: SPREADING THE WORD

With an unwavering focus on the patient and family, the CIC is a continuous quality improvement initiative. The process of getting ideas, education, and initiatives from the committee meetings to the entire staff was a daunting challenge until the concept of a unit blitz approach to disseminate information was conceived. This method of information spread was done by educating the members of the CIC on a given topic and then providing them with a script, prepared by the members of the committee, so that they could "blitz" the staff on that same topic. Each member would blitz the information to their colleagues while working alongside them when there was an opportune time. A central list was kept to ensure that all staff members were reached with the needed information.

The first, and probably most influential and groundbreaking blitz that the CIC embarked on was in 2007, as we were preparing for the TJC visit. The CIC became proficient and knowledgeable about TJC National Patient Safety Goals, conducted a mock TJC survey, and then conceived the blitz concept to spread the information. With a goal of informing 100% of the day staff and as many staff as possible on the night shift, the CIC members brought this important, need-to-know information to the nurse at the bedside. They met their goal of reaching 100% of the day staff and their efforts and success were validated when the tracer survey method used by TJC traced a patient to our ICU. When the nurse chosen to present the patient was asked to speak to her practice and how that practice is captured in her documentation, even though she was terrified, she was able to speak intelligently; she was organized and comprehensive in describing her practice and the exceptional care she was providing her patient and that patient's family.

SIGNIFICANT ACHIEVEMENTS

Two CIC achievements stand out, the first for the external validation it gave us, and the second for our role as a BWH leader in quality and safety. The Massachusetts Department of Public Health (MDPH) has designated BWH as a primary stroke center, a status that requires recertification every 2 years. CIC has been instrumental in our quality initiatives to meet MDPH performance and quality measures, one of which is discharge teaching of stroke patients. As our content expert, Vince, in collaboration with the stroke program manager, Linda Bresette, and the clinical educator of the neuroscience intermediate unit, Heidi Doucette, developed an educational module for this purpose. Their goal was to increase the completion of stroke education prior to discharge for patients diagnosed with stroke and their families. They presented their plan to the CIC for review and feedback. They inquired about use of the blitz format for dissemination and the CIC approved. From the beginning of this educational program, yearly improvements have been recorded and BWH was awarded the MDPH Gold Performance Award for 2009.

The use of physical restraints to control agitated patients and prevent their premature removal of tube lines and drains in the critical care setting has come under intense scrutiny in recent years. Restraints must be clinically justified. In addition, TJC and the CMS have standards that are very specific regarding the need for approved protocols and a practitioner's order as requirements for the application of physical restraints. We realized that restraint reduction would require a cultural change in the way critical care nurses perceive the safety of their patients. This topic was discussed in the CIC meeting. It is not hard to imagine nurses' skepticism about any restraint reduction program working with any success in the neurologically impaired patient population. Willing to take on any challenge, though, the team went to work.

As the team started to strategize about the approach to restraint reduction, they worked closely with Mary Antonelli, the quality program manager for surgical nursing. This strategy of bringing resources and content experts to the CIC to assist in their initiatives has proven to work very well, and this method was applied to restraint reduction. Changing historic practice and cultural norms regarding restraint usage in the unit was going to be a huge endeavor. The CIC's educational blitz taught the staff about new policies and regulatory agency mandates. More significantly, the blitz shifted staff's thinking about restraints, emphasizing the importance of starting with the least restrictive restraint first. The CIC was attempting to change an attitude and culture regarding restraints. In September of 2009, a hospital-wide restraint prevalence survey showed that our unit had become by then, and continues to be, the hospital leader in restraint reduction.

We all take pride in these two achievements; however, the CIC has tackled several other major initiatives focused not only on patient safety but also on family satisfaction and patient flow challenges. Reading the curriculum vitae for the team gives a true appreciation of the tremendous work that has been done to improve the quality of care in the unit.

PATIENT SAFETY INITIATIVES

Handoff Report: Communication between staff members is essential to knowing your patient and having the ability to address the needs of your patient and family. Adapting a strategy comparable to that used in the airline industry, a handoff tool/checklist that was specific to the neuroscience ICU was designed and implemented (see Chapter 18.1).

Safety Pause: This applies to every invasive procedure, including those performed at the bedside. The operating clinician is responsible for conducting the pause immediately prior to incision or beginning the procedure. Again adapted from the airline industry, during the pause, the entire team must confirm the following using a checklist: correct patient identity using two identifiers, correct side and site, procedure about to take place and site marked, if appropriate. Audits were done by CIC to ensure that all procedures done in the ICU included a safety pause, and the results were shared with the physician leadership of the unit for any needed remediation.

Hand Hygiene: An organized, systematic approach that ensures adherence to hand hygiene policies reduces the transmission of pathogenic microorganisms to patients and personnel in the health care setting. The CIC kicked off an education and awareness blitz on hand hygiene. They used an educational theme of a football tailgate party, kicking off the season of hand hygiene. They educated the staff regarding the policies and benefits of hand hygiene, periodically monitored and recorded adherence, and then provided feedback to the staff regarding their performance, both individually and as an overall unit. Hand hygiene is a never-ending improvement initiative, and the team is always looking for novel approaches to improve compliance.

Critical Labs: The process of receiving, documenting, and reporting critical lab values was standardized by hospital policy in accordance with TJC National Patient Safety Goals. CIC introduced, educated on, and audited the new process with all members of the nursing staff.

Vaccinations: Assessing patients admitted to BWH on their pneumococcal and influenza vaccination status is a hospital-wide nursing responsibility.

Capturing this in the nursing admission form was and continues to be a challenge for a number of reasons, ranging from nurse omission to the patient's inability to verbalize vaccination status. Audits and continuous remediation are both parts of the team's approach to this topic.

PATIENT AND FAMILY SATISFACTION

Signage: During open conversation at a CIC meeting, a team member described how a patient's family member was very frustrated with the poor signage in the hallway and waiting room. CIC evaluated the current signage, agreed it was poor, and designed and made new signage for the hallway and waiting room. They elicited feedback from families, all positive. The temporary signs are being made into permanent signs.

Welcome Package: CIC was concerned that patients and families were overwhelmed with the amount of medical information they were receiving during a stressful hospital experience and while being subjected to a collection of unfamiliar hospital and unit rules. They researched and gathered literature specific to the neuroscience patient population, to BWH, and resources in the surrounding area to make these available to patients and families.

Overnight Guide: Our physical plant is very limiting in some aspects, including patient room size. Recognizing the constraints of the room size, and balancing it with the belief that the family is an important component of a patient's hospital experience, CIC is currently developing guidelines for overnight stays.

EXPANDING OUR HORIZONS

While we took great pride in the achievements of the CIC and the effectiveness of our blitz disseminations, we realized that this approach only involved nurses; we were operating in a silo. We invited our social work and nutrition colleagues to join us and they enthusiastically accepted. We initially hoped that they could help nursing fully understand the contributions they make to the care of our patients. This multidisciplinary collaboration with our new partners was short lived, as it quickly progressed to a transdisciplinary collaboration style. Time was devoted at each meeting for both of our new members to enlighten and teach the full team about their discipline so that their expertise would be integrated into the care of the patients (Hamric, Spross, & Hanson, 2005). As the CIC adds new members and strives to improve patient care, we believe the true winners are the patients and families who are cared for in our ICU.

This moved us to our next expansion. We realized that all of the terrific work done by the CIC is shaped by health care professionals. We use evidence-based literature to plan and deliver our care, but there was still something missing. That missing piece was input from patients and families. After a team of nurses, physicians, and social workers atttended an Institute for Family-Centered Care conference, it was clear that we had some work to do in this area. Collaborating with patients and families to ensure that our quality improvement work is patient and family centered was the next step.

As the team began to realize the importance of involving patients and families in our work, they also felt that the name of the team should reflect this idea. The team's name was changed to the Partners in Care (PIC) team and the search for a past patient or a family member to join our team was started. At this point, after suggestions and recommendations from team members regarding patients or family members who might be appropriate, we have reached out to two patients and both have agreed to join our team. Although they have not become fully active in the work of the unit, this combination of the health care team's professional expertise and the unique perspective of patients and families will create a partnership that will enhance delivery of health care for patients and families.

Because I hold the position of nurse director at BWH, I was strongly encouraged to become a master's-prepared nurse. During the development and creative achievements of the PIC I have described here, I have been enrolled concurrently at Boston College in the School of Nursing as a Haley Scholar (see Chapter 7), working toward an advanced degree as a clinical nurse specialist. Under the tutelage of my professors, particularly Dorothy A. Jones and Rosanna De Marco, I have been able to immediately apply what I am learning in my graduate studies to my everyday practice and to the quality improvement efforts at BWH. Thus, they too play a role in our ongoing work toward excellence in patient care.

I think the work of the CIC and now the PIC has been amazing and this team of committed colleagues has been phenomenal because the focus is always on the safety and well-being of the patient and family. I decided it was a story worth telling.

REFERENCES

American Association of Retired Persons (AARP). (2007). *Leading a multigenerational workforce*. (2007). [Pamphlet]. Retrieved from http://assets.aarp.org/www.aarp.org_/articles/money/employers/leading_multigenerational_workforce.pdf

Benner, P. (1984). *From novice to expert: Excellence and power in clinical nursing practice*. Menlo Park, CA: Addison-Wesley.

Berwick, D. M., & Leape, L. L. (2005). Five years after *To err is human*: What have we learned? *Journal of the American Medical Association, 19*, 2384–2390.

Hamric, A., Spross, J. A., & Hanson, C. M. (2005). *Advanced practice nursing: An integrative approach* (3rd ed.). St. Louis, MO: Elsevier Saunders.

Institute of Medicine. (1999). *To err is human: Building a safer health system*. Washington, DC: National Academies Press.

National Academies. (2000). *Roles of the committee chair*. Retrieved from http://www7.nationalacademies.org/committees_chair_roles/Roles_PDF.pdf

Porter-O'Grady, T. (1999). Quantum leadership: New roles for a new age. *Journal of Nursing Administration, 29*(10), 37–42.

Sherman, R. (2006, May 31). Leading a multigenerational nursing workforce: Issues, challenges and strategies. *OJIN: The Online Journal of Issues in Nursing, 11*(2), Manuscript 2. Retrieved from http://www.nursingworld.org/MainMenuCategories/ANAMarketplace/ANAPeriodicals/OJIN/TableofContents/Volume112006/No2May06/tpc30_216074.aspx

Sullivan, E. J., & Decker, P. J. (2009). *Effective leadership and management in nursing* (5th ed.). Upper Saddle River, NJ: Prentice-Hall.

Changing and Enhancing Nurses' Roles

19.1 *Transitioning New Nurses Into Acute Care Practice: Our Journey of Program Redesign*

Ellen Bergeron, Dorothy Bradley, Diane M. Campbell,
Miriam Greenspan, Carol J. Luppi,
Mary Pennington, and Laura Mylott

Nurses entering acute care settings are challenged to quickly achieve competency in a broad set of skills and knowledge. In addition to mastering a multitude of clinical technologies and therapeutics, they must acquire and refine clinical judgment and critical thinking skills and learn to communicate and collaborate as a member of an interdisciplinary care team. Newly licensed nurses (NLNs) face a particularly steep learning curve. Reported turnover rates as high as 29.5% (Halfer, 2007) validate that the first year of practice for a new graduate nurse can be a time of great stress and vulnerability. Mentored transition programs that provide opportunities for experiential learning and ongoing guidance and support can greatly facilitate the transition into practice settings for new graduates and experienced nurses alike. Evidence suggests that such programs are associated with higher levels of satisfaction and promote retention among newly hired nurses as well as unit-based clinical staff (Beecroft & Kunzman, 2001; Halfer, 2007; Schloessler & Waldo, 2006b).

The Center for Nursing Excellence (CNE) provides three programs that facilitate the entry of professional nurses into clinical settings. One of the programs is designed to meet the unique needs of NLNs, another supports the entry of newly hired experienced nurses into general units, and the third supports Brigham and Women's Hospital's (BWH) clinical nurses entering critical care practice. Because all of the programs partner new nurses with experienced preceptors, the CNE also provides a special program designed to help nurses who serve as preceptors develop critical teaching and coaching skills.

In this chapter, we discuss guidelines that inform the design of these important programs and describe how we redesigned each program to incorporate innovative, evidence-based teaching strategies that promote clinical practice development, socialization into professional practice, and integration into the broader organization. Collectively, we believe that the programs illustrate how CNE nurse educators support clinical nurses in developing safe, evidence-based, compassionate practice. Although this is only one way in which the CNE advances the vision and mission of the Department of Nursing (DON), it is one that touches on all the dimensions of the vision statement: *"Excellent care to patients and families, with the best staff, in the safest environment."*

BACKGROUND

As described in Chapter 6, supporting the successful transition of experienced and NLNs into practice is one of the CNE's primary goals. Soon after we created the CNE in 2006, we began evaluating transition programs supported by the DON. In reviewing the content, methods, and structure of each program, we found that the transition programs offered important opportunities for contextually based, peer-supported learning and acculturation, and were valued by participants, clinicians, and leaders on the units. We also learned from this review that we could strengthen our existing transition programs by introducing new teaching methodologies and enhancing the preceptor component. Additionally, we realized we needed to restructure the programs to minimize delays in transitioning nurses to their hiring units and to better accommodate the increasing number of nurses that were being hired to support an ongoing expansion in the hospital's clinical services.

We restructured each of the transition programs over the next 2 years. In our work to redesign the programs, we adhered to the following guidelines:

1. Partner with clinical leaders. Unit directors, educators, and clinical staff have a unique appreciation for the challenges nurses face when transitioning to a new practice area, and for the types of support needed to ensure a nurse's success. When redesigning each transition program, we worked closely with leaders and staff in the clinical areas. Together, we defined skills nurses need to acquire before working in practice settings and developed strategies for moving nurses quickly to their hiring units. Through our collaborative efforts, we also created a climate of partnership that promoted the development of supportive relationships among newly hired nurses, preceptors, and other staff. Such relationships are critical for successful transitions (Bridges, 2003; Ponte, Kruger, & DeMarco, 2004; Reising, 2002; Thomka, 2001).

2. Build on theoretical and conceptual principles. Researchers have observed that clinical practice development among nurses occurs through the incremental acquisition of situational and experience-based knowledge that builds on theory and occurs within a social context (Benner, 1984; Benner, Sutphen, Leonard, & Day, 2010). Nurses refine their clinical and caring knowledge and self-understanding as nurses through clinical experiences and in relationships with patients and colleagues. Building on existing knowledge and creating a relevant context for the learner further enhances the learning process (Knowles, 1980).

In redesigning the transition programs, we therefore emphasized experiential learning opportunities, including simulation-based experiences, reflection, skills laboratories, and provision of care under the guidance of a preceptor.

We wanted these to permeate the transition programs to ensure that our nurses would develop the technical skills and clinical judgment required for safe patient care. The experiential learning strategies also gave our CNE staff, preceptors, and nurse leaders opportunities to guide new nurses through predictable and seminal clinical situations that can affect a nurse's transition journey and acculturation to the unit. By supporting and guiding nurses through experiences such as the death of a patient or a medication error, preceptors and nurse leaders help ease the stress associated with the transition process (Schloessler & Waldo, 2006a, 2006b).

3. Use simulation to facilitate active learning.   Nurses have long used simulation-based education (SBE) to facilitate learning. In the past, methods were limited to conventional SBE, which typically involved the use of actors or role-playing and static manikins. Today, moderate- and high-fidelity human patient simulators or manikins are available that can be programmed to simulate a wide range of situations and illnesses (Seropian, Brown, Gavilanes, & Driggers, 2004). SBE allows educators to provide a standardized, reproducible, evidence-based learning experience that promotes rapid skill acquisition and facilitates the development of critical thinking and clinical judgment. SBE offers learners numerous advantages, as it allows them to engage in active learning in a realistic work environment without the threat of patient harm. Nurses can also practice important interpersonal skills, including communication and delegation techniques, through SBE (Chickering & Gamson, 1987; Eaves & Flagg, 2001; Jeffries, 2005; Larew, Lessans, Spunt, Foster, & Covington, 2006; Morey et al., 2002).

We incorporated role-playing and high-fidelity simulation into all of the transition programs. We begin sessions involving the high-fidelity human patient simulator with a preparatory briefing session, in which we assign each participant a role and share information about participating in the scenario. The briefing session is followed by the simulated clinical scenario, in which we offer multiple opportunities for experiential learning. At the end of the scenario, we conduct a facilitated debriefing session, which encourages individual reflection and group knowledge construction; this is where much of the learning occurs (Franz, & Breit, 2005; Jeffries, 2005; Kolb, 1984; Larew et al., 2006; Schön, 1987; Tennant & Pogson, 1995; Wiske, Franz, & Breit, 2005).

4. Support learning and socialization on the hiring unit.   In our previous transition programs, newly hired nurses spent time on a designated orientation unit where they learned about hospital systems and equipment while providing patient care under the guidance of a faculty educator and a "co-assigned" senior staff nurse. Afterward, the new nurses moved to their hiring units, where they were paired with preceptors for the remainder of their orientation. Having nurses spend time on a designated orientation unit presented a number of challenges. As the volume of new nurses increased, there was often not enough technology available on the orientation unit to support individual learning. The number of senior staff available for co-assignment was also limited. Additionally, equipment and technology used on the orientation unit were often different from those used on the hiring units, requiring nurses to "re-learn" technology once they began working with their preceptors. Delaying the nurses' transition to their unit of hire also negatively affected the socialization and acculturation process.

In the redesigned transition programs, we eliminated time on the orientation unit. Nurses now move directly from central orientation classes in the CNE to their hiring units and learn what they need to know through SBE and a dedicated preceptorship on the unit of hire. This new approach avoids the need for re-learning BWH systems and practices and facilitates the socialization and acculturation that is key to a successful transition experience.

5. *Promote strong preceptor–nurse partnerships.*   We designed each of our transition programs to recognize and support the preceptor–nurse dyad as the central learning relationship. The social support provided by preceptors is essential to the progression of learning and the development of a professional nursing identity (Benner, 1984). By working alongside nurses and offering coaching and guidance, preceptors help new nurses recognize patterns and discern shades of meaning and qualitative distinctions within clinical situations, thus facilitating the development of clinical judgment. BWH has long maintained an introductory training program for preceptors. In examining our data on this program, however, we discovered that less than a quarter of nurse preceptors had attended. Additionally, the curriculum had not been evaluated or substantially revised in years, and there was little coordination among the ad hoc program faculty. Given the importance of the preceptor role, we made improvement of the introductory training program for preceptors a priority for the CNE. In 2007, the CNE introduced a new program, "Building the Practice of Precepting," that helps new and experienced preceptors acquire and enhance skills that are required to guide new nurses and facilitate a safe transition to practice.

Having established our guidelines for the kind of programs we intended to create, we embarked on a change process with the goal of enhancing outcomes for all participants and making our expression of the department's vision a reality. In the following sections, we describe how we used these guidelines to redesign our transition programs for newly licensed and experienced nurses entering practice at BWH and for BWH nurses entering critical care. We also provide additional details about the program we created for nurses assuming the preceptor role.

NEWLY LICENSED NURSE PROGRAM

The DON first developed a special transition program for NLNs in 2001. Called the NLN Faculty Model, the program began with a week of central orientation in which new nurses were introduced to the organization, nursing culture, and key policies and expectations. After central orientation, the nurses were divided into smaller groups and spent 2–4 weeks on specially designated orientation units prior to transitioning to their units of hire.

The NLN Faculty Model was effective in improving the satisfaction, confidence, and retention of NLNs and eased the burden of nurse preceptors (Griffin, Hanley, & Saniuk, 2002). As noted earlier, however, the program was unable to keep up with the hospital's expanding clinical services and increasing volume of new hires, and encountered difficulty in exposing new nurses to technologies and systems unique to their hiring units. Additionally, NLNs reported that the time spent on the orientation units felt "like being in school" and negatively affected their transition to independent practice. Transitioning to their units of hire, where they developed a relationship with a second role model or preceptor, felt like "starting over." Given these challenges, we made redesigning the NLN Faculty Model a top priority.

Program Design

To begin the redesign work, we convened a work group composed of nurse specialists and educators from the CNE, and nurse directors, educators, and clinical nurses from units that had previously hired large numbers of new graduates. The work group was charged with evaluating the NLN Faculty Model in light of current best practices and findings from the literature and developing recommendations for program improvements.

Through its literature review, the work group identified key themes or factors that contribute to the successful transition of new graduates. These include socializing new nurses to the unit and creating a welcoming environment; facilitating a close and supportive relationship with a preceptor; creating an environment that supports teaching and learning; progressively and purposefully advancing assignments in a manner that allows new nurses time to reflect on their developing practice; and providing timely, respectful, and specific feedback (Casey & Fink, 2004; Schloessler & Waldo, 2006a; Tradewell, 1996). The work group then conducted on-unit interviews with senior clinical nurses and focus groups with new nurses to identify how well these themes were incorporated into the NLN Faculty Model and the orientation experience. Feedback suggested that although the NLN Faculty Model incorporated each theme, integration of the themes occurred informally and was highly variable. The work group recommended that the themes be embedded more explicitly in a redesigned program. This recommendation formed the basis for the creation of the unit-based NLN Program.

In creating this new program, we retained elements of the NLN Faculty Model, but also introduced changes to ensure a more immediate transition to the unit of hire and to help new nurses transition to independent practice. Key features of this unit-based NLN Program include:

- *Simulation-based introduction to hospital systems:* Following 1 week of central orientation, NLNs participate in a 1-day simulation experience that introduces them to the hospital's computer systems and equipment used in the clinical setting.
- *Learning systems and routines:* NLNs transition to the hiring unit immediately after central orientation. Upon arrival on the unit, the nurses are partnered with preceptors. The new nurse's first 2 weeks on the unit are designated as a "primer" period. During this time, the nurse and preceptor share a patient assignment. This provides time, space, and opportunities for the new nurse to learn hospital systems and unit routines. The hospital's computerized systems, medication administration and documentation systems, and routines specific to the unit's patient population are learned naturally and in "real time" while the nurse gains experience caring for patients and working alongside other

members of the health care team. Research suggests that introducing systems within the context of the patient experience facilitates learning and helps the new graduate begin to think like a nurse (Tanner, 2006).

■ *Ongoing guidance by the preceptor and unit leadership:*   Following the 2 "primer" weeks, the new nurse continues orientation in partnership with one to two primary preceptors for the next 7–9 weeks. The length of the orientation varies depending upon the nurse's progress toward meeting specific unit-based clinical and learning goals. The preceptors provide support and guidance, helping the new nurses achieve competency in required skills and supporting their introduction and socialization to the unit and unit colleagues. The number of patients and the complexity of the patient care assignment are gradually advanced to promote learning and organization. The preceptor, with guidance from the NLN Program coordinator, the nurse director, and unit-based educator, monitors the continuity and complexity of the assignments with the goal of facilitating the new nurse's skill development and role transition.

Program Implementation and Evaluation

We piloted the NLN Program on an intermediate care unit and on several oncology units that were experiencing an influx of new staff due to an expansion of the oncology service. In preparation for the pilot, managers, educators, and preceptors on the pilot units worked with the CNE program director to learn about the NLN Program and develop resources for NLN preceptors. These included a manual describing the process of professional development, topics covered in central orientation, and suggestions for supporting new nurses during their transition experience.

Throughout the 6-month pilot period, we maintained the original Faculty Model to support new graduate nurses hired on other units. Part of our evaluation of the new NLN Program involved comparing retention rates associated with the two programs after 1 year. We also asked nurses from each program to complete a survey after their first 2 weeks of orientation on their hiring unit. Through the survey, we assessed new nurses' confidence in managing hospital systems. Our evaluation results indicated that both programs were associated with a 1-year retention rate of 90%. We also found no difference in the confidence level of nurses. Given these results, and a reassurance that our new model equaled the prior in outcomes, we decided to expand the new NLN Program, because it allowed us to accommodate an increasing number of new nurses and streamlined nurses' transition to the unit of hire.

In January 2009, we extended the NLN Program to all nurses entering intermediate care and oncology. As part of our continued evaluation, we asked 60 nurses to complete a survey rating their overall satisfaction with their unit-based orientation and providing feedback on how well the NLN Program facilitated socialization, preceptor relationships, learning in a professional practice environment, and effective feedback. Thirty-three nurses (55%) completed the survey. Among the respondents, 87% indicated that they were highly satisfied or satisfied with their orientation and the resources available during their transition to practice; 91% indicated that they were confident they could independently provide safe, competent care to their patients. Respondents also gave favorable ratings to the way in which the NLN Program facilitated socialization, precep-tor relationships, and learning. Retention rates associated with the NLN Program also remained high, with analyses indicating an 18-month retention rate of 94%, a modest increase from our prior results.

Additional Supports for New Graduate Nurses

The stress of transition and the transition experience for NLNs does not end with the conclusion of formal orientation. Rather, it continues for the next 12–18 months as the nurse moves from the advanced beginner to the competent stage of development (Benner, 1984). The CNE offers a variety of programs to support NLNs throughout this transition period and facilitate their ongoing learning and profes-sional development. Several of these programs were developed in conjunction with the original Faculty Model. We introduced others more recently in response to sug-gestions from new nurses and to supplement the unit-based NLN Program. The offerings include:

- *Monthly discussion sessions:*   These monthly, 4-hour sessions offer new nurses an opportunity to discuss their transition experiences. We use appreciative inquiry, which emphasizes building on good experiences, as a context for discussion, and use presentations, case studies, and narratives to encourage reflection and sharing.
- *Novice Simulation Day:*   In this simulation-based program, new nurses practice communicating with physicians and other members of the health care team while acquiring knowledge and practicing skills needed for bedside emergencies. We developed the program in response to a survey in which new nurses identified communicating with physicians, and uncertainty in their ability to recognize and respond to changes in their patient's condition, as particular sources of stress. Nurses are encouraged to attend this program after practicing independently for 3–6 months.
- *Novice Class Day:*   This program supports new nurses in examining pain management practices, end-of-life decision making, and ethical issues encoun-tered in practice. Although the knowledge presented is not "new," nurses' lived practice experience gives it more meaning.
- *Leadership and Case Study Day:*   This session brings new nurses together after 9 months of practice to share clinical stories about situations that have been clinically or personally challenging. Nurse educators from the CNE use a vari-ety of exercises and strategies to help nurses identify their individual manage-ment and leadership styles and acquire conflict resolution skills.

FACILITATING THE TRANSITION TO PRACTICE FOR EXPERIENCED NURSES: THE SIMULATION-BASED ORIENTATION PROGRAM

In 2008, we introduced the Simulation-Based Orientation Program (SBOP) to help newly hired experienced nurses transition to independent practice on their hir-ing units. Nurses participate in SBOP after completing our centralized classroom orientation session and before they transition to a preceptorship on their unit of hire.

SBOP replaced an older "bridge" program, called the Faculty-Based Program (Griffin et al., 2002), which involved a 4-day clinical experience on an orientation unit, where newly hired experienced nurses learned about BWH policies, practices, and technologies while providing patient care under the guidance of a faculty educator and a co-assigned staff nurse. At the end of the 4 days, the faculty coordinator completed an individualized evaluation and action plan for each nurse, sharing it with the nurse and his or her nurse leader; the newly hired nurses then proceeded to their hiring units to complete orientation. Although we knew the Faculty-Based Program was useful in introducing nurses to aspects of BWH nursing practice, a variety of structural limitations hampered its effectiveness. Patient populations, clinical technologies, and systems encountered on the orientation unit were often different from those on the hiring units, limiting the usefulness of the bridge experience. Additionally, newly hired nurses participating in the program often worked with several different co-assigned staff nurses, resulting in a lack of continuity. Nurses in the co-assigned role also experienced a lack of support and training. These factors, combined with our acquisition of a high-fidelity human patient simulator, led us to develop SBOP as a new bridge program.

Simulation-Based Orientation Program Design

Nurse educators in the CNE developed SBOP in collaboration with nurse directors, nurse educators, and preceptors from the clinical units. The goals of SBOP are consistent with those of the Faculty-Based Program, and include introducing newly hired nurses to the health care culture and nursing work flow at BWH; facilitating the integration of universal safety systems and technology into nursing practice; and providing new nurses with an opportunity to practice and apply what they learn during centralized orientation. An additional goal that distinguishes SBOP from the Faculty-Based bridge program involves ensuring a timely and efficient transition to the unit of hire. This goal is achieved by using a simulation-based approach to learning that capitalizes on SBE's effectiveness in helping nurses rapidly acquire new skills and enhance their critical thinking abilities.

SBOP is conducted over 2 days. On day 1, nurses participate in three simulation scenarios that build on content presented in the centralized orientation program, and are designed to help newly hired nurses learn to use BWH clinical systems and technologies and integrate them into safe patient care. On day 2, nurses participate in two additional scenarios. These emphasize emergency preparedness (i.e., Code Blue and Rapid Response) and practices promoting a safe work environment (i.e., SBAR (Situation-Background-Assessment-Recommendation), handoff reporting, closed-loop communication, and mutual respect). In each simulation scenario, nurses interact with a computerized, human patient simulator in a mock patient room. The scenarios proceed in three phases. Phase 1 involves a briefing period, in which participants are given information about the simulated case. Phase 2 involves a 15- to 20-minute simulation, in which participants respond to a defined situation and to programmed physiologic changes manifested by the manikin. The last phase, phase 3, involves a 15- to 30-minute facilitated debriefing session. The debriefing session is widely acknowledged as the most beneficial phase, as it allows participants to engage in collaborative, reflective dialogue through which they harness the collective wisdom of the group and integrate their new knowledge (Gordon, Wilkerson,

Shaffer, & Armstrong, 2001; Henneman & Cunningham, 2005; Holcomb et al., 2002; Jeffries, 2005; Seropian et al., 2004).

After the 2-day program, nurses transition to their units of hire. The SBOP program coordinator facilitates the transition by remaining available to preceptors and newly hired nurses and serving as an additional source of consultation and guidance.

Factors Contributing to SBOP's Success

Nurse educators in the CNE routinely obtain formal and informal feedback from SBOP participants and clinical stakeholders and use it to refine and improve program elements. SBOP faculty also modify the program as needed to reflect changes in nursing practice and the clinical settings. Feedback obtained from participants consistently indicates that SBOP provides nurses with a unique and essential opportunity for synthesizing the vast amount of information presented in the core orientation. Participants report that SBOP sessions increase their confidence and understanding of BWH nursing practice and facilitate their transition to the hiring units. We believe a variety of practices have contributed to the program's success. These include:

- *Faculty training.* Before SBOP was piloted, all faculty members attended a 3-day simulation faculty development course that reviewed debriefing techniques and modeled ideal simulation-based education. The course helped the SBOP faculty appreciate the importance of the debriefing sessions and how they provide a unique opportunity for reflective, collaborative discussion. Faculty members continue to build on the skills they acquired through the faculty development program by reviewing the simulation literature and networking with other nurse educators involved in simulation-based instruction.
- *Participant preparation.* Although learners adjust to SBE quickly, SBE is a different kind of learning and requires a different level of engagement and participation. To ease the simulation lab learning curve, we ask program participants to complete an online introductory course prior to attending SBOP. The online course introduces nurses to the principles of simulation, capabilities of the manikin and lab environment, and program-specific objectives. We reinforce this material during a brief classroom introduction and also give participants a tour of the simulation lab immediately before the first simulation scenario. We have found this helps learners focus on the clinical learning activities, rather than the simulation equipment and setting.
- *Role clarification.* Initially, many SBOP participants reported some confusion about the role they were expected to play in a simulation scenario. To resolve this, we clarified role definitions and expectations for functioning in the simulation lab. We also began introducing nurses to the simulated patient in the context of their role and encouraged them to ask questions whenever they were confused. Because most nurses want to play an active role in a simulation scenario, we also maximized opportunities for participation. For example, we choreographed multiple variations of an "active observation" role, in which participants perform designated tasks related to the activities in the simulation while also observing the central action. Our goal in making each

of these changes was to maximize experiential learning and promote shared reflection during the debriefing sessions.

■ *Tailoring to group needs.*   Our philosophy is that SBOP provides a unique and valuable foundation for each newly hired nurse's entry into practice at BWH. We have therefore accommodated groups as small as one participant and as large as 16. During our pilot program, we invited nurses in the NLN Program to join a small group of newly hired experienced nurses. However, we found that separate sessions are more effective, as they allow us to better individualize classroom content and tailor simulation scenarios to match each group's learning needs.

Nurses participating in simulation-based learning are its greatest advocates, as illustrated by the following comment from an SBOP participant: "I thought that the simulation lab really put together every piece that we learned last week. Working with eMAR/Alaris/and patient care together in a critical situation helped me feel more at ease when I got on the floor. I also liked the group work and feedback." Nurses' enthusiasm for simulation-based training led us to change other aspects of orientation and introduce more opportunities for experiential learning. For example, we added an active learning element to our documentation instruction, began to actively involve participants in our session on smart infusion pumps, and developed learning labs for a variety of other skills.

CRITICAL CARE NURSE INTERN PROGRAM

Over the years, BWH, like other hospitals, has experienced an increase in patient acuity. This has led us to expand our critical care units, and to change our critical care hiring practices: from hiring only nurses with critical care experience to also hiring BWH nurses with a medical–surgical background. This change in hiring practices prompted us to evaluate our critical care orientation program to ensure that it met the learning needs of medical–surgical nurses, and that it was consistent with our guidelines for transition programs and with our commitment to advancing the DON vision and goals.

A work team consisting of the critical care nurse program director in the CNE, critical care nurse leaders and educators, and clinical nurses from each critical care unit led the effort to evaluate the existing critical care orientation program and develop a new program suitable for medical–surgical nurses. The work team realized that bringing medical–surgical nurses on staff was a cultural and paradigm shift for the critical care areas, and multiple changes were needed to ensure the nurses' successful transition to critical care practice. After reviewing the existing orientation program, the team identified two key areas that had to be addressed: First, the orientation content had to be expanded and enhanced by experiential teaching strategies; second, the preceptor role had to be strengthened, as preceptors would now be challenged to guide and support nurses with a very different set of learning needs. Additionally, the work team recognized that they needed to engage all members of the critical care units in creating a welcoming environment and supporting the new nurses' learning and socialization.

Developing the Program

As a first step, the work team reviewed the literature to identify best practices and recommendations for ensuring a successful transition to practice. Building on their findings, they developed the Critical Care Nurse Intern Program (CCIP), which includes a classroom component and a 10-week preceptorship. This orientation program for nurses new to critical care is based on a robust educational foundation that incorporates experiential, reflective, and transformative learning theories (Mezirow, 2000; Brookfield, 1993). The program is limited to four to eight nurses at one time, which allows the instructors to assess each nurse's learning needs and tailor their instruction accordingly.

The CCIP curriculum is consistent with standards and guidelines developed by the American Association of Critical Care Nurses (2008). The program curriculum covers key physiologic processes and interventions, using a blended approach that combines didactic presentations with clinical experiences (Morris et al., 2007). Hands-on experiences are incorporated into each lecture or session. For example, one session, "Caring for a Patient on Mechanical Ventilation," begins with a low-fidelity simulation of a patient requiring emergent intubation. A staff nurse from the surgical intensive care unit (SICU), who is an experienced instructor in Advanced Cardiac Life Support, presents this segment. In addition to presenting didactic content, the SICU nurse teaches, preps, coaches, and mentors the nurse interns through the simulated patient crisis. Through the simulation, the nurse interns gain exposure to managing an unstable airway, assisting with intubation, and engaging with a patient in crisis. After the simulation, they attend patient ventilator rounds conducted by expert nurses in the ICU. At the end of the day, the instructor facilitates a discussion session in which the nurse interns reflect on what they learned. This approach, which is used for other topics as well, breathes life into the simulated experience of a critical care patient.

Expert critical care nurses serve as faculty throughout the program. This is a deliberate strategy that fosters leadership among clinical staff and promotes multiple levels of learning among new nurses. It also helps clinical staff connect with the new nurses and feel accountable for their learning and success. In their presentations, the clinical nurses present specific content and also introduce new nurses to the culture of ICU practice, facilitating their socialization. They also give new nurses a vision of advanced ICU clinical practice and of nurses as clinical leaders.

The CCIP Preceptorship

The 10-week preceptorship is an essential part of the CCIP and critical to a successful transition experience. To prepare preceptors for their role, the work team conducted a special, 4-hour preceptor retreat. The CNE's program director for critical care reviewed teaching methodologies and facilitated discussion among the preceptors by having them write narratives describing situations with orientees that went well or in which a breakdown in communication occurred. By sharing their experiences, the preceptors gained insight into their role. They also learned the value of using reflection as a teaching tool and gained exposure to multiple perspectives on what "competent/expert precepting" looks like. Based on the retreat's success, we began offering it annually as a way of helping preceptors keep their skills finely honed. We also created preceptor teams to facilitate dialogue and sharing among preceptors. Over time, these have become an important source of ongoing support.

As the medical–surgical nurses began working with their preceptors and transitioned to independent practice, they experienced a groundswell of support from clinical nurses, nurse leaders, and other staff in the critical care areas. This support was critical to making the new nurses feel welcome and helping them become socialized to the unit culture. The support of clinical nurses was especially important. We believe that having clinical nurses help create the CCIP and serve as teachers and preceptors helped them appreciate the stresses new nurses face, and strengthened their commitment to ensuring the medical–surgical nurses' successful transition to practice. Through their involvement, clinical nurses also discovered the important role they play in helping the DON vision become a reality.

BUILDING THE PRACTICE OF PRECEPTING

Preceptors and the preceptorship are critical components of each transition program. In addition to helping new nurses gain technical and clinical competence, preceptors facilitate their socialization to the organization, unit of hire, and their nursing profession. As noted earlier, the DON offered an introductory preceptor training program. In evaluating this program, we found that many preceptors did not attend it, the curriculum had not been updated in years, and there was little coordination among faculty. Given the importance of preceptorship, we resolved to create a new program focused on helping nurses gain an understanding of the preceptor role and advancing their precepting skills.

The CNE's program director for precepting practice development led the program redesign effort with the help of several different task forces. As a first step, the program director convened a task force consisting of preceptors, educators, and managers from various practice areas, asking them to describe the goals of a preceptored clinical experience and review the literature to identify best preceptor practices. The group established that precepting is a practice, not a project, and requires education, judgment, skill, and experience. Goals of the preceptor–orientee relationship include supporting the orientee in achieving clinical practice competency, acquiring familiarity with the specific work environment, and becoming socialized into the unit culture and as a member of the health care team. The group identified research by Benner (1984), del Bueno and Beay (1995), and Woodring (2004) as providing the best evidence for precepting practices. The work of this task force provided a foundation for the next steps in redesigning the introductory preceptor program.

The program director next conducted focus groups of preceptors and educators to obtain their input and recommendations for the content and structure of the new program. A key recommendation emerging from the focus groups was to replace the ad hoc preceptor program faculty with a committed and dedicated preceptor faculty team composed of individuals selected for their knowledge, experience, diversity, and commitment to preceptor practice development. Based on this recommendation, the program director identified a faculty group to define the program curriculum. The team met frequently over 6 months, deepening their expertise and knowledge of preceptor needs and creating a curriculum that used innovative and interactive teaching strategies to meet the needs of new and experienced preceptors.

Our new program, "Building the Practice of Precepting," was offered for the first time as a pilot. Program participants gave the pilot high marks and encouraged their colleagues to attend; enrollment soon exceeded capacity. With the demand for preceptor education established, the CNE began offering the program on a regular basis.

Program Description

Coaching and facilitation are the essence of precepting, and are the primary focus of the "Building the Practice of Precepting" program. One of our primary goals is to instill confidence in preceptors, help them "own" their practice of precepting, and learn to empower orientees to own their practice of nursing. We find that as the preceptors begin to understand their roles as mentor, coach, and role model, they are released from the myth that they "need to know everything" and begin viewing the preceptorship as a dynamic, mutually respectful, and trusting relationship in which both parties are active participants and learn and grow throughout the experience.

At the start of the program, participants create a list of their own learning needs. This models the concept of self-directed learning and highlights the importance of creating a teacher–learner partnership. We repeat, model, and discuss the theme of self-directed learning throughout the day and again at the end, when participants provide verbal feedback about program content and strategies they found beneficial.

We use a variety of teaching methods, including discussion, small-group work, role-playing, and narrative and video reviews to promote learning. The faculty work to create an environment of respect and safety so that participants are comfortable sharing experiences. Specific topics addressed through the program include:

- Enhancing compatibility in the orientee–preceptor dyad
- Generational differences in learning and communicating
- How nurses learn and develop their clinical practice, and using these concepts to inform goal-setting and teaching
- Communication, feedback, and conflict resolution skills
- Strategies for teaching critical thinking at the bedside
- Managing work flow
- Facilitating socialization and the integration of new nurses into the unit culture and health care team
- Strategies for self-renewal, respite, and re-energizing

In addressing each topic, the program faculty begin by asking participants to share their precepting experiences. They then weave these experiences into the session and use them to provide context and promote a deeper understanding of preceptor practice. As the discussions unfold, participants begin to recognize and appreciate the knowledge and experience they already possess and the diversity of practice and precepting concerns represented by the group. Throughout the day, faculty emphasize the importance of preceptors and their practice to the overall practice of nursing at BWH. They also laud preceptors for their courage in opening their practice to scrutiny during the preceptorship experience. Since its introduction, "Building the Practice of Precepting" has become a critical part of our transition program strategy.

SUMMARY

All nurses at BWH share the responsibility of ensuring the successful transition of new nurses into practice. Through the transition programs described here, CNE staff and nurse directors, educators, and clinical nurses on the units partner to support new nurses, helping them achieve competency and become socialized to their roles as members of the health care team and acculturated to the organization. In addition to facilitating the successful transition of new nurses, the programs have helped foster a renewed commitment to creating a welcoming and supportive environment for nurses—one that promotes leadership, continued learning, and ongoing professional development. In this way, the CNE is able to meet its mission and commitments and advance the vision of the DON: *"Excellent care to patients and families, with the best staff, in the safest environment."*

REFERENCES

American Association of Critical Care Nurses. (2008). *Scope and standards of care for acute and critical care nurses.* Aliso Viejo, CA. Retrieved January 17, 2011, from http://www.aacn.org/WD/Practice/Docs/130300-Standards_for_Acute_and _ Critical_Care_Nursing.pdf

Beecroft, P., & Kunzman, L. (2001). RN internship: Outcomes of a one-year pilot program. *Journal of Nursing Administration, 31,* 575–582.

Benner, P. (1984). *From novice to expert: Excellence and power in clinical nursing practice.* Menlo Park, CA: Addison-Wesley.

Benner, P., Sutphen, M., Leonard, V., & Day, L. (2010). *Educating nurses: A call for radical transformation.* San Francisco, CA: Jossey-Bass.

Bridges, W. (2003). *Managing transitions* (2nd ed.). Cambridge, MA: Perseus Books Group.

Brookfield, S. (1993). On impostership, cultural suicide, and other dangers: How nurses learn critical thinking. *Journal of Continuing Education in Nursing, 24,* 197–205.

Casey, K., & Fink, R. (2004). The graduate nurse experience. *Journal of Nursing Administration, 34*(6), 303–311.

Chickering, A., & Gamson, Z. (1987, March). Seven principles of good practice in undergraduate education. *AAHE Bulletin,* 1–10.

del Bueno, D., & Beay, P. (1995). Evaluation of preceptor competency and cost in acute care hospitals. *Journal of Nursing Staff Development, 11,* 108–111.

Eaves, R. H., & Flagg, A. J. (2001). The U.S. Air Force pilot simulated medical unit: A teaching strategy with multiple applications. *Journal of Nursing Education, 40*(3), 110–115.

Gordon, J. A., Wilkerson, W. M., Shaffer, D. W., & Armstrong, E. G. (2001). "Practicing" medicine without risk: Students' and educators' responses to high-fidelity patient simulation. *Academic Medicine, 76,* 469–472.

Griffin, M., Hanley, D., & Saniuk, C. (2002). Lightening the burden for preceptors: Consider adding a "Faculty Model" week to orientation. *Journal for Nurses in Staff Development, 18,* 322–326.

Halfer, D. (2007). A magnetic strategy for new graduate nurses. *Nursing Economics, 25*(1), 6–11.

Henneman, E. A., & Cunningham, H. (2005). Using clinical simulation to teach patient safety in an acute/critical care nursing course. *Nurse Educator, 30*(4), 172–177.

Holcomb, J. B., Dumire, R. D., Crommett, J. W., Stamateris, C. E., Fagert, M. A., Cleveland, J. A., ... Mattox, K. L. (2002). Evaluation of trauma team performance using an advanced human patient simulator for resuscitation training. *Journal of Trauma, Injury, Infection, & Critical Care, 52,* 1078–1086.

Jeffries, P. R. (2005). A framework for designing, implementing, and evaluating: Simulations used as teaching strategies in nursing. *Nursing Education Perspectives, 26*(2), 96–103.

Knowles, M. S. (1980). *The modern practice of adult education.* Englewood Cliffs, NJ: Prentice-Hall/Cambridge.

Kolb, D. A. (1984). *Experiential learning: Experience as the source of learning and development.* Englewood Cliffs, NJ: Prentice-Hall.

Larew, C., Lessans, S., Spunt, D., Foster, D., & Covington, B. G. (2006). Innovations in clinical simulation: Application of Benner's theory in an interactive patient care simulation. *Nursing Education Perspectives, 27*(1), 16–21.

Mezirow, J. (2000). *Learning as transformation: Critical perspectives on a theory in progress.* San Francisco, CA: Jossey-Bass.

Morey, J. C., Simon, R., Jay, G. D., Wears, R. L., Salisbury, M., Dukes, K. A., & Berns, S. D. (2002). Error reduction and performance improvement in the emergency department through formal teamwork training: Evaluation results of the MedTeams project. *Health Services Research, 37*(6), 1553–1581.

Morris, L., Pfeifer, P., Catalano, R., Fortney, R., Hilton, E., McLaughlin, J., . . . Goldstein, L. (2007). Designing a comprehensive model for critical care orientation. *Critical Care Nurse, 27*(6), 37–60.

Ponte, P., Kruger, N., & DeMarco, R. (2004). Reshaping the practice environment. *Journal of Nursing Administration, 34*(4), 173–179.

Reising, D. (2002). Early socialization of critical care nurses. *American Journal of Critical Care, 11*(1), 19–26.

Schloessler, M., & Waldo, M. (2006a). The first eighteen months in practice. *Journal for Nurses in Staff Development, 22*(2), 47–52.

Schloessler, M., & Waldo, M. (2006b). Organizational infrastructure to support development of newly graduated nurses. *Journal for Nurses in Staff Development, 22*(6), 286–293.

Schön, D. A. (1987). *Educating the reflective practitioner: Toward a new design for teaching and learning in the professions.* San Francisco, CA: Jossey-Bass.

Seropian, M. A., Brown, K., Gavilanes, J. S., & Driggers, B. (2004). Simulation: Not just a manikin. *Journal of Nursing Education, 43*(4), 164–169.

Tanner, C. A. (2006). Thinking like a nurse: A research-based model of clinical judgment. *Journal of Nursing Education, 45*(12), 204–211.

Tennant, M., & Pogson, P. (1995). *Learning and change in the adult years: A developmental perspective.* San Francisco, CA: Jossey-Bass.

Thomka, L. (2001). Graduate nurses' experiences of interactions with professional nursing staff during transition to the professional role. *Journal of Continuing Education in Nursing, 32*(1), 15–19.

Tradewell, G. (1996). Rites of passage: Adaptation of nursing graduates to a hospital setting. *Journal of Nursing Staff Development, 12*(4), 183–189.

Wiske, M. S., Franz, K. R., & Breit, L. (2005). *Teaching for understanding with technology.* San Francisco, CA: Jossey-Bass.

Woodring, B. C. (2004). Clinical nurse leaders: New roles, new responsibilities, new preparation. *Journal for Specialists in Pediatric Nursing, 9*(4), 129–134.

19.2 *A Collaborative Teamwork Approach to Unit-Based Nursing Orientation*

Christine Smith

*I*n thinking about a change story I wanted to include in this book, I immediately wanted to share with everyone the enormous amount of energy and work that goes into orienting new staff members. More importantly, I wanted to emphasize what a tremendous job the staff of my unit, Tower 14AB (where I work as the clinical nurse educator), does with new staff orientation. Even after the orientation period is complete, there is ongoing role-modeling of professional behaviors and accountability, and encouraging of autonomy in our next generation of nurses. My experience validates what researchers document. In the 8 years that I have been in this role, it has become more evident to me that the new nurses are more likely to develop excellent nursing practice and strive to become expert nurses when the transition from student to nurse is a positive experience with the help of expert nurses, role models, and mentors. We are fortunate to have many expert nurses, mentors, and role models on Tower 14AB that exemplify these qualities.

Although it has been more than 20 years since I was a newly licensed nurse (NLN), I can still vividly remember the anticipation, excitement, and anxiety that I experienced during my first days on a busy neuro-neurosurgical unit in a moderately sized teaching hospital. Brigham and Women's Hospital (BWH) is larger and the patients' illnesses are more complex today. Until recently, there had been a fair amount of nursing turnover on our high-acuity medical intermediate care unit. At times, we have 15–20 NLNs who go through orientation in a short period of time on Tower 14AB. Sometimes we have nurses at different intervals in orientation, too.

The NLN will spend the first 12 weeks of orientation with a primary preceptor. Every new RN to Tower 14AB receives either the NLN Orientation Resource Book or the Experienced RN Orientation Resource book during the first week at BWH. The resource books, which we developed for our unit, provide specific information regarding how to increase the new nurses' patient care assignment and patient complexity during orientation. During their first week in the hospital-wide nursing orientation sponsored by the Center for Nursing Excellence (see Chapter 19.1), I meet with the new orientees to go over the orientation schedule and provide them with the orientation resource book. It does help to ease some of the anxiety when they have a better understanding of what to expect during the orientation and what is expected of them. The primary preceptor receives a copy of the orientee's schedule and will make sure the orientee knows about any schedule changes. The orientee follows the preceptor's schedule for the entire orientation.

We have used a few different models for our unit-based nursing orientation program. Our most recent six new-nurse hires attended the hospital-wide nursing orientation and then worked with one of our expert nurses for the first 3 days on 14AB. The goals for the first week were discussed with the group. I work closely with the experienced nurse to make sure overall goals are met. During the first few days on 14AB, the new nurses become familiarized with the environment and the flow of the patient care unit. They also meet many of the 14AB staff. It is key that the new nurses be introduced to their preceptors before their first shift working together. During the 12 weeks, all of the new nurses participate in an all-day, unit-based orientation class with me. We review the nursing documentation system, navigate several resources available to the nurses on the computer, review some of the respiratory equipment, review the Code Cart, Zoll, and Code documentation. We care for the adult patients who have cystic fibrosis (CF) and work closely with the CF health care team. The nurse practitioner for the CF team does a presentation about the CF patients. The learning curve is steep, but the information provided is invaluable to their practice on 14AB! Over the years, I have repeatedly heard from new nurses that there is much less anxiety about using the emergency equipment when they are familiar with the functionality of the equipment before an emergency really happens.

Because the chief nurse educator has made changes in the initial nursing orientation, the new nurses come directly to the patient care unit after the hospital-wide nursing orientation. This makes it easier to tailor each nurse's orientation based on past experiences. For example, if we have a NLN who has never worked as a patient care assistant (PCA), he or she will work directly with one of our unit-based PCAs to better understand this role at BWH. It helps with time management and delegating appropriately, too. More importantly, it starts the development of a new relationship. New nurses often express anxiety about not knowing other team members' names. Our unit coordinators (UCs) explain where many of the forms and patient care supplies are located, and discuss the process for communicating patient transfers/discharges to the unit coordinator. Our UCs ensure that we have the equipment and supplies the nursing staff needs to appropriately care for our patients. We take pride that on our team, every member of our 14AB staff has something to contribute to a new staff member's knowledge. The new nurse also develops an appreciation for each team member's workload. Delegating to the PCA and/or UC is part of the nurse's role. It helps when the new nurse has a better understanding of what is involved in each role.

The entire health care team has a role with each new nurse, from the primary preceptor(s) to the nurse manager, educator, PCA, UC, rehab specialist, dietician, phlebotomist, unit associates, and physician colleagues. We are very fortunate to have many expert clinicians on our floor. Several of the nurses are preceptors, role models, and mentors to the new staff as well as to the less experienced nurses. An abundance of nursing literature validates that preceptors are integral to role-modeling of professional behaviors and facilitating nurses' adjustments to their role. Preceptors' major goals are to help their orientees acquire the basic nursing skills needed on our unit or further develop the basic nursing skills learned in the classroom. They familiarize the new nurses with hospital policies, protocols, and guidelines. They integrate the new nurses into the unit culture, too. The literature that guided the development of this orientation program validated that new nurses who do not develop relationships with peers and preceptors have lower job satisfaction. Often these are the nurses who leave their first nursing job within 2 years. In health care, teamwork is essential to provide safe, quality patient care. Health care teams that effectively communicate and collaborate have higher staff job satisfaction, increased patient safety, and improved quality of care.

Although time management is a factor to consider, I encourage the nurses on orientation, whenever possible, to accompany their patients to diagnostic tests and procedures, again to better understand the roles of other health care team members.

We are fortunate on Tower 14AB to have nurses in various stages of nursing practice. I encourage the NLNs to talk with other nurses on 14AB who have just finished their first year as a nurse. It is difficult for the new nurses to believe that they will have made such a huge amount of progress over the first year. In general, I tell the new nurses to give themselves about 1 year before feeling confident in their practice. We strongly encourage the new nurses and their preceptors to go to lunch and/or dinner breaks together. It definitely helps to strengthen the developing peer relationships. By the end of the orientation, the new nurses should be able to competently and safely care for their patients.

Being the clinical educator for these new, enthusiastic, energetic nurses has been rewarding but, at times, challenging. It is really enjoyable to work with the NLNs because they have so many questions and are always seeking more knowledge to help them best care for their patients. One facet of my role is to oversee the entire unit-based orientation process. We work closely with the preceptors for new staff. We make recommendations for improving time management, prioritization, and organization. There are many different personalities, and the preceptors try to accommodate each nurse's uniqueness and learning styles to provide the best orientation possible. Although we provide an extensive unit-based nursing orientation program, the new nurses may lack self-confidence, can be easily intimidated, and do not have the clinical experience to draw from for urgent patient care scenarios. Therefore, even after orientation is completed, the preceptor continues to support and mentor the newer clinical nurse on 14AB. The new nurses continue to develop critical thinking skills, improve prioritization, and manage time efficiently. We all have previous experiences that can affect our coping abilities and how we manage a conflict. We work with staff members who need to develop and/or change their coping skills to better care for our patient population. For the younger nurse who does not have a lot of life experiences to draw from and has not had to deal with much conflict, we work closely to help better manage these situations.

We have weekly or biweekly meetings with the orientee to discuss patient diagnoses, treatments, interventions, and patient plan of care. Each week, the preceptor and educator discuss the progress that has been made with each orientee. It is beneficial to the new orientee and the preceptor because they both gain a better understanding of where the new nurse is in his or her nursing practice development. We discuss areas of weakness in the nurse's nursing practice and emphasize his or her strengths. It is important to be approachable for the new nurses. Many new nurses over the years have requested verbal and/or written feedback from the preceptor and nurse educator. Because they lack confidence, they don't want to ask questions if the preceptor or educator shows negative facial expressions or body language. In particular, nonverbal body language that is perceived as negative by the new nurse can cause a barrier to learning. On many occasions new nurses have expressed anxiety about asking physicians questions. We encourage all nurses to be part of the patient care team rounds for each patient every day. When the nurses have a professional relationship with the physicians, there is more effective communication and collaboration.

New staff want honest, tangible, constructive feedback at intervals during nursing orientation. Even when delivering negative feedback, it is very important to consciously think about how to phrase it. Effective communication is key. Some new nurses become defensive, yet need to know that this feedback is essential to help develop their nursing practice to better care for their patients. Providing recommendations for improvement is needed when discussing weaknesses in the nurse's practice. There are times when I have developed an individualized, structured educational plan for the new nurse to follow. For some of the NLNs, it is beneficial to write out the daily and/or weekly educational plans. It helps with visually showing the progress the nurse is making; if there is a lack of progress, we need to identify the barriers immediately to make this a positive learning experience. During the first week on 14AB, the preceptor and orientee are given a 1-page form that they are asked to complete at least weekly. The new nurse is asked to write three things that went well during that week and three things that did not go as well as they could have.

There are nurses who may not be the right fit for the high-acuity medical patients we care for on Tower 14AB. Occasionally we have had nurses who were struggling on orientation even after following an individualized educational plan. In those cases we have had candid discussion about other options. If an orientee is overwhelmed and unable to provide safe patient care, the leadership team meets with the nurse and recommends that this individual get a few years' experience in a less acute environment and then come back to BWH so the learning curve will not be so steep. Although we do not want nurses to feel like failures, we cannot allow unsafe nursing practice to exist anywhere. Nurses are in a unique position because we have many employment options. Some nurses blossom and become expert nurses in a slower-paced environment, whereas others thrive in the fast-paced, high-acuity environment.

We continue to change our unit-based nursing orientation model as needed for each individual group of new nurses. As I noted earlier, there is continued growth and development for the newer nurses as well as the more expert nurses. I continue with educational inservices based on our patient population and the needs of the nursing staff. And as time goes on, our newer, less experienced nurses develop the nursing skills they need to be the role models and mentors for our future generation of nurses at BWH.

19.3 Off-Shift Nursing Administration: Shaped by a Vision

Judith Perron, Neha Thakkar, and Elvi Rigby

The nurse administrator is a professional nurse with advanced experience who provides direction, clinical resources, and hospital leadership to a health care institution during off-shift hours. The *off shift* is defined as those shifts not occurring during traditional business hours: This includes evenings, nights, weekends, and holidays. The focus of the nurse administrator is to combine and centralize knowledge throughout the institution, work that is typically distributed amongst numerous divisions of the hospital. As a result, the tasks and responsibilities of the nurse administrator on the off shift encompass those assumed by the various departments during shifts where their managerial personnel are onsite. Essentially, the nurse administrator role has evolved into the assignment of one or two individuals who "cover" the whole hospital, or, as we like to call it, "covering the house." In this chapter, we describe a typical shift for a nurse administrator at Brigham and Women's Hospital (BWH), addressing the key aspects of the position, as well as common events that arise which make this role unique.

The vision of the Department of Nursing (DON) has helped to guide all decisions, and the DON's vision provides a foundation that allows us to confidently make decisions with the patients' and hospital's interests in mind. These three components are:

1. Excellent care to patients and families
2. The very best staff
3. The safest environment

Each situation requires the nurse administrator to act quickly while ensuring that the safest and highest quality care is provided. By maintaining an understanding of and belief in the vision, the nurse administrator can handle the challenges encountered during any given shift.

At the beginning of a shift, our first concern is staffing throughout the institution. Upon entering the staffing office, we are given the basic knowledge of staffing needs at that time, as well as a list of available unit-based and float-pool nurses. We must quickly make decisions about how to allocate these nurses to areas of need. Problem solving is at the core of many of the tasks we undertake during a shift. The procedure and process of staffing can be compared to an analytical thinking section of standardized tests in which we are trying to determine where we will assign the float nurses. Where an individual nurse can be placed is based on clinical competency, floor preference by individual, and overall unit needs in the hospital. Similar decisions must be made regarding those individuals who will serve as our main clinical resources, such as the emergency (STAT) nurse (Box 19.1) and designated intensive care (DIN) nurse. These nurses are responsible for communicating important patient status information back to us throughout the shift.

BOX 19.1 *Focus: The Very Best Experienced and Seasoned Staff*

The STAT nurse responds to a diabetic patient situation. The crisis started due to the high ICU patient census that prevented immediate admission of the diabetic patient into an ICU bed. The STAT nurse utilized ICU protocols over a 4-hour period of time on a non-ICU unit to ensure that the patient received the best possible care available. At 4 hours, the patient stabilized and was no longer in a critical status, therefore no longer requiring an ICU bed.

The skills of the STAT nurse and the availability of the STAT nurse as a resource are essential to providing the *very best staff* available. The nurse administrator core group established the position of the STAT nurse after assessing the level of high acuity outside the ICU and ways in which the hospital could maintain the ability to provide the most knowledgeable and experienced staff in a safe environment for the patient in all situations.

This highlights another important aspect of the nurse administrator position. Communication is essential to identifying current areas of need, integrating information from several sources, and collaborating among various units and departments. This is accomplished through face-to-face conversations, phone calls, e-mails, and beepers. As a result, technology has become vital to the role in recent years. A nurse administrator, therefore, needs to be familiar with and capable of using up-to-date technology in the institution.

After establishing the staffing needs in the hospital and assigning available nurses to appropriate units, we start walking rounds in the institution. By walking to each unit, we are able to assess the impending needs of the institution, recognize urgent situations, and identify patient flow issues. We collect information from each unit and determine which issues have to be addressed immediately, while noting those that can be resolved at a later time. Rounds also serve as an effective means to establish high visibility for the nurse administrator during a shift. When hospital staff and personnel see us walking through the halls and managing issues, we reinforce our credibility and authority for decision making. The off-shift workforce of all hospital departments provides us with information needed to manage the hospital because they identify us as active and "on premises" administration (Box 19.2).

In recent years, we have found it helpful to start rounds by checking with a typically crowded emergency department, post-anesthesia care units, and departments that close during the off shift, in order to obtain a good indication of current conditions. These units act as informative surrogates of the overall status of the institution and provide us with an idea of potential challenges that may arise during the shift. In addition, we check with the intensive care units (ICUs). The ICUs give us a unique perspective of the hospital because they have 24/7 attending physician coverage and nurses-in-charge (NICs) who are at a higher experience and training level. We can get a sense of potential changes in the patient population, patient care ratios, and demands being placed on the ICUs from these and other departments. The information and data we gather includes key BWH units: seven specialty ICUs; a high-risk Labor and Delivery unit; a Level One Trauma/Burn center; and a 24-hour PACU/OR. This guides the decisions we must make to provide the safest and most appropriate care utilizing the expertise of the nursing and physician staff.

We continue rounds to visit every floor and every unit. We utilize the information obtained to analyze patient flow through the hospital so we can begin to formulate a plan to accommodate patients efficiently. Additionally, we can obtain subjective patient health statuses from the perspective of the nurses caring for these patients. These nurses are working closely with the patients and families, so they can give us the best description of their current health and potential needs.

BOX 19.2 *Focus: Safest Environment*

One evening, the nurse administrator—in this case Judy—was called to a Code Gray (security emergency). I arrived to find that an irate patient waiting for a psychiatric bed had thrown a chair at the nurse caring for him. She was not physically hurt; however, upon observation it was obvious that she had been emotionally traumatized by the event. Security officers arriving on the scene used appropriate actions to restrict the patient from inflicting further harm. While security dealt with the patient, my immediate attention was on the nurse. This was the first time that this young nurse had had an experience such as this one. After consoling the nurse and allowing her an opportunity to express her thoughts and emotions, we discussed strategies that she could employ if a similar situation were to occur in the future.

One of the main roles as an off-shift administrator is to take opportunities, especially when they occur with young nurses, to offer education in an approach that will improve their skills and work environment. Through experience and education, the institution ensures that a safe environment will be maintained for both patients and staff.

Completing rounds can be a daunting task at times. As we try to visit all the units in all of the buildings, we are constantly receiving pages on our beepers and calls to our nursing administrator cell phones. In addition, we receive forwarded page requests from other departments, as these departments do not have personnel onsite during the off shift. By way of example, in one night, routinely, we can be fielding an issue that would normally be addressed by Environmental Health and Safety one minute, and then acting as a liaison for Patient/Family Relations the next minute. In addition, high-level administration personnel are not available on the off shift. As a result, we are acting as the surrogate for the chief nurse and the hospital administrator.

Because BWH is a teaching institution, we also receive numerous pages from house staff (e.g., interns, residents, and fellows) or attending physicians who are not on site during the shift. They are looking to the nurse administrator for knowledge of a situation or advice on how to deal with a particular case or crisis. As a result, we often take on the role of mentor to numerous house staff, helping them develop their crisis management and problem-solving skills and coaching them about the resources available to them during the off shift.

Additional pages to our beepers and calls to our phones involve acute care situations, including traumas and codes. As nurse administrators, we are pivotal persons involved in all patient and institution-wide crises (Box 19.3). We are recognized formally as the hospital leadership on the off shift. During these circumstances, we must quickly assess and implement solutions using available resources, such as on-call hospital administration, onsite department supervisors, and staff throughout the hospital. The challenge for the nurse administrator is determining whether a situation requires the assistance of on-call hospital administration or other administrative hospital support not usually on duty during the off shifts. This challenge is met through the use of rapid decision making and solid problem-solving skills. The nurse administrator must determine the extent to which a situation demands additional resources not available on a typical off shift. Overall, all situations require the nurse administrator to convey any adverse events through written and verbal communication to hospital administration.

BOX 19.3 *Focus: Safest Environment—Code Hazmat/Incident Commander*

This example, recounted by Judy in her role as nurse administrator, highlights the safety challenges implicit in the role. As "Code Trauma—15 minutes" alerts through my beeper, I arrive in the Emergency Department (ED) to collect more information from the nurse-in-charge (NIC). I am informed that a burn victim is being transported to BWH ED. I learn that the individual has a chemical burn to 90% of his body. I quickly identify that the patient will need to be decontaminated due to the chemical exposure. I notify the page operator for a Code Hazmat to be activated. Due to this activation, I immediately become the Incident Commander, assuming the responsibility of coordinating resources and communicating with internal and external interested parties and community officials. This activation will alert a select group of trained individuals within BWH that decontamination will have to be available and performed upon arrival of the patient by EMS. Time is essential, as it takes approximately 15 minutes to activate and prepare the decontamination trailer and area. By activating the group, I summon assistance from a variety of departments, including Environmental Services, Security, Engineering, and Nursing.

Upon the patient's arrival by Med-Flight, the patient and EMS/flight crew are directed to the decontamination trailer, all the while maintaining trauma and life support. As this patient is a trauma patient, the ancillary services of social services and chaplaincy are also involved in the coordination of care efforts. They focus on the family as I continue to coordinate the admission of the patient to the Burn Intensive Care Unit.

After the patient is admitted, it is now my responsibility to coordinate cleanup of the area and then perform a review of the incident with all of the leaders of hospital incident control (HIC). I must also be sure that the Code Hazmat and implementation of the incident command model are written up and communicated to the administrator on call and the emergency director. Throughout the entire incident, I have also maintained the other responsibilities of my role.

In recent years, there has been an increase in physical and verbal abuse against nurses in acute care settings. As nurse administrators, we need to assure hospital staff that they have a safe working environment and have access to appropriate support during high-risk situations. In order to achieve this, we need to collaborate with Security to ensure direct support during threatening incidents, while also having resources in place to prevent violence and abuse at the unit level.

Another aspect of the nurse administrator role is involvement in community relationships. BWH is a major trauma center in an internationally diverse city. As a result, there is an array of cultures, religions, and languages in our surrounding communities. Our hospital must therefore provide the best-qualified staff to care for a diverse population of patients. We receive patients whose families are facing conflict while trying to make difficult decisions. Because the Department of Patient/Family Relations is not on site during the off shift, we step in as nurse administrators to help social workers, chaplains, and house staff support patients and families when needed, mediate conflicts, and support staff dealing with complex family dynamics that may affect patient care (Box 19.4).

BOX 19.4 *Focus: Excellent Care to Patient and Families in the Darkest of Times*

Frequently we are called upon to carry out a task that requires the utmost respect and dignity. We have the responsibility, on the off shifts and weekends, of bringing family members to view their deceased loved ones in the viewing room. It is our responsibility as nurse administrators to prepare the deceased body for viewing and to bring the body to the viewing room.

We see grief in all of its forms and have to be able to appropriately intervene in each situation. Some families are stoic and express very little, while others are vocal and extremely emotional. Some families' grief is very visceral and we need to physically support them.

The chaplain and social worker on call are often working in collaboration with us and offer their support and expertise. Each situation is unique. Although it is at a difficult time and a demanding aspect of our role, it is a privilege to support families at their most vulnerable.

After making rounds throughout the house, answering countless pages and phone calls, and responding to acute care situations, we have to prepare for the end of our shift. This involves preplanning for the upcoming shift by determining staffing needs, recognizing future patient flow, and following up on incidents that occurred during the shift that is just ending. Patients who might be high risk during the upcoming shift are identified and this information is communicated to the STAT and DIN nurses. Specific occurrences require follow-up communication. For example, Occupational Health must be notified by e-mail if a nurse experiences a needle stick; Patient/Family Relations will receive phone messages when problems have occurred with patients, families, or visitors. All events during the off shift are also summarized in a report and sent to executive directors in the nursing department, hospital administration, and Patient Care Services.

Ultimately, a nurse administrator must balance the needs of patients, families, staff, and various departments in order for the overall institution to work efficiently and effectively. In this chapter we set out to describe a typical shift for a nurse administrator at BWH. We think it also highlights the characteristics needed to be successful in this role. A nurse administrator needs to be an independent, critical thinker with good problem-solving and communication skills. To accomplish the wide range of tasks that must be dealt with on the off shift, a nurse administrator requires knowledge of the institution and an ability to utilize available resources effectively. The nurse administrator acts in the role of continuous quality improvement—improving on the patient/family experience, ensuring the very best staff in an environment of safety and quality care. Because nurse administrators take on an immense amount of responsibility, they need to be proficient under high-stress situations, capable of multitasking, and have the personality that drives them to work the off shift. As is perhaps apparent, they are uniquely situated to promote and implement the DON vision, ensuring a seamless congruence among all shifts at BWH.

20

Values and Vision

20.1 Authentic Leadership: Real-Time Application at BWH

Nancy Hickey and Eileen M. O'Connell

A leader leads by example, whether he intends to or not.

—*Author Unknown*

There is much in the literature today about "Authentic Leadership." Our Department of Nursing (DON) at Brigham and Women's Hospital (BWH) has explored and committed to this characteristic in support of promoting our vision of nursing practice: "Excellent care to patients and families with the very best staff and in the safest environment." While building an infrastructure for change as described earlier in this book, we collectively discovered the characteristics of authentic leaders that would shape that change. Here, we describe our practical application of leading authentically. We both have nursing leadership positions that make that application a daily learning experience.

The DON of the BWH is probably like many other large academic nursing departments. Our nursing staff have significant experience and tenure and are accustomed to working in complex environments that are both exhausting and rewarding. Those of us in nursing leadership positions are responsible and hold ourselves accountable for supporting clinical staff, innovation, and operational and financial efficiency, and for ensuring that patients and families are well taken care of with a constant focus on quality. Perhaps only those in leadership roles can fully understand the complexity and difficulties of this responsibility. Many of us have learned that the best way to lead is to learn from our own experiences, as well as the experiences of others. We describe our lessons here. To really learn these lessons requires a tremendous amount of self-reflection, openness, honesty, sincerity, and commitment. This commitment to continuous self-improvement can be exhausting. However, it allows us to reach expanded self-awareness and a higher level of self-confidence, which becomes possible when we are open to the journey.

Authentic leaders generally have good senses. We have found it as important to be good listeners as it is to be good communicators. One interesting skill is to hear not only what is being said but also what is not being said. For example, we have found that our nursing staff reacts negatively when "told" what to do. This, we believe, is because our staff most often knows exactly what to do and, more importantly, wants to do the right thing. Both of us have come to realize that staff members experience the leader who prescribes to them what to do and how to do it as clumsy and ineffective. However, when faced with a problem and invited to join in the decision-making process, clinical, frontline staff are frequently able to identify the solution and the best way to get there. The keys are trust, respect, and openness. An excellent example is managing critical care flow through our busy organization. Despite high occupancies and regionalized intensive care units, our staff often will work out the best patient-centered solutions when they feel their voices are being heard and their contributions recognized.

Authentic leaders stay engaged in the mission. In our case, understanding our responsibility to ensure the well-being of our patients—friends, family, and neighbors—who seek tertiary, expert care at BWH is paramount. We are dedicated to the good work we seek to do; we also are inspired by and seek to influence the good, compassionate work of others. Our inspiration comes from our patients, our frontline staff, and our colleagues within and beyond the nursing department. We further believe that being keenly observant and demonstrating steadfast fidelity to the DON vision is critical. We work toward this vision in an organization that is committed to providing care to our local community and to a very large number of patients transferred from other organizations, both near and far. While this is an enormous responsibility, embracing and committing to the characteristics of an authentic leader has helped us navigate and make decisions that affect the organization on a regular basis. Rather than being overwhelmed, truly understanding and embracing the responsibilities of our leadership roles keeps us balanced and focused.

We have come to learn that authentic leaders are adaptable. BWH has grown in complexity and size over the years: Change is constant. Learning to embrace, recognize, and expect change rather than avoiding change is the key. Openness to new opportunities to learn, grow, and improve our skills is a must. However, it requires a commitment to avoid personalizing of difficult situations, inviting feedback, and constantly engaging in self-reflection and adaptation. Under pressure, we have experienced tense and difficult conversations. Rather than retreating, we have found this is the time to fully engage, remain open, and seek to understand before being understood.

We have learned that sincerity, compassion, insight, tolerance, and avoiding hypocrisy in our discussions and decisions ensures us that we are leading both authentically and effectively. Just as importantly, we have found that these values are both a demonstration of personal and professional integrity and help us put the work before our own self-interests. For example, we have learned that judgment must be suspended and blaming others is destructive. We have an unwritten rule, "No Monday-morning quarterbacking." Therefore, when situations are discussed, input from others is sought, and respectful dialogue is expected. There is zero tolerance for hostile or disrespectful communication. We understand that situations minus the emotion look different after the fact, and trust that well-intended decisions are made in the moment. As a result, most often our colleagues are willing to explore and openly discuss these challenging decisions. They are also open to feedback and discussion, with the emphasis on learning and improving their decision making and optimizing patient outcomes.

Last, but most importantly, we believe that we are inspired and strive to inspire others as authentic leaders. As we gained tenure in our organization, we have talked about our future legacy work and what we call "building the bench." We have recognized that roles in nursing leadership can be viewed as unappealing by staff members with high leadership potential. Nonetheless, we are hopeful that the next generation of nurse leaders will be inspired by the sincerity, courage, and genuineness of our enthusiasm for nursing, and by our DON's vision, thus motivating the best to take on new leadership opportunities. We have seen this in many young nurses who are in graduate school or recently entering advanced practice and looking for opportunities to be coached and mentored in leadership. We are confident that the best is yet to come.

20.2 *True Collaboration: A Multidisciplinary Model*

Kristin Alt Styer

---

*F*or the past 3 years, as the nursing quality program director for Perioperative Nursing, I have participated in many quality improvement (QI) projects. Several of these projects have involved members of the anesthesiology and/or surgical leadership teams. While all patient care requires nurse and physician teamwork, the operating room setting is unique not only in the number of people, but also the number of disciplines required at any one time. All these disciplines depend upon one another for optimal care of any given patient, specifically keeping the patient safe during a high-stress procedure.

When I was asked to help oversee a pilot of the World Health Organization (WHO) Surgical Safety Checklist, with the Department of Anesthesiology vice chair for clinical practice (S.E.) as my clinical partner in the pilot, I did not think this was going to be any different than the multiple improvement projects I had worked on in the past during my time in this role. My anesthesia partner and I met several times to formulate a plan for the pilot, which we implemented over a 2-week period. The lessons we learned during those 2 weeks and the discussions that followed proved to be a turning point in our approach to true collaboration among all disciplines for QI in the operating room.

Upon completion of the pilot, S.E. and I needed to complete the evaluation process, not only of the project, but also of the process. We were interested in making the WHO Checklist a permanent part of practice in the operating room. We needed to determine how we could spread this from a pilot project involving a few operating room teams to an institutional rollout, which would include all 42 operating rooms—no small task! We had more than 200 registered nurses, 250 anesthesiology attending physicians and residents, and countless surgeons, including attending staff, fellows, residents, and interns. Every person needed to be educated appropriately on this checklist to ensure its successful adoption.

My anesthesia colleague and I developed a list of requirements for a successful rollout. Although we had initially planned for equal leadership of the pilot, I became increasingly more involved in the education, communication, and onsite observation. My anesthesia colleague and I agreed that this could not happen during the global rollout. As we reviewed the lessons learned from our pilot project, two stood out:

1. The WHO Checklist required active participation from the three major disciplines in the operating room: anesthesiology, nursing, and surgery.
2. The pilot leadership had involved only two of those disciplines; we were missing a surgeon partner.

At the top of our "list of demands," as we jokingly referred to them, we wanted a surgeon partner. The choice of word was intentional: *partner*. We learned from the pilot that we required a surgeon who would agree to equal "ownership" of this project along with us, and who was fully committed to it. Having a name or face attached to a project of this magnitude, without the day-to-day participation and decision making involved, was not going to be enough. We were looking for someone who would dedicate the time required and hold himself or herself responsible to communicate and coordinate education to the department of surgery. And we had someone in mind.

The vice chair of surgery, who was very involved in other QI projects we had worked on over the preceding years, fit the bill perfectly. When I presented him with our proposal, he barely paused before jokingly asking, "Do I get to yell at other surgeons?" He was in. As a nurse, I had not realized this would be considered his payoff for agreeing to join with us on this venture toward safer, systematic care!

Once we had presented our plan to our chiefs of departments and received their endorsement and approval to proceed, we built our team: a project manager (a nurse who would oversee the day-to-day operations), an administrative fellow (for measurement of documentation compliance), and the Tri-Leaders (my anesthesia and surgery partners, and myself). We would meet weekly at a set time.

Over the first few weeks of our meetings, we worked diligently to develop a plan for a 14-week staggered rollout to include all 10 surgical services. Each service would receive a week of communication and education, a week of "Go-Live" with daily, in-room monitoring, and a week of follow-up. Each service would essentially require a 3-week process. The communication and education responsibility lay with each of the Tri-Leaders. We were to coordinate and ensure that the communication and education occurred prior to the week of Go-Live. I ensured this through service-specific, nurse staff meetings to provide this education. Our anesthesia partner presented at grand rounds and e-mailed the service-specific anesthesiologists when it was their designated week. Our surgery partner presented at grand rounds and personally e-mailed each surgeon the night before their Go-Live and scheduled in-room observation, to remind them of their required participation in the checklist the following day.

As we proceeded into the 14-week rollout, our weekly meetings morphed from predominantly planning into an ongoing evaluation phase. Each of the Tri-Leaders, myself included, wanted to make sure our discipline "had a voice" in this process. During in-room observations, we heard feedback and/or questions from staff and this allowed us to address concerns in real time. We brought that feedback to the weekly meetings and updated the leadership team on what was actually occurring in practice, not just on paper.

Staff had a variety of concerns we needed to address: a surgeon being uncooperative with performing his section at the proper time; a nurse not reading the debriefing questions aloud for the whole team to hear; an anesthesiologist giving medication before leading their pre-anesthetic checklist section. Feedback that was timely and specific afforded us the opportunity to evaluate the process of putting the checklist into practice, determining if further clarification, education, or even changes to the checklist were needed. If these problems could not be solved this way, the leader for the person at issue was to address behavior immediately (i.e., we each dealt with members of our own discipline). Never did any of us balk at having to speak to a member of our discipline. This was our role and we needed to maintain oversight and accountability if we believed in this. Otherwise, the project would fail.

I learned a lot from the process. Often while teaching and training, you take more away than you ever give. What had been missing from other QI projects was the oversight. We often rolled out projects and then started on the next one. We had also lacked follow-through from engaged, dedicated leaders, such as we had in this project. As a nurse leader, I have often asked nurses to "give us names" of the people involved in counterproductive behavior so that we could address this issue specifically. However, nurses often lacked confidence in the "system" to truly follow through with their physician counterparts. This time was different! It did not take long before people were hearing that Dr. M or Nurse Y had been asked to explain their actions with the checklist, or sometimes their lack of action with the checklist. What followed was an overall change in culture to not only one of accountability and responsibility, but also one where behavior was addressed in real time and expectations were made clear.

Nearly a year after completion of the rollout to the entire operating room, very little has changed from the actual checklist process, but truly, much has changed in our ORs! The Tri-Leaders still regularly e-mail any concerns with any staff member or general discussion on the checklist. Our anesthesia partner has since left BWH and has been replaced by an equally dedicated anesthesiologist. We meet as needed, to reevaluate the checklist practice or address any issues we have heard about. This has been the most enjoyable and successful project I have been involved in to date.

I sometimes struggle to determine why it was so very different, and realize it is because we worked as a team. We talk about the importance of teams in health care all the time. This is why. I learned a model system for every project moving forward, specifically looking at involvement of multiple disciplines. For me, this was, and remains, true collaboration.

Leadership Stories

21.1 *From Groupthink to Action Teams: Changing How We Solve Problems*

Eileen Molina

A consulting group, Crotty and LaJeunesse, employed by Brigham and Women's Hospital (BWH) to help us explore high levels of staff dissatisfaction in the workplace, introduced me to the idea of action teams in 2003. As I understood action teams (as they described them), they involved getting the staff and directors together to collaboratively work on solutions or resolutions to a specific identified major problem, including the multiple issues involved (see www.odyssey-consulting.net). We believed there were not enough written rules regarding staffing and scheduling; this, coupled with high management turnover and poor staff longevity, the staffing and scheduling on the service was disorganized and sometimes chaotic.

Frustration with the lack of cohesiveness between staff and management was a major concern. Staff identified the staffing/scheduling on the Hematology-Oncology/Bone Marrow Transplant Service as an important area for improvement. With more than 200 staff members and within the context of a joint venture between the Dana-Farber Cancer Institute (DFCI) and BWH, there remained a great deal of inconsistency, with people making their own rules to suit their needs. Along with this, some staff from both sides of the joint venture were not happy with the new policies and the seniority changes because of the joint venture. Adding to this confusion was a very strong union for nurses, with contract provisions that further influenced the experiences of the staff and could be interpreted in a variety of ways.

I spoke to Paul Crotty, one of the consultants, who told me verbally how to pull together an action team. He suggested I bring together a group of diverse staff and allow people to speak freely about their ideas. I took his advice and modified his suggestions to fit our needs, making adjustments with time. The directors of our service have since adapted this method to tackle any difficult problem we have encountered, although here I will use the original staffing/scheduling action team to describe the process and the impact. Since the creation of the original action team, we have developed numerous other teams when a major issue arises. By way of example, we have had discharge action teams, chemo action teams, transfer action teams, and other action teams focused on other identified problems. All our action teams have yielded success grounded in a strong commitment by staff, and have resulted in improvements concerning the addressed problem or issue.

CONFRONTING GROUPTHINK

Groupthink is a term coined by social psychologist Irving Janis (1972, 1982). It occurs when a group makes faulty decisions due to group pressures. This can lead to a deterioration of "mental efficiency, reality testing and moral judgment" (Janis, 1972 p. 9).

Groups affected by groupthink can ignore alternatives and tend to take irrational actions that dehumanize other groups. A group is especially vulnerable to groupthink when its members are similar in background, when the group is insulated from outside opinions, and when there are no clear rules for decision making (Janis, 1972).

I believe groupthink was engrained in our former culture on both sides. Staff did not feel free to speak up about the issues, but instead went along with the most powerful staff and their opinions. After BWH and DFCI created a joint venture, nursing staff from both sides thought the other side should conform to their way of staffing and scheduling. Walls were set up between the two sides and they did not want to open up to the other side. Neither side wanted management's input at all.

Most of the staff are confident and feel empowered, and do not respond well to top-down management styles. Thus, they found action teams an ideal venue to solve problems. A commitment from all levels of administration was evident as we established these teams. The hospital administration supported us with time, money, autonomy, and the confidence to know we were accomplishing great work. Over the next few months, the positive work was reflected in a more organized approach to staffing/scheduling, as well as increased staff satisfaction. These action teams were recognized by staff and administration for their legacy building, for their capacity to help us meet our mission and vision.

MY FIRST EXPERIENCE USING ACTION TEAMS

As noted earlier, the first action team I tried was designed to address the issue of staffing/scheduling. To start the process, we put out an e-mail, requesting that staff who were interested in joining this team let the designated leader know. In this e-mail, we stated that we would not be taking all volunteers, but instead would look for a group that represented each unit, each shift, and each role (nurse, patient care assistant, and unit secretary). We were looking for staff interested in identifying issues and developing recommendations. We would also keep the numbers down to a workable group of 10–12 people (anything larger, we believed, would not be able to reach decisions and would foster too much debate and not enough decision making).

We carefully chose team members we felt would best represent the staff, choosing one staff nurse from each unit (nurses were the majority of the staff, but we also made sure we had representation from other ancillary nursing staff). We then sent out another e-mail announcing who would be the representatives from each unit. We asked the entire staff to bring any issues they had identified to their action-team representative for discussion. We requested that the staff honor any decisions that the representatives made on their behalf. Also included on the team were a union representative, the staffing scheduling coordinator, and the operations coordinator. This way, they could speak out if they believed that the group veered off track with its recommendations. The union contract provisions were sometimes interpreted in a variety of ways, so we developed specifics that worked for the service, the budget, and so on within these guidelines.

The entire action team met for one full day to identify issues and develop recommendations for improvement. This was done in a round-table fashion, with flip charts to record the "problems/issues" and the "recommendations." We included the union representative, we had a union contract to refer to, we pulled all appropriate hospital policies; in short, we worked diligently to make sure the recommendations were fair and equitable for everyone and did not break any hospital or union rules.

A set of ground rules was established prior to the meeting by the director leading the team, which established the expectation to respect and honor all participants. We believed it was important to post these rules. We also believed the most important rules were commitment to the team, as well as respect for other team members' opinions. Honesty and sharing thoughts were important. Debates and opposing thoughts, with respect, were encouraged. We wanted team members to speak out, and discouraged groupthink.

STEPS IN CREATING OUR OWN ACTION TEAM

Our first step was to make sure the "team" understood the process of scheduling. We met with the financial/budget director. Team members visited the computer learning center to be introduced to BWH's way of scheduling through "One-Staff" and to make sure they understood how it worked. The director of Labor and Negotiations met with the staff and answered any questions, as did a Human Resources generalist. Now that everyone knew the background and expectations, we were ready to get the work group in motion. We met in a large room and everyone was given a chance to talk about issues they brought to the table, with recommendations. One director served as the group leader. We maintained documentation through a flip chart, which was later transcribed into meeting minutes, labeled as "problems" and "resolutions." The director was responsible for keeping everyone on track, maintaining order, and doing follow-up after the meeting. At the end of the day, everyone was mentally exhausted, but felt good about the changes for the better. We all felt that great work had been done.

Following the meeting, minutes were sent out to the entire staff. They were received very well. The team met quarterly for 2-hour meetings until there were no more issues to be discussed. Any issues that staff brought up after the meeting were filtered through the representatives. Staff respected their coworkers for their decisions and often had discussions with them about the issues. The staff had become invested in their work, their decisions, and their future. When the directors made decisions about staffing/scheduling, they came from the recommendations, as all at the meetings had agreed to them. If something came up that people did not believe to be fair or equitable, staff spoke up.

We had worked within the hospital guidelines and the union contract to develop a plan that worked for most people. The rules were applied to ancillary staff also, who were not part of the union bargaining unit. These recommendations were fair and equitable to everyone. The directors were working with the union and the union admired and appreciated this. It was a "first" to most who had not witnessed collaboration between the groups in the past. The staff were the stakeholders, and wanted this structure to work. Decisions were made that everyone could live with and follow.

The directors would then take some of the recommendations (as needed) and work with various people, departments, and so on to see what would or would not work; the directors brought this back to the group until the final minutes were accurate and complete and the final rules had been distributed. All of this work stayed within hospital policy and within the guidelines of the union contract. This action team was so popular, and produced such positive results, that it is not uncommon to hear staff or directors state: "We should put together an action team for this problem."

There have been times when issues start arising again. We pull out the minutes and get the team back together to look at problems and their resolutions, although these follow-up meetings usually only need 1–2 hours of time. Sometimes they may require quarterly meetings until all problems and issues are resolved.

Data can be collected to determine improvement. Sometimes we notice that the complaints at staff meetings have diminished and see this as a validation of our efforts. Once these issues were resolved, we discovered we all had more time to work on other projects and the ability to bring our staff to a higher level of professional competence. We discovered we had more time for research or presenting scholarly work, because the major underlying basic problem that was taking all our time and energy had been resolved. Action teams made it possible for us to focus on the Department of Nursing vision and achieving its ideals.

CONCLUSION

The work accomplished in our original action team has carried over to other successful action teams. The requirements to build a strong action team are an open leader, committed staff involvement, and a group that will represent the various groups involved in the issue, including various senior levels of staff, various shifts, and different positions. The group members need to feel relaxed and empowered enough to speak.

I now believe that groupthink is something of a past at BWH. The participants in these action teams realize how important it is to have diversity of opinions on the team, to allow the positive power of helping to establish change and break down barriers. The group learned that they could work with directors, who are an important part of the team, equally important as all the other members. All barriers that stop people from working together have been removed. Everyone on the team takes pride in his or her workmanship. Respect from coworkers as the representative on an action team has meant more than any award or monetary increase.

Commitment and action from both directors and team members who are dedicated to improving quality and productivity in the workplace are valued and respected. Members of the teams enjoy being the solution, not the problem. Everyone in the workplace has something important to say and should be valued. Allowing the staff to be stakeholders in the system leads to improvement and productivity in the workplace. Although at times these action teams may not lead to 100% improvement, they do lead to a great deal of improvement. And the staff is heard. We have listened to them. They are part of the solution. A high level of trust and bonding developed between the staff and the leaders of the action teams. The time that has been devoted to these action teams has created outcomes that have established a longstanding legacy. Rarely have we needed to regroup and bring the team back, but if needed, we have done so with the same commitment to improvement. Our journey from groupthink to action teams has been a constructive and successful one for all of us.

REFERENCES

Janis, I. L. (1972). *Victims of groupthink*. New York, NY: Houghton Mifflin.

Janis, I. L. (1982). *Groupthink: Psychological studies of policy decisions and fiascoes* (2nd ed.). New York, NY: Houghton Mifflin.

21.2 *Choosing the Best Place to Work*

Joan M. Vitello-Cicciu

I have done it all in nursing. I have been a staff nurse, a unit-based educator, a clinical nurse specialist in critical care, a nurse manager, a nursing director, a chief nursing officer (Chief Nursing Officer), and (for a brief stint) a chief operating officer. I have worked in academic and community-based settings and for faith-based and secular systems. When I left my role as a CNO of a health care system north of Boston in January of 2009, I began an exploration. What was next in my career? For the past 12 years I had worked for several community hospitals. I realized I felt a longing to go back to an academic health care center.

When I received a phone call from a search firm asking that I consider doing some leadership consulting for the Brigham and Women's Hospital (BWH), I initially declined the offer. I realized that it was a hospital where a nursing union had been present for decades, and there had been contentiousness with this union in the past. I didn't know what I could expect from nurses and the care they were providing. But the president of the search firm happened to be my former CNO, and she said, "Joan this is a great place for you to work while you look for another permanent position and you are really needed there." So I accepted the opportunity to come and work on a cardiac surgical intermediate unit as the interim nurse manager.

My primary responsibilities were to be involved daily with the operations of the unit, to have a presence with the staff, to help reduce the expenses, and to assist with getting a new nurse director on board who would be taking over the management of this unit in 14 weeks. What an opportunity to be back in my clinical specialty and to do coaching of a new nurse director! And so my journey began . . .

What impressed me from the very beginning at BWH was the caliber of the nurse directors and the nursing executive director whom I had the chance to interact with on a daily basis. They were dedicated nursing professionals who had the same values that were important to me: striving for patient-/family-focused care, emphasizing nursing leaders knowing their staff and the patients on their units, and working to make the environment safer for patients and staff.

The highlights of my 14 weeks there was witnessing firsthand the exceptional patient-/family-focused care that was being delivered by the majority of the staff and having the opportunity to role model for the new nurse director a rich array of skills, which included resolving conflicts among the nursing staff and interdisciplinary staff, chairing a meeting, engaging in disciplinary action, writing a performance evaluation, giving critical feedback, and exploring ways of reducing expenses. He was such an engaged learner and a joy to work with and I just knew that this unit would be led by an upcoming star performer.

The 14 weeks flew by and I was back to being in search of another position. Less than a month passed before I received another phone call, this time from the CNO, Mairead Hickey, asking me to once again come back to BWH as another interim, this time as the executive director of Perioperative Services. Thus began another interesting aspect of my career journey at BWH.

I started in the fall of 2009, while I was actively interviewing for other positions elsewhere. In less than 2 months of working with high-caliber surgeons, administrators, and excellent nursing staff, I realized that this was indeed a service line that was very important to the success of the BWH. I also realized that it was in need of my skill set around mentoring nursing leaders, creating a participatory nursing culture, and co-creating a healthy workplace environment. Further, I was inspired by the exceptional nursing leaders who quickly became my peer group and the visionary leadership of Mairead Hickey and Trish Gibbons. So I decided to apply for the permanent position. After doing a national search, BWH selected me as the new executive director for Perioperative Services and I began my new job in January of 2010.

Why did I want to stay and work permanently at BWH? I have asked myself this many times. After some reflection, I realized that I have been searching for an environment where I could not only teach but learn as well, where I could give and receive in return, and where I could make my optimal contribution to patient- and family-focused care as a nursing leader and know that others are equally committed to creating this environment. That place is truly BWH in the Department of Nursing. I have come home.

The Nurse Educator

22.1 *The Impact of the Clinical Nurse Educator*

Ronna E. Zaremski

What is a nurse educator, and why are they essential to nursing? In this chapter, I share some of my convictions about the influence a nurse educator can have. Defining the role of the nurse educator is no simple task. Our primary work, providing quality educational experiences to staff nurses, also is critical in maintaining and strengthening the workforce. Although nurse educators have individual styles, all educators share the passion to work side-by-side with staff, as mentors and motivators.

Establishing myself as the nurse educator on my floor was a challenging and rewarding process. Because I did not begin my career at Brigham and Women's Hospital (BWH), the nurses on my unit did not know my skill set, my nursing practice, and my passion for education. I had to earn my stripes by demonstrating that I was capable of providing education in times of need and in preparation for future endeavors. Coming from another institution also allowed me to examine the systems and the processes of BWH very closely. I had to read the details of the policy manuals and learn the intricacies of the computer systems. The expert was now the novice. But I took pride in remembering I had knowledge on my side, and my knowledge was certainly my power.

BWH orients new nurse educators by pairing them up with other nurse educators in similar practice settings. The mentoring process was very important to me. I knew that understanding the BWH culture and that of the educator group and the staff nurses would be vital for a smooth transition. I was fortunate to have a supportive mentor, one who still supports me daily.

I work in a medical intermediate unit. The patients we care for are incredibly complex, with a variety of medical diagnoses and require frequent monitoring, in contrast to those with a more limited range of needs. Some of the nursing staff chose to work on our floor because they preferred this variety. Still, a limitless number of medical diagnoses can generate a limitless number of questions. I took the job of a nurse educator in this environment because I knew it would allow me to share my knowledge and to advance my learning. I am comfortable admitting to my staff nurses that I may not be able to answer all of their questions. Together, we search for the answers.

At BWH nurse educators report to the unit's nursing director. Staff nurses often view the nurse educator–nurse director team as the leadership of the unit. It is imperative that they share a good communication system and be in constant collaboration. Soon after I joined the staff, my nurse director and I met to craft future goals and discuss aspirations we had for the staff and the unit. We used this vision to help motivate and mature our staff. I have respect for and admire the challenges my nurse director faces, and feel this makes it easier for her to share her thoughts and ideas on how we can improve care on our unit. We work well as a team, and the staff appreciates knowing that their leadership is working hard to support their nursing practice.

KNOWING MY STAFF

The staff nurses working on any particular shift influence the role of the nurse educator for that shift. Familiarity with each staff nurse, his or her personality, and level of experience at the bedside is essential. Of course, the blend of staff nurses is rarely the same day to day or shift to shift. Thus, on my floor, I try to find that delicate balance between knowledge and practice. Does the staff nurse need more education about a disease process? Do I check and see if the documentation is correct? Is this a time when I can stop this nurse for a moment to ask questions? Will this nurse even want my help? Does this nurse need my help but does not recognize it? Is this nurse refusing to interact with me?

Nurse educators must willingly place themselves in situations that may be uncomfortable. Safe patient care is our shared responsibility. I ensure that best practices are occurring and, if they are not, I lend my support to make the necessary changes.

As the nurse educator, I try to take a holistic approach with each nurse. I pay attention to all aspects of the staff nurses: their emotions, thoughts, and feelings. The staff nurses in return need to have faith and comfort in my ability as a nurse. I feel that I am both a teacher and a mentor. In offering support and guidance, I do what I can to ensure that the staff nurses know they are appreciated. As a result, the majority of the staff nurses welcome my thoughts and suggestions.

WORKING WITH MY UNIT STAFF TO IMPROVE PATIENT CARE

Much like the staff nurse, a nurse educator often has an unpredictable shift. My daily routine involves checking in with staff nurses to assess who may require my assistance, responding to clinical questions, and perhaps seeking out experts for answers. I try to make myself visible on the unit as much as possible. Although I retreat to my office when I need to focus on a specific project, the staff nurses know that my door is always open: I will stop and provide assistance. Beyond this daily routine, my role gives me numerous other opportunities to have an impact on patient care. The following examples demonstrate what I mean.

Orienting New Staff

When a nurse is interviewed for a position on our floor, I am an active participant in the process. Observing interviews of possible staff members allows me to hear the confidence or trepidation the nurses have about the possible job. Is the candidate nervous or calm? One can gather so much information from a nurse describing what it is like to take care of a challenging patient or what it takes to deal with a confrontational situation.

Once a nurse is selected for, and accepts, a position, I am responsible for the planning and implementation of a (hopefully) successful orientation. One of the first actions is to select a preceptor to pair with the new nurse to help with the transition. Creating this dyad means more to me than just matching a qualified preceptor with a new nurse. Given the opportunity, I take into careful consideration the personalities of both individuals. As I introduce the idea of mentoring a new staff member to the prospective preceptors, I also assure that person that, after thinking about it, the final choice is his or hers. My hope is that staff will feel pride when asked to precept. Ideally, a preceptor should be chosen because of his or her work ethic, communication skills, and clinical competence. I have become a strong proponent of an organized and effective system in preceptor selection.

After creating a preceptor-new nurse dyad comes the orientation schedule. During the orientation, I integrate into the schedule meetings with the new nurse and preceptor to ensure their constant communication. I observe the interactions of the dyad on the unit and use the information as feedback at our meetings. During the orientation process, it is part of my job to ensure that nurses are exposed to the various technical skills they will need once they transition to caring for patients on their own. Novice nurses can certainly get caught up in the daily tasks for the patients assigned to them. The dyad needs occasional reminders to review what has not yet been learned. Preceptors will often request that patients with specific disease processes that require certain skills (like peritoneal dialysis) be assigned to the dyad. Even experienced nurses acclimating to the unit need to adjust to possible differences in procedures or equipment. While I have found that most dyads are delightful to work with, some dyads are not as successful. It is then my job to create a smooth transition to the next preceptor. Orienting new staff is time consuming, but providing the right path sets the stage for a successful outcome.

Providing Inservice Education

Changes in technology, requirements from accreditation bodies, and hospital-initiated quality and safety programs continually reframe the staff nurses' environment. Thus, part of my job involves preparing, presenting, and reviewing items that the nurses must incorporate into their nursing practice due to these changes. This can be extremely challenging. Waiting for a staff nurse to have a lull in the flow of his or her shift to review material is almost impossible. Although educating multiple nurses at the same time would be ideal, staffing patterns on the patient care units rarely allow for group discussions. Nurse educators (such as myself) balance the importance of the topic with the risk of slightly throwing off the work flow of a busy staff nurse.

I find that the staff nurses on my patient care unit adjust well to the frequent changes they encounter. I encourage them to provide feedback, positive or negative. It certainly can be difficult if the process I am introducing does not fit into the work flow. Because staff nurses have enormous demands placed on them during their work shift, adding more to their to-do list is the last thing that I want to do.

Educating staff nurses can be extremely rewarding. Some of the learning that occurs is through review sessions at lunch. Observing that "aha" moment is something special and one of the reasons I became a nurse educator. Moving the staff nurses through the learning process and witnessing a positive outcome feels wonderful and keeps me energized. Of course, I also deal with the frustrations of poor planning, bad timing, and uninterested staff nurses; for me, the more important point is to figure out how to make adjustments that may improve these situations.

Auditing

As a nurse educator, I play a vital role in evaluating nursing practice. By auditing the nursing care we provide, we can identify patterns for improvement. These patterns lay the framework for the nurse educators' work on the patient care unit. Critical elements of documentation in the medical record are assessed frequently and captured in an institutional database. On my unit, the nurses-in-charge assist in assessing the charts and providing feedback to the staff. Much of the work is reviewing the positive aspects of the chart along with the areas to improve. If a deficiency trend develops on our unit, we work as a team to find out why the deficiency exists and how we might fix it.

I have found that conversations with the staff nurses often provide invaluable information about a deficiency and why it exists. They will easily share their frustrations with me and make helpful suggestions. I then work with my nursing director to determine what action we can take to address the deficiency.

It can be difficult if deficiencies continue despite ongoing educational efforts. One of the techniques that we use on our unit involves dedicating an entire month to one issue. Continuous discussion and instruction to the point of exhaustion has changed practice. With success here, I feel that I can relax a bit and focus on other important issues. Sustaining best practices is always a challenge for me. I find that motivating the staff and occasionally providing nourishment (often chocolate) help somewhat, but there is always more that can be done.

Quality Improvement Initiatives

As the nurse educator, through auditing and observation, I notice how systems can be improved. One quality improvement project our unit worked on concerned documentation and administration of vaccinations to patients who require the pneumonia and influenza vaccine. The work was important for a number of reasons: meeting Centers for Medicare and Medicaid Services requirements, preventing disease transmission, and improving a partially broken process.

Our unit worked in parallel with other task forces in order to improve the documentation process. A fun, creative process was designed to increase vaccination compliance rates. As the nurse educator, it was important for me to understand the reasons why such an important, simple task—such as giving a vaccination—was not occurring. Talking with staff and continuously receiving their input was vital in improving the system. After a few months, our unit, along with similar units, had increased the compliance rates to 100%, and compliance continues to remain high. This demonstrates that a well-planned change can help improve patient care on the unit.

Promoting Progressive Care Certification in Nursing

One of the unique accomplishments on our patient care unit has been promoting certification with the American Association of Critical Care Nurses' Progressive Care Certification (PCCN) examination. My nurse director and I agreed to make it a goal and a priority that our staff would successfully pass and maintain certification as the standard for our unit. We both understood, as certified nurses ourselves, the value and pride certification could bring to our unit, and hoped to lead by example. We believe that obtaining this certification builds confidence in the staff nurse and improves clinical competence. Soon after we presented the concept of certification, a staff nurse on the unit decided she would prepare for the examination. With her hard work and dedication, she passed. It was a joyous moment for the nurse, but for the entire staff as well.

Soon after, it felt like all of the nurses were knocking on our doors, asking for more resources. What books do I read? Am I ready for this certification examination yet? PCCN resources are limited, but we found a handful of helpful resources for the staff. Study groups were formed and test dates were chosen. The BWH Department of Nursing provides financial assistance for the examination costs and for yearly continuing education classes, but this did not appear to be what motivated our staff. The achievement of proving their knowledge to patients and staff seemed to be enough.

What has promoting certification done as far as outcomes on our unit? We have had nurses realize that they want to continue to learn in the classroom, and now many are enrolled in master's classes. Our patient satisfaction (Press-Ganey) scores are consistently high. Our quality scores for bad outcomes remain relatively low. Many of our nurses have become involved in nursing research and patient outcomes improvement projects. I am sure that staff nurses will continue their excitement in their journey toward certification. It demonstrates without a doubt that the staff nurses (the best staff) are providing the best care for their patients. As the educator, it makes me so proud that the staff independently, outside of work, took the time to further enhance their nursing practice.

Research Projects

The unit has been involved in numerous research projects over the years. A few years ago, leading nurse researcher Patricia Dykes invited our unit to become one of four sites for her research on fall prevention. As the nurse educator, I became the link between the nursing staff and the research team, and the advocate of the project with staff, helping to explain how important it was and why a fall prevention program could be so powerful. We selected three interested nurses to help keep the staff motivated. The falls project combined a well-known fall scale, interactive computer programming, and follow-through on accurate fall prevention signage. Fall prevention is a national nursing issue and our unit led the way in creating nursing driven changes and outcomes (see Chapter 14.3).

The program also paved the way for my three nurses and I to feel more involved in the research process. The nurses worked tirelessly on their first poster presentation. I accompanied the nurses to multiple national conferences focusing on falls and fall prevention. I was invited to speak at a citywide conference on the project and one of the staff nurses spoke at an informatics conference as well. These educational experiences helped me express to my nurses how nursing research can change practice. It showed them how rewarding poster presentations can be when nurses from other institutions continuously approach you and want to hear more about the research.

MY ROLE BEYOND MY UNIT

Part of my time is dedicated to committee work, task forces, and group meetings. It is important that nurse educators be active participants in these gatherings, where they can represent the voice of nursing, bringing the nursing perspective to the table. Other disciplines may not think the way nurses think about a specific issue.

Our nurse educator group meets monthly, as do the intermediate care nurse educators, and meetings are often filled with discussions about hospital-wide initiatives, new products, and practice updates. These meetings are important to attend, not only to remain informed, but also to assist in the outcome of projects, ensuring excellence in all our shared educational endeavors. These meetings provide opportunities to change the trajectory of a project if need be. We work collaboratively to achieve the best outcomes.

Nurse educators, led under the direction of two wonderful advisors, also attend a policy meeting twice monthly. Policy work is an important aspect of the educator role. Policies dictate practice. Staff nurses often turn to these policies when they encounter an unfamiliar procedure. The information that is provided must be accurate, clearly written, and regularly updated to stay current with practice standards. Integrating evidence-based practice into the policies improves the quality of care.

Our work as nurse educators is not only to write, rewrite, and present these policies, but also to make our staff aware of significant changes. I think it is important to speak with staff about policy meeting outcomes. It is interesting how these conversations often lead to another policy. Many staff do not realize that we can rework confusing sections or add more information to a policy. I find that sharing my work actually leads to improvements in other areas.

This chapter has focused on the role of the nurse educator on the patient care unit. Our institution also has nurse educators who work with us to help promote quality patient care. Many of the central nurse educators assist with the orientation of new staff. Others work with our computer systems and patient education materials. Many of these nurse educators have contributed to this book. They are considered part of the nurse educator family at BWH.

To truly encompass all the roles of the educator would take thousands of pages. Nurse educators work incredibly hard to make sure the staff nurses have all the knowledge they require at their fingertips. It is my hope that my description demonstrates that the role is complex and full of interesting pathways. The nurse educator role has certainly made enormous contributions to the nursing community at BWH. The vision of nursing would not be complete without the impact of a nurse educator.

22.2 Nurse Engagement: Rekindling the Passion

Cynthia F. Loring

What does it take to revive and re-energize a wilted workforce? In recent years the health care system has asked so much of nurses that some of them have lost the desire to give back, to invest, to engage in their practice. On Center for Women and Newborns (CWN) 10, we have provided an environment that promotes, rewards, and sustains nurse engagement. This is the story I would like to share.

INTRODUCTION

In 2005, I took the position of clinical nurse educator on CWN 10, a 30-bed postpartum/nursery unit. As I got to know the nursing staff, I had two impressions. First, the unit was blessed with an incredible depth of specialty knowledge and experience; many of our nurses had been working there for several years. Second, there was virtually no participation in professional activities beyond bedside nursing care, and very little appreciation of why such activities would be important. Typical remarks I heard from staff included statements such as these: "I don't see why we need to change the newborn documentation. What we have has worked for 20 years." "We're always running out of these supplies on weekends, but what's the point of complaining, it won't change anything." "The pediatricians tried to do a clinical research project a few years ago, but they couldn't get anyone to participate."

It was my sense that somehow these nurses had become disengaged, feeling that they were not active participants in shaping the work of the unit, that their voices were not being heard. The saving grace for me was that most of them were still very concerned about providing safe, competent care; educating families; and advocating for their patients. I knew that through this devotion to their patients, we could find the flame of passion that was burning low and reignite it. I also knew that this was a process that was going to take time and patience. Changing the culture of a work environment cannot happen overnight. I was fortunate, however, in being hired about the same time as our new chief nursing officer, Mairead Hickey, and it was clear that her focus was on culture change. I believed my efforts could be part of that larger organizational shift.

I also knew that there have been many studies supporting the notion that workplace environments where nurses do not feel empowered or engaged in their practice lead to staff burnout, poor staff retention, and (eventually) practices that negatively affect patient safety (Fasoli, 2010; Spence Laschinger & Leiter, 2006; Spence Laschinger, Wilk, Cho, & Greco, 2009). What could we do to reverse this trend on CWN 10? Again the literature was helpful to me in answering that question, indicating the elements that are crucial to staff engagement:

- Leadership that empowers (Kerfoot, 2007; Wong, Spence Laschinger, & Cummings, 2010)

■ Organizational structure that empowers (Freeney & Tieman, 2009; Simpson, 2009)
■ Coaching and mentoring (Harmon, Sey, Hiner, Faron, & McAdam, 2010; Locke, 2008)
■ Teamwork (Kalisch, Curley, & Stefanov, 2007)

BEGINNING THE CHANGE PROCESS

On CWN 10, my director and I started with modest first steps. We reinstituted monthly staff meetings on all three shifts, which we called practice group meetings. At these meetings we designated time for staff to bring to the table any issue that they wanted to discuss. We also scheduled time to present information and updates to the staff. After the meetings, we typed up the notes and made them available to the staff. We wanted to establish open communication, let the nurses know we were listening.

I began publishing a monthly newsletter for the unit, to make sure all staff were updated on and informed about changes happening on the unit and in the division. The newsletter was also a vehicle for raising staff awareness about standards of practice; our specialty organization, the Association of Women's Health, Obstetric and Neonatal Nurses (AWHONN); and recent clinical research that related to our patient population and practice. In addition, we used the newsletter to build a sense of team on the unit, by publishing examples of staff participation in professional activities and including pictures of the staff and unit in each issue.

Fortunately, concurrent with our first steps, over a span of 2 years, the leadership of Women and Newborn's Nursing and Clinical Services sponsored team training for all postpartum staff (nurses and support staff) from each of the three postpartum units. The clinical focus of this training was the management of postpartum hemorrhage; however, the fundamentals of team training were embedded in the program, and this experience became an important foundation for later initiatives that required teamwork.

A second concurrence was the impact of changes the Department of Nursing (DON) was implementing throughout the hospital. One of these initiatives was a focused effort to include staff nurses in work groups, team meetings, and standing committees. At first, these responsibilities sometimes were met with resistance from coworkers when an assignment required coverage for the nurse attending the meeting. But as staff began to see this kind of participation as an expectation instead of a burden, and eventually as an opportunity to have voice, the attitudes changed. Currently, approximately 20% of the unit staff are involved in committees and projects on all levels of the nursing organizational structure.

COACHING AND MENTORING

We were beginning to see our culture shift happening, and that shift led to more change. In early 2006, several nurses from all three shifts came to me individually to express concern about care of one our most vulnerable populations, the late preterm infant. The theme of concern was consistent: "The late preterm infants are 'mixed in' with the regular-term newborns in the nursery and I am afraid they are falling through the cracks."

This was the spark I had hoped for: a way to relate a real patient care issue to professional practice activities that would eventually improve patient care. This project had all the elements that could promote staff engagement:

- It was patient centered.
- The issue was brought forth by staff from all shifts.
- The staff brought the issue forth to the educator, in the hope that something would be done about it.
- This was, and still is, a topic of great concern to nurses and providers all over the country.
- This was not going to be solved with a quick fix; it was going to require a lot of staff time and effort.
- With the support of leadership, this project could be the starting point for practice change, clinical research, and professional presentations and publications by staff nurses.

Because the nurses themselves initiated this change, I assumed the role of mentor and coach. Bringing the staff nurses into the process of planned change and coaching them through the initial stages of participation and eventual change, implementation was accomplished using several strategies and messages:

- *Take action:*   I arranged a meeting with these nurses.
- *Validate the nurses' concerns:*   I assured them that they were not alone in their concern, that this is important, and a practice change is required to achieve best practice.
- *Acknowledge perceived challenges and staff resistance:*   I accepted the realities of the situation without judgment.
- *Make a study plan:*   I planned to review the literature to make sure that any proposed practice changes were evidence based. I modeled the appropriate first step in a professional approach to solving the problem.
- *Keep the patient's and family's welfare at the center of all discussions:*   I supported the values and vision that were shaping the BWH DON change process.
- *Be inclusive:*   Inform and collaborate with the rest of the unit staff, the other postpartum/nursery units, stakeholders, and any other interested parties in the division.
- *Reward accomplishments of the staff:*   I made certain that the positive behaviors were rewarded.

The process we collaboratively initiated is now in its fifth year. During that time, a core group of nurses has been involved in all of the late preterm infant projects that emerged from this staff concern. Table 22.2.1 lists the timeline of events associated with the late preterm infant initiative on CWN 10 and thus tracks the professional development of these nurses. Our research study on thermoregulation in the late preterm infant is a perfect example of how we were able to use the research process to engage staff nurses. Remarkably, this research study was conceived and completed by CWN 10 staff nurses. In addition, because this well-established group of staff nurses had been working on improving the care of the late preterm infant since 2006, they were recently asked to serve as part of the multidisciplinary effort to update the care of the late preterm infant throughout the division. Part of their

TABLE 22.2.1 *Late Preterm (LPT) Infant Initiatives on CWN 10: Task Force Accomplishments*

Year	Milestone	Professional Development
2005	Staff expressed concern	Validating staff concern
2006	Task force formed	Learning how to function as a task force
	Defined issues for LPT	Researching literature, standards of care
	Projects: crib cards, folders	Introducing practice change to staff
	Poster display in lobby	Sharing professional knowledge
	Joined other committees	Collaborating with other units/disciplines
2007	Nurse scientist hired	Consulting with research specialist
	Study question identified	Validating critical thinking
	Successful grant application	Learning how to obtain funding
	Poster display in lobby	Building on/sharing knowledge
2008	CITI training completed	Learning re protection of human subjects
	IRB proposal accepted	Learning re research protocols
	Paper presented, AWHONN	Appreciating professional organizations
2009	Research study started	Learning re recruiting subjects, informed consent, data collection
	Poster presented, AWHONN	Preparing for dissemination of findings
2010	Research paper presented at AWHONN	Presentation of original nursing research
	A new model of care for the late preterm infant	Interdisciplinary, divisional project collaboration
2011	Anticipating publication of research study in professional journal	Contribution to the body of nursing literature on care of the late preterm infant

mission is to involve as many staff as possible in the planning, every step of the way. Having learned from their own involvement, they are now engaging others in their process of rekindling.

FIVE YEARS LATER

Today, the CWN 10 staff has a new look. Nurses who were never involved in professional activities now are. Nurses whose first response to change was to reject it now contribute to the process of change. Our project to implement a new model of care for late preterm infants has incorporated input from all CWN 10 staff and has served to provide yet another avenue for participation. In the past, it had been difficult to find nurses who would participate in a work group or committee, or sometimes even give an opinion about a proposed change. That is not the case now. We continue to enjoy support from our unit and division leadership. Most importantly, the more the staff engage in the work of the unit, the more possibilities they see for improving practice. Typical remarks from staff now reflect this change: "I have noticed that we keep running out of this piece of equipment. How can we make sure there is a backup supply for the weekends?" "In the next news flyer, would you please remind the staff how to perform this assessment correctly?" "How are you doing on that research project? When will we know the results?" "How can I get onto a committee? I want to be involved."

CONCLUSION

Staff engagement is a necessary component of successful nursing practice. Ensuring this engagement is like caring for a garden: It needs constant attention and care. As educators and managers, this is one of our greatest challenges: to establish and maintain work environments where nurses can grow and thrive.

REFERENCES

Fasoli, D. (2010). The culture of nursing engagement: A historical perspective. *Nursing Administration Quarterly, 34*(1), 18–29.

Freeney, Y., & Tieman, J. (2009). Exploration of the facilitators of and barriers to work engagement in nursing. *International Journal of Nursing Studies, 46*(12), 1557–1565.

Harmon, K., Sey, R., Hiner, J., Faron, S., & McAdam, A. (2010). Successful nurse engagement: One health care system's story. *Nursing for Women's Health, 14*(1), 43–48.

Kalisch, B., Curley, M., & Stefanov, S. (2007). An intervention to enhance nursing staff teamwork and engagement. *Journal of Nursing Administration, 37*(2), 77–84.

Kerfoot, K. (2007). Staff engagement: It starts with the leader. *Urology Nursing, 27*(5), 451–452.

Locke, A. (2008). Developmental coaching: Bridge to organizational success. *Creative Nursing, 14*(3), 102–110.

Simpson, M. (2009). Predictors of work engagement among medical-surgical registered nurses. *Western Journal of Nursing Research, 31*(1), 44–65.

Spence Laschinger, H., & Leiter, M. (2006). The impact of nursing work environments on patient safety outcomes: The mediating role of burnout/engagement. *Journal of Nursing Administration, 36*(5), 259–267.

Spence Laschinger, H., Wilk, P., Cho, J., & Greco, P. (2009). Empowerment, engagement and perceived effectiveness in nursing work environments: Does experience matter? *Journal of Nursing Management, 17*(5), 636–646.

Wong, C., Spence Laschinger, H., & Cummings, G. (2010). Authentic leadership and nurses' voice behaviour and perceptions of quality of care. *Journal of Nursing Management, 18*(8), 889–900.

22.3 Brigham and Women's Hospital From a Nursing Instructor's View

Patricia Normandin

The purpose of this chapter is to highlight my experience as a nursing instructor at Brigham and Women's Hospital (BWH) over the past 5 years as the Department of Nursing (DON) has pursued a vision: *"Excellent care to patients and families, with the best staff, in the safest environment."* BWH has deep roots as an academic setting, and is internationally recognized as a leader in excellence in patient care. From my personal experience, however, I became convinced that BWH's commitment to the education and training of nurses had taken on new life and enthusiasm. In addition, evidence-based research was continually discussed and practiced by the BWH nurses.

They can "walk the walk" as they describe and create an environment of excellent care for patients and families from all walks of life. Early on, I noticed that Mairead Hickey, the chief nursing officer at BWH, was always visible and accessible to all staff nurses. It seemed to me that her vision and positive attitude toward the entire nursing staff was an essential foundation of nursing at BWH. Nursing leadership also welcomed and respected cultural and individual diversity in patients, families, and staff at BWH.

THROUGH THE EYES OF A NURSING INSTRUCTOR

For me, the Center for Nursing Excellence (CNE) clinical and administrative staff provide a glimpse through the window of BWH. As a large academic, tertiary care hospital, BWH's responsibility to ensure proper credentials and expertise of nursing instructors can be a daunting assignment. The CNE staff is charged with credentialing not only nursing instructors but also every nursing student. Before students are approved to give care at BWH, they must complete mandatory educational training that includes confidentiality rules and computer access protocols. The CNE staff are the foundation for successful experiences for nursing instructors and students. I have developed a deep appreciation for their professionalism and tireless work to ensure a smooth transition for the instructors and nursing students. Most recently, they have streamlined the credentialing process of nursing instructors, which is a welcome change. I feel that no matter how busy they may be with orchestrating the student nursing experiences, the key principles of providing high-quality and safe patient care are always at the forefront.

Being a nursing instructor at BWH gives me behind-the-scenes knowledge of the daily caring and collaboration by all disciplines. The friendliness, professionalism, and warmth displayed by the secretaries and personal care assistants on each unit make me feel like I am working among family. The information desk personnel, receptionists, housekeeping staff, security, nursing, technicians, and physicians all display BWH's dedication to patients.

My nursing students make me smile. I feel proud that I am their nursing instructor; it is truly my pleasure and honor. In preparation for writing this chapter, I reread the student nurses' journal reports related to their learning experiences at BWH. I did this to give readers the opportunity to see the high quality of student nurse precepting and patient care through the eyes of student nurses learning from their preceptors, guided by the BWH's nursing vision of professional excellence.

The influence of Florence Nightingale is our nursing foundation. As a nursing instructor, I feel it is important to reflect on the values of BWH in relation to Florence Nightingale's principles that still hold true today. She stated that the very first requirement in a hospital is that it should do no harm. Student nurses experience this principle through BWH's collaboration among multiple disciplines during patient care rounds on the different units. As I reflect on this principle of Florence Nightingale's, I see it expressed in hospital hygiene, sanitation, and a strong emphasis on evidence-based practice grounded in statistical knowledge. I feel that BWH exemplifies Florence Nightingale's beliefs and goes beyond them.

Cultural diversity within BWH staff and patients is embraced and recognized under the new nursing leadership. Student nurses have the opportunity to actively engage in learning opportunities that recognize cultural diversity. Nursing students and their instructors are also invited to the many educational offerings provided by BWH.

NURSING STUDENT EXEMPLARS

As a nursing instructor, I am able to witness in practice BWH's mission, vision, and values through descriptions in my student nurses' clinical journals. After each clinical experience my students e-mail to me journal entries describing their experiences. It is one way for me to hear about their experiences and plan appropriate teaching responses. These exemplars are from a few of my nursing students' experiences on a Center for Women and Newborns postpartum unit.

"I had a great clinical day! My postpartum patient was a woman who is a multi gravida from Santa Domingo. She is homeless and an illegal immigrant. Social services and her nurses were making arrangements for her and her daughter. It was great to see these processes and services in place." In fact, this particular student went on to write her required research paper on the many barriers involved when caring for homeless women. This is a good example of what makes me love teaching nursing at BWH.

Another student nurse wrote: "My nurse 'A' was fantastic. I made a point to tell her that I could help her if she needed it with other patients too, so she grabbed me to help with the perineal care of another patient. That was interesting, because as simple as it seems now, I had never thought before about how to actually remove the underwear of a woman who had a Foley catheter. If I'd come across that on my own I probably would have taken the tube out of her instead of passing the underwear all the way down the tube and over the bag!" This example demonstrates how this BWH nurse not only provided high-quality, safe patient care, but also gave a student a valuable and practical experience.

One student nurse wrote: "I also had trouble getting the baby's heart rate. I felt like it was beating so fast. The nurse in the nursery told us that it is a skill that just comes with experience so I'll definitely have to practice listening to more infant heart rates. The nurse in the nursery was very friendly and receptive to having students." This is another thread that I have found in my student journals, as they share how BWH nurses integrate their work with students needs, are supportive, and thus maintain strong academic partnerships.

The following student nurses' journals describe experiences while on BWH Towers units. "I want to start off my journal entry by writing how much I like my nurse 'S' and the unit I am on. I have had a great experience here so far. The nurses have been nothing less than nice and supportive. Even other nurses on the unit approach me and ask if I am okay or needed help with anything. If given the opportunity, I would definitely consider working at BWH."

"Today I worked a 12-hour day shift, 7 AM to 7 PM, with 'C.' We had three patients, one of which I had the previous shift on 8A and overall we had an excellent day. I am truly getting the hang of assessing which patients I should see first, pass medications to first, and my mornings have been flowing well. I have been organizing my time nicely and I am generally caught up between 9 AM and 10 PM."

This same student nurse wrote: "For nursing core competencies I saw leadership this shift when the charge nurse determined we were over staffed and she decided to float one nurse to another floor and another nurse got to go home at 3 PM. I saw evidence-based practice when a nurse utilized proper procedure in removing a Foley catheter by letting the 10-cc balloon empty on its own into the 10-cc syringe. I saw safety when I made sure every patient's bed was in its low and locked position and that the call bell was within reach every time I left one of my patient's rooms. I saw informatics utilized when one of the nurses on the floor printed out a strip from the monitor for one of her patients who was on telemetry monitoring and she analyzed the strip to determine if her patient was in normal sinus rhythm. Overall this was a very good shift. I had 'C,' my nurse, go over how to measure out the wave PR, RS, and RT intervals [wave intervals on the monitor strip] and that was very good practice. I am looking forward to my last few shifts and am very happy with my experience on this floor thus far!"

The following paragraphs are from a nursing student's journals regarding her experiences in the Shapiro building. My nursing student was fortunate to have "H" as her preceptor. Her journal shows the magnitude of learning, application, and synthesis of her learning experience, a slight glimpse into the phenomenal facilitation of learning that occurs daily by the nursing staff with student nurses and patients at BWH.

"The four competencies I used today are: Patient-Centered Care, Informatics, Safety, and Quality Improvement. Patient-Centered Care was demonstrated with the patient in recognizing and trying to respect his desire to be left alone. I tried to cluster his care as much as possible and was able to check in on him often enough because he had medication due every 2–3 hours. If I happened to be walking past his room I would peek in to make sure he was okay but didn't say anything. Informatics was utilized when I used the computer to look up medications I was not familiar with before handing them out to my patients. By doing this I was able to safely distribute anti-rejection medication. In this case the safety was for me too because some of the pills should not be handled by women of childbearing years without gloves because they are teratogenic. Quality Improvement fits into today in a different way. When teaching patients about their medications, one of the better ways to teach is to bring all the medications into the room and allow the patient to choose which pills to take when. Unfortunately, TJC [the Joint Commission] does not allow this so the back-up plan is to have the patient keep a log and have pictures of their pills. Given the situation that we could not use the best teaching method, we went to the next best option. This seemed to be working. This was a great day and I was very excited to have a heart transplant patient. I learned a lot today and was able to experience new things. I pulled out my first central line and watched chest tubes pulled for the first time as well as external wires. I have been very fortunate to be placed on this floor and everyone has been very pleasant and willing to help me and teach me."

Because, as a nursing instructor, I am grateful for all the time and commitment the nursing staff give my students, I encourage the students to give back to the staff nurses. Cultural diversity recognition and active learning of specific traditions of the different cultures of the patients we care for are competencies I incorporate into my teaching with all my clinical groups. One group of Simmons College students developed a rich collection of professional information on how to provide culturally competent care for women and their families from diverse cultures. At the end of their clinical rotation, they gave the collection to the nurses on the unit where they had clinical rotation. Another group of Simmons College students developed, with my help, an in-depth report on cultural considerations when caring for Chinese women and their families. This report was published in BWH's in-house nursing newsletter in February 2008.

OBSERVATIONAL EXPERIENCES

One of the reasons I love nursing and being a nursing instructor at BWH is that the opportunities and possibilities for observational experiences are endless. I think the opportunity my nursing students have to observe in different areas is phenomenal. Each area provides unique learning opportunities. These learning opportunities display BWH's core values and demonstrate to my students the interdisciplinary relationships that are crucial to ensuring safe, reliable, evidence-based nursing care. I have made so many good friends that my professional colleagues seem like family. I teach my students that when they are in the clinical setting or observational areas, they always should look and act professional. I teach them that they are to be respectful and act as you would if you were a guest in someone's home.

My students have the opportunity to observe cutting-edge health care orchestrated like beautiful music. They have observed state-of-the-art mammography, maternal-fetal medicine procedures, caesarean sections, and high-risk antepartum testing. Other nursing students have had the opportunity to observe radiation oncology procedures, surgical procedures, and cardiac catheterizations. The nursing students have had observational learning experiences in multiple intensive care units, including the neuroscience, surgical, medical, cardiac, and burn/trauma units. I have developed close friendships with many of my professional BWH colleagues who have been gracious enough to precept and mentor these future nurses.

NURSING INSTRUCTOR IMPLICATIONS

In the past 5 years as a nursing instructor, I have seen increased professionalism and infusion of evidence-based practice at BWH; evidence-based professional nursing practice is always in the forefront. My nursing students and I have been invited to many educational offerings. Nursing students have witnessed firsthand various evidence-based nursing projects or changes in policy related to new scientific information. World-renowned physicians work at BWH and always take time to discuss current scientific evidence or new procedures with my nursing students. Teaching at BWH stimulates learning and student inquiry concerning nursing practice and the highest quality of nursing care.

Nursing research has blossomed under the new nursing leadership. The nursing staff consistently provide an academic teaching environment that fosters vision and the values of the nursing. Personally, I feel there are no limitations for a nursing instructor at BWH. I only wish there were more hours in the day and I could clone myself to be able to teach on multiple nursing units.

CONCLUSION

BWH'S professional nursing growth in the past 5 years has provided me with many professional nursing instructor opportunities. Evidence-based research is the key to learning, and it is professionally rewarding to be involved in the cutting edge of health care and nursing where this key is valued. The DON's vision of *excellent care to patients and families, with the best staff, in the safest environment* is exemplified daily in my experiences at BWH. I am honored to be a nursing instructor in this world-renowned academic teaching hospital.

Beyond Our Borders

23.1 *His Name Is Samuel*

Patricia C. Powers

I was flattered to be asked to write a nursing narrative about my experiences in Haiti. Although I have told my story of Haiti many times, it has been difficult to put the most life-changing 2 weeks of my life onto paper. There are just too many heart-wrenching stories that should be told. Where do I begin? I could describe the exhilaration we as nurses felt about the newborn baby we saved. Or I could describe the despair we felt as we carried a young girl back to her tent on a stretcher post-op, knowing that she would wake to the news that her leg must be amputated. Perhaps the account of the woman who was 8 months pregnant with bilateral lower leg fractures, who would not consent to a below-the-knee amputation for 2 days until she understood that her unborn baby's life was at stake, best illustrates my Haiti experience. I now find myself ashamed that I do not even remember her name or know her fate, yet I cried with this woman and operated on her twice.

Maybe individual stories are simply inadequate and I could describe the utter and total destruction I witnessed in Port au Prince. However, the written word cannot properly describe the smells of the mass graves burning, or the sounds of the suffering—the wails of family members who lost a loved one—throughout the city.

Therefore, it seems that the best way to tell my story is to start at the beginning, when I realized that I was going to do my job as a nurse no matter the circumstances. It was in my first 12 hours in Haiti that I met Samuel, and he gave me the confidence that I could do what I needed to do as a nurse to help the Haitian people.

I had been in Port au Prince for less than 12 hours and was standing inside one of the few remaining standing structures at Haiti University General Hospital waiting to speak with the nursing supervisor, Mrs. Thompson, a quake survivor herself. The entrance had a wrought-iron gate and was being manned by a guard. Beyond the gate was the yard, or "Forest" as we would call it in the coming days. The Forest was where hundreds of patients, all in need of urgent medical care, were lying on the grass with tarps draped from tree to tree to protect them from the hot Haitian sun.

Suddenly there was a very loud noise like an airplane or helicopter overhead. The noise got louder and people started to run toward the gate. I felt myself being pushed up against the wrought-iron gate and just when I was about to panic, the gate burst open and I was pushed outside. I soon learned that the noise was not an airplane but a strong aftershock.

As I stood outside trying to regain my composure and digest what had just happened, a young man with panic in his eyes grabbed my arms and gestured for me to follow him. I followed him around the corner and he pointed to an emaciated man on the ground, lying on a makeshift cardboard stretcher. As I got down on my knees, the young man pointed to his leg that was covered with a blanket.

I removed the blanket and was immediately hit with the smell of gangrene. The leg was black all the way up to the knee; bone was visible with flies engulfing the wound. It was immediately clear that the man would need an amputation, and by the looks of him we could only hope it was not too late to save his life. As I worked to orient myself and get the sick man some help, a reporter from the *Miami Herald* introduced himself and told me that he spoke Creole. As I got down on my knees and took the patient's hand, I asked the reporter if he could tell the patient that my name was Trish, I was a nurse, and I was going to try to help him. I watched as the reporter told him this. The man squeezed my hand, communicating that he understood.

I then asked the reporter to ask him his name. The reporter asked the question and the man replied, in English, "Samuel." Through the reporter, I told Samuel it was a pleasure to meet him and that we were going to transfer him to where the doctors could take a look at him. We carried him to where we were instructed. I went inside the tent and asked if there was a doctor who could come take a look at the patient I had outside, since I thought he needed urgent attention. I brought a doctor over to the makeshift stretcher, got down on my knees, and lifted the blanket so that he could see the leg. I looked up and he stated, "That leg needs to be amputated!"

The doctor ordered the people who had helped me carry him and told them to bring Samuel over to the OR immediately so that they could amputate—and started to walk away. I stayed down on my knees, grabbed Samuel's hand, and asked the reporter if he could translate for me and he agreed. I told Samuel that he needed to have his leg amputated because it was infected. I told him that if his leg was not amputated, the infection would go to the rest of his body and would kill him. I asked Samuel if we had his permission to do the life-saving surgery and, as he started to cry, he agreed.

The doctor was impatient to do the surgery and yelled at us to "get him in here now!" I answered the doctor as calmly as I could: "His name is Samuel and he consents to have his leg amputated." I squeezed Samuel's hand, and asked the reporter to tell him I was sorry he had to have his leg amputated and that I would pray for him.

I never saw Samuel again, but I think of him often when I look back on my days in Haiti and hope and pray he recovered from his ordeal. As they carried Samuel away, I thought to myself, "I may not have all the material things that I need here in Haiti, such as gloves, drugs, instruments, or state-of-the-art facilities, but what I do have is what I've had my whole nursing career: compassion for my patients and a desire to give each one the best care possible no matter the circumstances."

23.2 *Lessons Learned in Haiti*

Elizabeth A. Samson

On January 12, 2010, an earthquake with a 7.0 magnitude hit the country of Haiti. More than 250,000 people were killed, more than 350,000 were injured, and more than 1,000,000 people lost their homes. The people of Haiti were desperate and called out for help—and the world responded.

Seven days later, I was aboard a private plane along with 14 other people, all but one strangers, to begin a medical relief tour in Port au Prince. We arrived in the dead of night to our makeshift tent-city homes. We laid out our sleeping bags on the concrete ground and tried to sleep.

The next day we arrived at the Port au Prince hospital to find chaos. There were people everywhere trying to help the thousands of people who were lying around on makeshift beds, on the ground, or on cots, needing help. There were people in every space and even more outside the hospital, looking for medical attention. Even with health care people from all over the world ready and willing to work, we still needed to find supplies to do surgeries, change dressings, and so on. While we waited for supplies, I decided to do the next best thing. I realized quickly that my job was to do whatever was needed of me at the time. Soon, I began to unload the supply trucks, help transport people to makeshift operating rooms or wards as they were made available, to play with the boys and girls who were looking for a friend, or to pray with the people looking for comfort. My service was to be more than a nurse: It was to be a compassionate multitasker and do whatever was needed.

Many people ask me about my experience in Haiti and why I went. I worked closely with more than 40 people from Haiti every day, each one directly affected by the earthquake. Still, as much as I would like to share my experiences about what I witnessed in Haiti, it is difficult to do so. I can sum it up this way: It was like combining some of the most horrific pieces of history. The way we had to operate was like a scene from Vietnam. The amount of death was like an image from a concentration camp. The destruction was like that of 9/11. And when you use all your senses, as you imagine these images, you get a small glimpse of what is was like, and is still today, for many Haitian people.

What I would like to share with you about my trip to Haiti is what I learned.

1. Teamwork. I believe that teamwork is vital in anything we do. Without all of us working together, no mission could be truly accomplished to its fullest potential. It did not matter that we were strangers, or that we all spoke different languages, or that we came from different walks of life; we pulled together to do what was needed to make the most impact and get the job done.

2. Resilience. I was amazed by the Haitian community's resilience to move forward. Each day as we drove through Port au Prince, I noticed change, people trying to rebuild, going to work, and trying to return to life before the quake. Many people still slept in the streets next to their homes that were destroyed. They wanted to reclaim their property or, even worse, their dead. Many tried to get back to work to support their families. Living on $2.00 a day just got worse with limited water, scarce food, and no jobs to make money. Try to imagine that: If we just did not drink our Dunkin Donuts coffee for a day, we could feed a whole family.

   3. *Faith.*   Each day we not only did surgeries, but did dressing changes on the people we had operated on. Without the use of much pain medication, we had to improvise—use general anesthesia, if we were lucky—to put them at rest so we could change their dressings. One day I was changing a young woman's dressing; her leg was badly damaged and she was in a lot of pain. We were surrounded by people who were crying and screaming in pain. It was very nerve-wracking for both of us. A young woman came into the tent and began singing a hymn in a low voice. Within minutes we were able to change the dressings and the patients were singing with her.

   When this patient was regaining consciousness, I thought she was scream-ing. I was concerned about her pain. Through a translator, I asked if she needed anything. The translator informed me that she was praying, not in pain. She was asking me if I believed in Jesus and telling me what a wonderful man he was; how great he was. She was thankful that he saved her during this earthquake. She was not angry with him that she had lost most of her family or her house. She believed that they would rebuild and that they all would be safe. To say I was awestruck is an understatement. The amount of faith the Haitian people showed me was amazing. From praying and thanking me daily for helping them, to watching them pray and sing every night in the parks, I could see that their faith was unshaken.

   I will share one other story with you. On my first day at the hospital, we helped a mother and her 3-hour-old daughter. The daughter was in distress and needed to be transported to the Navy ship to seek medical attention from the pediatricians onboard. In the late hours of the night, we were able to accomplish that task. What we could not do was bring the mother with the baby. For the next 12 days, she asked me daily, through a translator, where her daughter was. Even though I felt confident enough that the daughter was still safe and alive aboard the ship, I was unsure. This mother cried herself to sleep every night, wondering if she would ever be able to see her baby again. Even though there were many people who worked on her baby that night, it was me that she and the local Haitian physician depended upon to take care of this baby and reunite her with her mother. I would ask many people in charge of this disaster relief to find out where the baby was. I tried des-perately to get them reunited. Each day was a challenge. It was not that people did not want to help me find the baby; it was that there was so much to do and no one knew where to start. Finally, I took matters into my own hands. I hounded the 82nd Airborne daily to help me find out if the baby was on board the ship and still alive. I borrowed a phone from a colleague and placed a call back to a friend in the United States. I met this friend, 19 years ago, while giving birth to my son Zachary, as his wife was giving birth to his son Jonathan.

   I asked for his help by having him call his cousin, Admiral Fitzgerald, the second in command of the Navy, and see if he could find out any information for me. (The ship, the *Comfort*, was a Navy-run floating hospital in the Port au Prince harbor.) Unsure if this would work, I prayed. Within 10 hours, the admiral's assistant, Cindy, who was on a ship in the harbor, contacted me. She helped me find the baby on one of her ships. The next day, together with the men and women of the 82nd Airborne, we found a way to get the mom and baby reunited. The mom, who was discharged from the hospital with little hope that I could help her find her baby, was called back. When she arrived, we put her on an ambulance to the helicopter pad where the Navy would later take her to the ship her daughter was on. I put her on a helicopter with only faith that the Navy would help her find her daughter on the ship. Four days later, I received a picture of them together, which confirmed their reunion.

Teamwork, faith, resilience! Mother Marlana and baby Angela are now a family. They are Haiti's future.

We all live very busy lives. We wake at early hours to come to work. We work long hours and then go home to our busy families. Life is a very fast roller coaster to many of us. I ask you to slow down. Take the time to meet your patients, to realize that being a nurse to them may involve more than our basic skills and services we do each and every day. Take the time to find out about them and help their whole body heal.

What I will tell you is that if you go into work with your mind open and willing to help at any cost and to do whatever is needed, you will be rewarded 100 times over by your sense of accomplishment. Later in life, you may find out that this meeting today helped you do something great even 20 years later. You may even meet someone who will tell you a story of their life and a hardship. You may find out that this 1 day of work was the day that changed someone's life.

23.3 *The Global Health Nursing Fellowship: Beginnings*

Patrice K. Nicholas

The Global Health Nursing Fellowship (GHNF) was a central initiative of the Brigham and Women's (BWH) Department of Nursing (DON) in collaboration with the Division of Global Equity, managed by the Center for Nursing Excellence (CNE). It was designed both to bring BWH nursing expertise to developing countries and to give BWH nurses an opportunity to experience clinical rotations and expand nursing's role in global interdisciplinary care projects. As Director of Global Health and Academic Partnerships in the CNE, I had the opportunity firsthand to see this initiative take shape.

The GHNF program formally began in 2008 when we deployed our first nurse mentor, Emily Hall, to Rwinkwavu, Rwanda, the primary site of a Partners in Health (PIH) project as implementing partner to the Clinton Foundation HIV/AIDS Initiative. Her role in the program was to facilitate and guide nurse fellows as they were introduced to Rwinkwavu Hospital and set goals for their fellowship. Emily quickly established strong connections upon her arrival in Rwanda. Her first 6 months were spent learning about the many aspects of the project, establishing relationships with the clinical staff, and planning for the first nurse fellow from BWH. This introductory period was key to assessing needs in clinical care areas and determining how an experienced clinician could best be utilized.

We created a rigorous screening process and attracted several qualified applicants to be our first GHN Fellow. In June 2008 we announced our inaugural fellowship recipient, Kate Sullivan, a certified midwife with more than 30 years of experience in patient care and education. Three months later, she arrived in Rwinkwavu, eagerly welcomed by staff. Though there are frequent clinical visitors to Rwinkwavu who contribute to patient care and mentor clinicians, this was a rare event in the maternity department.

Kate accomplished many things during her first 3 months, which were primarily spent in Rwinkwavu. She attended many births and was able to get an accurate understanding of clinical decision-making techniques and the care methods being used. Kate provided feedback to PIH leadership about equipment and staffing needs in the department, advocating for better resources and extra hands when a number of nurses were on maternity leave. These actions helped the department in the short term, but also modeled behaviors that will serve these nurses in the long term. Nurses make up the majority of health care clinicians in rural settings in Rwanda, and Kate was able to show how they might better advocate for themselves, both to increase resources and, over time, to demonstrate their readiness for leadership positions in health care systems.

Kate gradually began focusing on training goals she had identified as vitally important. Postpartum hemorrhage is a major risk for women delivering children in rural settings. Maternal mortality is high in areas where women experience poorly managed, prolonged labors and where there are no operating rooms, staff, and equipment to do cesarean sections when necessary. Kate identified two potential nursing actions responsive to this problem and focused training efforts on them. The first was the safe and appropriate use of an underutilized medication that can prevent blood loss in postpartum women. The second was the use of a safe and easy manual technique to stop postpartum bleeding. These concepts were taught through a combination of classroom training and clinical mentoring during patient cases. Kate's dynamism and her extensive knowledge of maternity care allowed her to be creative in her approach to training her Rwandan colleagues.

After the initial 3-month period of her fellowship, Kate began to split her time among the three hospitals where PIH was engaged. Her early experiences informed her approach to these other facilities and enabled her interventions. At Kirehe District Hospital, Kate attended weekly clinical meetings, which gave her a forum to raise important issues and learn about the day-to-day challenges the maternity department faced. Kirehe Hospital is a new facility, and many of the nurses working in the maternity department were new to the area and to PIH. Kate provided initial support to those nurses as they transitioned and provided feedback to the medical director about their needs.

The Burera District Hospital is the newest PIH facility in Rwanda, having opened just 6 months before Kate arrived in Rwanda. With the help of a Burera-based obstetrician, Kate facilitated a 3-day training course for the maternity nurses working in the clinics surrounding the hospital. The course provided an overview of concepts and skills used to manage women in the late stages of labor that can help prevent adverse outcomes, such as the need for cesarean sections. Kate focused on rural clinic nurses in order to better manage labor at the clinics and detect warning signs for timely and appropriate referrals. Kate emphasized practical guidance so the nurses could quickly transfer the concepts introduced in the training setting into their clinical care setting.

The contributions our first Global Health Nursing Fellow made to Rwinkwavu Hospital and the maternity programs at PIH facilities throughout Rwanda were invaluable in terms of patient care, training, and system improvement. Kate's success demonstrated to us that this innovative program met our goals with positive outcomes for the fellow, the participating institutions, and most compellingly, the patients in Rwanda.

24

Why Do People Aspire to Work at Brigham and Women's Hospital? A View From Business Services

Leo F. Buckley, Jr.

For 15 years, I have occupied, both literally and figuratively, an extraordinary vantage point from which to observe the comings and goings of hundreds of Brigham and Women's (BWH) clinical care staff. As Executive Director of Business Services for Patient Care Services (PCS) and the Department of Nursing (DON), my office is situated in the center of the PCS and Nursing Administration suite. Each day a steady stream of staff nurses, nursing directors, operations supervisors, and patient care assistants can be found passing by or stopping in my office on their respective ways to obtain shift assignments, participate in departmental meetings, schedule appointments with nursing leadership, attend entry and exit interviews, or simply offer a quick hello. In addition, my job portfolio and committee assignments place me in strategic and daily contact with clinical staff, hospital administrators, and union representatives as we strive to create respectful partnerships through which the very best patient- and family-centered care can be achieved. In my work as co-chair of the Nursing Recruitment and Retention Committee, as well as in my collaborative efforts with executive leadership and nursing executive directors on issues such as budgets and staffing, I have been granted the privilege of a front-row seat from which to make a few observations about the changes we have all shaped during the past 5 years, and what makes this institution so special.

One of the most impressive hallmarks of BWH, I believe, is its attractiveness as a place of employment for those searching to make a difference in the world of health care. People aspire to work at BWH because of its well-earned reputation for providing quality care to patients, accompanied by compassionate support to patients' families; it has been recognized by *U.S. World & News Report*, *Becker's Hospital Review,* and *The Leapfrog Group* as one of the premier hospitals in the United States. BWH employees take great pride in their work and many have shared with me the feeling that they consider themselves "blessed" to have had the opportunity to make a personal contribution to the outstanding legacy of care that the hospital has carefully nurtured and developed over the years. Our employees are proud to tell people that they work at a top-notch academic medical center positioned at the cutting edge of health care.

Fortunate to have what I consider to be an unparalleled clinical staff, BWH has little trouble recruiting or retaining competent employees. The hospital rewards its employees with extremely generous and competitive compensation and benefits packages. Staff contributions and achievements are regularly spotlighted throughout the year with various award and recognition programs. An annual Nurse Recognition Week is celebrated each May, culminating in a formal dinner reception held to honor the recipient of and finalists for the Essence of Nursing Award.

In addition to recognizing the professional achievements of its staff, BWH strongly encourages its employees to further their educational and professional development and provides a very generous tuition reimbursement program to support this goal. To further facilitate staff's participation in lifelong learning, BWH has entered into academic partnerships with several area colleges that provide access to nursing degree programs that include an option for direct payment of tuition. This creative structure, which I had an opportunity to help develop and implement, allows nurses enrolled in either undergraduate or graduate-level studies to have monies from their annual professional development stipends paid directly to the institution in which they are enrolled, thereby eliminating initial out-of-pocket payments (which ordinarily would be reimbursed at the conclusion of courses) and streamlining the administrative paperwork associated with the tuition payment process. For those staff members not enrolled in degree programs, the Nursing Department encourages staff to use the annual professional development funds for training seminars, professional conferences, and certification.

A logical consequence of BWH's significant investment in the professional development of its staff is its equally determined commitment to employing state-of-the-art health care technology in providing the best patient care possible, thereby making this acute medical center second to none. One example of this commitment has been the expansion of the Electronic Medication Administration Record application to all inpatient units. The purpose of this application is to ensure that the right dose of the right medication is dispensed to the right patient, by the right route, at just the right time. By staying abreast of advancements in health care technology and having the opportunity to use the latest technology, BWH nurses simultaneously raise the standards of care and find more time to be present for their patients.

Clinical experience at BWH prepares staff for professional advancement, opens them up to a world of career possibilities, and can influence virtually every sphere of life itself. Staff members are constantly challenged to learn something new every day and are provided exposure to a diverse range of clinical issues. Part of the prestige of practicing nursing at an institution with the name recognition of BWH is the opportunity to care for patients with complex medical conditions. This is the greatest experience a nurse can hope for on the journey to becoming an expert clinician. Supported by a strong preceptor program, clinical education at the unit level, and instructional opportunities in the Center for Nursing Excellence, the BWH staff member is counted among the very best of health care professionals.

The greatest evidence to illustrate why people aspire to work at BWH comes from the patient care community itself, both past and present. Gert Glode, RN, began her career in 1951 at what was then known as the Robert Breck Brigham Hospital. Today, at 92 years young, Gert returns regularly to BWH to visit the friends and the institution she has loved for more than half a century. When I asked Gert what she most cherished about her time at the hospital, she noted the great satisfaction she felt in knowing so many staff members by name. After many years as a staff nurse and manager, Gert rounded out her service at BWH as a hospital volunteer and, in the days before direct deposit, as the official distributor of nursing employee paychecks. It was then that she truly got to know everyone by name! Detta Quigley-Lavoie, RN, recently retired as nurse manager of the Gynecology/Oncology unit in the Center for Women and Newborns after more than 30 years of service to BWH. Detta noted, "I believe that my confidence in providing care was due in great part to the fact that this was Brigham and Women's Hospital, and here, all the support and guidance I needed was readily available." Furthermore, after many years as a staff nurse, Detta was delighted to find that accepting a position in nursing leadership did not signal the end of her involvement with patient care: "I found that it was not patient detached at all, and that frequently I could influence a whole unit practice as opposed to just a few patients." In a final example, Leigh Bozzi, RN, a recent newly licensed nurse, commented, "I worked at the Brigham before I went to nursing school and during it. I knew from the start that obstetrical nursing was my passion and that it was the field I was meant to be in. People I admired mentored me, supported me, and believed in me. During those years there were staff members who went out of their way to teach me. I saw what these people did, how they did it, and witnessed firsthand how good they were at doing it. I am proud to say that I became a BWH nurse!"

While some might point to its international reputation or national ranking, and others to its history of clinical excellence and innovation, a strong argument could be made that what really attracts health care professionals to BWH is much more personal. It's the opportunity to work among colleagues whose passion for patient care and service to others is not just a job, but a life's work. How else can one explain the need to establish a waiting list for the surplus number of staff members volunteering to be deployed as rescue workers in the aftermath of the 2010 earthquake in Haiti? Whether it's donating benefit time to a colleague on a leave of absence because of illness, or rallying support for the 115 members of "Team Brigham" as they train, fund-raise for, and run in the Boston Marathon to raise half a million dollars for community health programs, at BWH the proof is in the people.

In the end, there's a pretty simple answer to the question of why people aspire to work at BWH. It's an opportunity to provide unrivaled patient care, alongside the most qualified and best-prepared clinicians the health care community has to offer, in a world-class institution whose leadership values, supports, and nurtures the professional expertise of its staff. But it's also something more: It's a chance to work side-by-side with those who see health care not as a way to make a living, but as a way to live one's life.

The author extends thanks to David McMahon, who provided input into this chapter.

PART FOUR

Summary and Conclusions: The Journey Continues

25

Lessons Learned:
The Journey Through the Rearview Mirror

Phyllis Beck Kritek

Many authors in this book would tell you, some bemusedly, that I campaigned for this book. As an observer of the change process Mairead Hickey set in motion, I had amassed reasons to do so. I was then, and am now even more, convinced that we need to hear the voice of practice more often in our literature; that our students should be studying, at least part of the time, from textbooks that tell the story of nursing as lived and reported by those actually doing the work of nursing. They tell a story that only they can tell. I believe this book validates my conviction.

I also believe that if we want the voice of nursing to be heard, we have to become intentional about that desire. We have to create the opportunities and support systems necessary for nurses to find voice, to master the use of voice, and to do whatever is necessary to get the story out. We have to be persistent, insistent, and focused. We have to be in it for the long slog. Brigham and Women's Hospital (BWH) was willing to make that investment. And again, I believe this book validates my conviction.

The insistence on attending to nursing voice is purposeful first out of simple justice: Nurses have the right to be heard. There are other reasons, however, in some ways equally compelling. Nurses also have something important to say. Nursing voice exercised, and heard, creates change. That change, as this book documents, improves patient care and creates healthier work environments. Nurses have grounded their self-definition and their code of ethics in patient advocacy. We may want voice first for ourselves, but most nurses also know that it is essential to the delivery of quality health care. Our patients count on it. And once more, I believe this book validates my conviction.

Taken as a composite, I think this book offers some key messages to its readers, in particular, nurse leaders overseeing change processes (which is pretty much every nurse), and nursing students, particularly those in graduate programs. Although the book is rich in information, the key messages speak more to our communal search for wisdom. Economy counts. I list these messages, words of wisdom, for your consideration.

1. Find the Good. Nurses are natural problem solvers. It is what we do, and I think we do it singularly well. Hence, when we want to create a change, we tend to direct our gaze to the problems we want to address, the ones we anticipate, the ones we fear. Mairead's approach was in this sense counterintuitive. She started with a search for what was good in the organization. She saw this as her richest resource and her best point of departure. She built on it. Most organizational development experts would affirm this decision, yet it is rarely made and acted upon. The outcomes tell the story.

2. *Know the Context.*   The process of change was grounded in a prior assessment of the context for the change, both at the institutional and the departmental levels. The ideological drift toward change as an idea rather than an embedded process leaves many good ideas adrift—or dead. By assessing context, planned change proceeded with a nuanced sensitivity to the forces surrounding, and yes, resisting the process. Context provides the guidelines for balancing the inherent tensions between the ideal and the pragmatic. Context counts.

3. *Synergy Succeeds.*   Early change theories posited a linear process, and that mindset has shaped many ill-fated change efforts. Chaos theory offers a more robust, promising, and realistic approach, where the minute-to-minute shifts in all the relevant forces in a field are seen not as problems but as opportunities. Keeping all the balls in the air is not easy, but it works. Rather than using a step-by-step process, this change experience catalyzed numerous processes, stood back and let them feed one another, capitalized on gains in one place to further the process in another, built on success. Interestingly, roadblocks in one venue became catalysts for others. Seeing the whole is always more informative than obsessing about the parts. The "we" is inherently more creative than the "I."

4. *Relationships Trump Policies.*   We in nursing have a great affection for our policy manuals, hoping they will provide roadmaps to the "one right way." Policy is important, even critical; however, it will only take one so far, then it stalls. *People* create change, and relationships are the arena where people, individually, in groups, and throughout a department or institution, shape one another's responses. Creative and constructive relationships make change happen, accelerate it, reward it, and stabilize it. Partnerships carry their own deep possibilities, often exceeding the imagined possible.

5. *Having Voice Engages.*   As I noted earlier, we nurses have spoken often, and with passion, about the importance of having voice in our work world. The historic silencing of nursing's perspective rankles, and we notice when that familiar inattention rears up. Having voice doesn't just happen. One must create the conditions to ensure it, and once heard, the voice must be heeded. This change process built in numerous opportunities for nurses to have voice, and the voice had an impact. Changes often happened because they were the changes everyone had asked for, not the ones imposed upon them.

6. *Development Is Demanding.*   Corporate America provides some powerful exemplars of what happens when you invest in your employees. Although the impact of this practice has been well documented, investment in nurses in the service setting has often been reduced to mandatory continuing education (CE) or new equipment programs that neither engage nor involve the learner. The developmental needs of the nurse are made secondary to the needs of the organization. In addition, nurses are often encouraged to seek further education in environments that not only fail to support them, but also can create substantive deterrents. If you want your workforce to pursue self-development and succeed, you have to accept the demands this places on your system . . . and your budget.

7. *Professionalism Pays Off.*   Nurses take pride in the work they do, and want it recognized for its intrinsic worth, value, and power. Professionalism is an ideal pathway to pursuing and achieving both. The change process described in this book was grounded in the assumption that BWH nurses were consummate professionals. It was grounded in the demands this conviction placed on nurse leaders, and ensured that the leadership, programs, practices, and rewards followed through on the commitments implicit in affirming professionalism. It paid off, as this book documents.

8. *Values Shape Vision.*   The vision that ensured energy and commitment to the change process described in this book worked because it emerged from the deepest values nurses hold and manifest. Nurses are ultimately a value-driven community of professional caregivers, and when the vision claims, supports, reinforces, and rewards those values, they become enthusiastic proponents of that vision.

9. *Discovery Disrupts.*   Extinguishing prior patterns of behavior rarely works. Rather, the introduction of new options draws attention to the new, the previously unknown, and creates the possibility for new behaviors. The use of narrative and reflective practices gave the BWH nurses the opportunity to engage in discovery, to find their own solutions and their own voice within. The changes described here were thus more organic, personal, and likely to persist. Not everyone embraced discovery, but those who did introduced new options to the total community, creating the conditions for others to embrace discovery on their own.

10. *Cultures Can Be Created.*   The introduction of the new, grounded in the good already in place, created the opportunity for new cultures to emerge. It is noteworthy that they were *created*, not imposed, required, or mandated. Rather, the community itself moved toward a new culture by grappling with the present and its implications, exploring alternatives, and testing out new options. Where the new options produced preferred outcomes, shifts occurred. Champions, super users, and first adopters help; a culture that attracts and rewards them is essential to spread that emerging culture.

I imagine that the usefulness of this book is apparent to many readers. Nurse administrators can find herein a roadmap for change. Nurse educators have a textbook that can enrich any course, and can make a leadership course a whole new adventure. Nursing students just beginning have a window into their futures, a real-world snapshot of how things are "out there." Advanced practice nurses (APNs) can find validation of the promise of improved care they offer nursing and health care. For the many DNP students in these rapidly emerging programs of study, the book provides a virtual menu of potential capstone projects. For the PhD student, it seeds the imagination, with studies to be developed or programs to be tested and validated.

At the beginning of this book, we issued an invitation, essentially one to join us in the story of a journey of change. That story, as told here, is a proposed antidote to the fable about the six blind men describing an elephant, each telling of their individual perceptions. The obvious solution: Ask the six men to have a conversation, share information, and create a composite description. That has been our intent: If you hear a story from a variety of perspectives, you have a richer and more nuanced understanding of the tale.

Stories sometimes get unexpected validation. As the production of this book neared its conclusion, my co-editor, Mairead Hickey, was promoted to Executive Vice

President and Chief Operating Officer of BWH and Faulkner Hospital. Sometimes the change process catalyzed in nursing gets noticed and affirmed. Another story begins.

Stories are time bound: they have a beginning, middle, and end. Ours spans 5 years, yet points to the future, to the emergent next stories, the next change that will move the nurses at BWH to make that which is today's best even better tomorrow. And so, we end by looking forward, to the next chapter, the next leg of the journey, provided by the new Senior Vice President of Patient Services and Chief Nursing Officer of BWH, Jacqueline Somerville.

26

The Journey Continues . . .
Just Follow the Yellow Brick Road

Jacqueline G. Somerville

"My! . . . People come and go so quickly here!"

—Dorothy, *in* The Wizard of Oz

I have been most fortunate to follow Mairead Hickey as the senior vice president of Patient Care Services and chief nursing officer. I began this journey in January of 2011. During the interview process, I was frequently asked what my vision was for the department. I joked with staff that once I decided to become a chief nurse, it felt like folks made an assumption that you had some sort of out-of-body experience that gave you the power to see the future. I clarified over and over again that my job was to witness the practice and celebrate and maintain the gains, and that collectively we would continue on this path called clinical excellence.

There was a real fear that the new chief nurse would come in with an agenda and dismantle the foundation that had been so thoughtfully laid. I had learned some valuable lessons over my years as a nurse executive. First and foremost, celebrate the legacy you have been given and care for it with the utmost respect. Second, surround yourself with bright people who have lived the history of practice evolution and work with them to continue to shepherd the work into the future, however, that might unfold. As long as we keep patients and families at the core of all of our decisions, we will maintain our "true north" as a profession and department.

Handoffs, as we have heard throughout this book, are a time of risk and vulnerability. Mairead, and her associate chief nurse, Trish Gibbons, and I agreed to structure this transition based on the same principles we have learned are effective in patient care. My research focused on patients' perceptions of feeling known by their nurses, and these patients taught me a lot about transitions. They identified four themes when they felt known: They felt recognized as a unique human being, felt safe, felt a meaningful personal connection with their nurse, and felt empowered by their nurse to participate in their care. The parallels for me during this transition have struck me as so similar. Staff and leadership at Brigham and Women's Hospital (BWH) are proud of their practice. They want the uniqueness of it to be understood, valued, and preserved; they want to feel that they practice in an environment that promotes excellence, safety, and effective teamwork; they want to feel that their leadership values them as unique human beings; and they want their voices to be heard. They want to be empowered to make decisions about their practice locally and organizationally.

To be an effective chief nurse requires enormous humility. The task of representing patients, families, and such committed nurses is enormous. I believe that the trust they place in me to do this well is sacred. It matters less who sits in the seat, because we will all come and go. What matters most is that each chief nurse has the humility to build on what has been accomplished and the creativity to recognize that, in service of our patients and staff, learning is lifelong and the possibilities are endless. I can't wait for the sequel! I hope it won't be entitled "Wicked!"—although, being a Boston native, "Wicked Good" would be just fine.

The journey continues . . .

Index